UNDERSTANDING AND TREATING ADULTS WITH ATTENTION DEFICIT HYPERACTIVITY DISORDER

UNDERSTANDING AND TREATING ADULTS WITH ATTENTION DEFICIT HYPERACTIVITY DISORDER

BRIAN B. DOYLE, M.D.

Clinical Professor of Psychiatry and of Family and Community Medicine, Georgetown University Medical School, Washington, DC

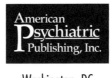

American **Psychiatric** Publishing, Inc.

Washington, DC
London, England

Note: The authors have worked to ensure that all information in this book is accurate at the time of publication and consistent with general psychiatric and medical standards, and that information concerning drug dosages, schedules, and routes of administration is accurate at the time of publication and consistent with standards set by the U.S. Food and Drug Administration and the general medical community. As medical research and practice continue to advance, however, therapeutic standards may change. Moreover, specific situations may require a specific therapeutic response not included in this book. For these reasons and because human and mechanical errors sometimes occur, we recommend that readers follow the advice of physicians directly involved in their care or the care of a member of their family.

Copyright © 2006 American Psychiatric Publishing, Inc.
ALL RIGHTS RESERVED

Manufactured in the United States of America on acid-free paper
10   09   08   07   06   5   4   3   2   1
First Edition

Typeset in Adobe's Palatino and Futura.

American Psychiatric Publishing, Inc.
1000 Wilson Boulevard
Arlington, VA 22209–3901
www.appi.org

Library of Congress Cataloging-in-Publication Data
Doyle, Brian B., 1941–
  Understanding and treating adults with attention deficit hyperactivity
  disorder / Brian B. Doyle.-—1st ed.
      p. ; cm.
  Includes bibliographical references and index.
  ISBN 1-58562-221-4 (pbk. : alk. paper)
  1. Attention-deficit disorder in adults. 2. Attention-deficit-disordered adults.
  [DNLM: 1. Attention Deficit Disorder with Hyperactivity—therapy. 2. Adult.
  WM 190 D754u 2006] I. Title.

  RC394.A85D69 2006
  616.85'89—dc22

                                                              2006005232

British Library Cataloguing in Publication Data
A CIP record is available from the British Library.

CONTENTS

PREFACE

> What good is like to this?
> To do worthy the writing, and to write
> Worthy the reading and the world's delight?

SO WROTE SAMUEL DANIEL IN "Musophilus," his eloquent poem in defense of the intellectual life. His words, written in 1599, aptly express my hopes for this book, *Understanding and Treating Adults With Attention Deficit Hyperactivity Disorder*.

The good news is that today attention deficit hyperactivity disorder (ADHD) in adults is getting the attention it deserves. Information about the disorder and its treatment is growing rapidly. With that comes enhanced life prospects for the many people who have ADHD. Treatment methods successful in children with ADHD also help adults who have the disorder. New medications enlarge the available range of options. A variety of human and technological interventions help adults with ADHD structure their lives and become more productive. The combination of available treatment approaches allows them to use their resources consistently in order to be at their best. Working with these patients is intellectually stimulating and personally rewarding. When treatment works, adults with ADHD thrive. Their lives can suddenly and dramatically change for the better. It is gratifying to catalyze that change.

Yet ADHD is still a controversial diagnosis, even more controversial in adults than in children. It is not yet listed as a diagnosis for adults in our current system, DSM-IV-TR. Clinical experience shows daily that many adults have ADHD. Some resourceful, talented individuals who have the disorder live successfully and creatively. Many others have diminished life prospects and are subject to anxiety, affective disorders, and substance abuse. Many fail to reach their potential. There is a high cost in human suffering as well as in lost productivity.

The book begins with a discussion of ADHD in children and adults. The clinical story of ADHD begins, and continues, with children. Knowing the evolution of the concept and treatment of ADHD in children illuminates current thinking about the disorder in adults. Chapter 2 ("Diagnosing ADHD in Adults") concerns diagnosis of the disorder, first in children and now in adults, and discusses the validity of the diagnosis, which is still controversial. Because of the strong neurological underpinnings of ADHD, Chapter 3 ("Biological Basis of ADHD") focuses on the biological bases of the disorder.

Chapter 4 ("Allies in Treatment") deals with the therapeutic alliance. When the clinician is working with adult ADHD patients, as with any patient, a strong therapeutic alliance is desirable. However, ADHD presents the clinician with special challenges: working actively with patients who have special characteristics; taking into account specific cultural, ethnic, and racial issues; and thinking in specifically legal as well as medical terms. Adult ADHD patients stir strong reactions in the clinicians who care for them, and thus countertransference also requires more than the usual attention.

Chapters 5 through 7 ("Treating Adult ADHD With Medication: Introduction," "Treating ADHD With Central Nervous System Stimulants," and "Treating ADHD With Nonstimulant Medications") deal with medication issues. Here is detailed information about using medication, with specific information about the central nervous stimulants and other effective medications. These chapters also discuss medications that are ineffective, albeit highly touted. Chapter 8 ("Comprehensive Treatment of the Adult With ADHD") covers comprehensive treatment, which involves far more than using medication. The detailed clinical example, with material drawn from several patients, illustrates the issues involved in treating adult ADHD patients over time.

Chapter 9 ("Comorbid and Treatment-Refractory ADHD") includes a full discussion of comorbid and refractory ADHD. This chapter deals with the clinical reality that in adults, ADHD rarely occurs by itself. These are complex patients. Because of their ADHD, they are even more likely than other persons to have a full range of psychiatric disorders. Comorbid conditions may require treatment before the ADHD can be addressed. Similarly, missed or overlooked ADHD can complicate or impede the treatment of other disorders, especially affective disorders and substance abuse. The chapter also contains approaches to the treatment for adult ADHD patients who fail to respond to standard interventions.

Chapter 10 ("ADHD Issues: Work, Women, and Family") reviews special issues that pertain to adults with ADHD. These include issues related to work, an important life domain often affected by the disorder. The chapter contains information as well about women and ADHD. Until recently, women were comparatively neglected as ADHD patients. However, because of their biology and their social roles and the effects of ADHD on these aspects, women deserve fuller discussion. Finally, the chapter provides information about the impact of adult ADHD on families. Although this book focuses on the individual ADHD adult patient, the disorder is a family problem. An affected adult has problems with intimate relationships and is likelier than other persons to have children with the disorder.

The Appendix indicates how to help patients use the Internet for high-quality information about ADHD. Clinicians can use this information to develop an electronic prescription, or "e-prescription," to supplement standard ones.

My aim is to provide accurate, timely information about the nature of ADHD and its treatment in adults. The material is largely evidence based, with an intermingling of clinical experiences. While I have fully documented clinical research literature and scientific data, I have tried to maintain a collegial, reader-friendly style. With this in mind, I have included figures and tables as quick reference guides. The clinical examples are set off from the text. As well as acknowledging the special challenges of adult ADHD patients, I want to convey the rewards of working with people who are often resourceful, creative, and persistent.

Brian B. Doyle, M.D.

ACKNOWLEDGMENTS

I HAVE SO MANY PEOPLE TO THANK in writing this book. First are my patients, whose struggles stimulated me to embark on this project. I appreciate their entrusting their care to me. I have tried to convey their experience, often in their own words, while protecting their privacy. All of the names are pseudonyms; clinical examples are composites from several individuals.

I appreciate the skilled help of Professor Ellen Detlefsen at the University of Pittsburgh for her help with the Appendix. Her work helps patients, and the clinicians who work with them, to find accurate, up-to-date medical information.

My thanks go next to my family: First, to my wife, Marg, for her patience with a word-addicted husband. To my daughter Mairin, who inspires us all with her tenacity in coping with the traumas of brain tumors and their treatment. To my daughter Cavan, whose knowledge of health law buttresses the section on legal aspects of ADHD. She is my model for steady, disciplined writing. To my son, Colin, whose success in overcoming ADHD informs my clinical work. He seamlessly integrates the computer with his daily function. He researched and assessed Web sites for the Appendix. My thanks go also to my dear mother, who in her late 90s engages fully and zestfully with life. Her love for learning keeps her young in spirit.

Thanks also go to the colleagues who provided support and clear thinking. Eleanor A. Sorrentino, M.D., got me started and helped me stay on course. Many colleagues reviewed the manuscript, offered helpful suggestions, or both. These colleagues include Diane Choate, L.C.S.W., Arnold Matlin, M.D., Margaret Anne Matlin, Ph.D., Brian Cross, Ph.D., Dolph Arnicar, M.D., and Meredith Cary, Psy.D. I completed this book with the help of Julie Flynt, T.C.L., whose computer wizardry repeatedly rescued me.

The editorial staff at American Psychiatric Publishing, Inc. (APPI), deserves great credit for their support, critical reading, and technical know-how. From the start, the leadership at APPI of both Bob Hales and John McDuffie has been steadfast. I appreciate their generosity in sharing their experience. The reviewers provided close reading and invaluable comments and suggestions for improvements, which I have tried to implement. The shortcomings of the text are solely mine.

Knowledge of the field is advancing rapidly. I welcome comments and suggestions from readers as I look toward a second edition of this book. In the meantime, I hope you learn from, and enjoy, this one.

CHAPTER 1

ADHD IN CHILDREN AND ADULTS

THE RECOGNITION AND TREATMENT OF ADHD in children is one of the great success stories of modern psychiatry. Added to this story is the explosion of interest in the disorder as it affects adults. With that new attention comes the prospect of enhanced life for many thousands of people.

Yet few psychiatric diagnoses stir as much controversy as the diagnosis of ADHD. Securing public acceptance for the diagnosis, even in children, is still problematic. This difficulty persists despite the decades that clinicians have diagnosed ADHD in children and treated them successfully. Resistance to the concept of ADHD continues not only in the United States but also in other cultures and societies around the world. ADHD in adults is even more controversial. Part of the difficulty lies in the original criteria: by definition, the diagnosis affected only children and adolescents. For years that assumption blinded psychiatrists to the fact that symptoms can and do persist into adulthood. Fortunately, some alert clinicians saw that reality, and they continued treatment for affected patients. Parents of children with ADHD realized that they had some, if not all, of the symptoms of their offspring. When we examine the lives of adults who struggle and fail, repeatedly, sometimes we find symptom patterns like those of children with ADHD. Some patients with decades-long difficulties with anxiety, depression, and substance abuse often have unrecognized and untreated ADHD. Once they have a proper diagnosis and full treatment, adults with ADHD can change their lives profoundly.

Many claim that what we call ADHD symptoms in children or adults is the result of a dysfunctional family, poverty, poor education, environmental toxins, or bad child-rearing (Barkley 1998). They think the diagnosis is a cop-out for lazy adults and bratty children (Johnston and Freeman 2000). Many parents still believe that ADHD symptoms in children deserve strict punishment, not treatment (Johnston and Patenaud 1994). Many people still regard the diagnosis with suspicion.

Is ADHD a fad? Is its name invoked to explain away the bad behavior of a spoiled generation? What we now call attention deficit hyperactivity disorder has been recognized for many years. In the eighteenth century, philosopher John Locke described students who "try as they might…cannot keep their minds from straying" (Amen and Goldberg 1998, p. 76). In 1902 the English pediatrician Still described children who were overactive and could not sustain their attention. He hypothesized that their deficits in inhibitory volition, "moral control," and sustained attention were causally related to each other and to an underlying neurological deficiency (Still 1902). After the encephalitis epidemic in 1917–1918, many children presented with behavioral and cognitive sequelae. Many of their symptoms are those now regarded as characteristic for ADHD: impaired attention, impulsivity, and socially disruptive behavior (Stryker 1925). As early as 1937, clinicians saw that central nervous system (CNS) stimulants improved the behavior and academic performance of such children (Bradley 1937). As the twentieth century advanced, clinicians increasingly invoked the concept that such children had "minimum brain damage" (Strauss and Lehtinen 1947). By the 1950s, clinical researchers had described a hyperkinetic impulse disorder in children, suggesting a CNS deficit in the thalamic area (Denhoff et al. 1957). Increasingly clinicians moved away from the focus on brain damage to hyperactivity. Many regarded the disorder as mild and self-correcting by adolescence (Chess 1960). In the 1970s, clinician researchers focused on attention deficits as central to the disorder (Rie and Rie 1980). Since the 1980s, our understanding of the disorder has deepened, and our diagnostic criteria have become more complex. Although what we call the *disorder* has changed over time, the *syndrome* of ADHD remains the most common psychiatric, learning, and behavioral problem in childhood. It affects between 5% and 10% of children (Amen and Goldberg 1998).

Reports on the syndrome of what is now regarded as ADHD in adults appeared as early as the 1960s (Menkes et al. 1967). However, serious and more rigorous scientific research into the clinical condition in adults only came in the 1990s (Wender 1995). This research continues to flourish today.

PROBLEMS DIAGNOSING ADHD

Researchers and clinicians are trying to define ADHD more exactly and reliably. The current name, *attention deficit hyperactivity disorder,* is unsatisfactory. How can we say the problem is an attention deficit, when many patients with this diagnosis focus intensely on subjects that interest them? They can hyperfocus, disappearing for hours into whatever appeals to them, whether soccer, the stock market, or video games. It is hard for them *not* to pay attention once they become involved in something they enjoy. Patients with ADHD can pay attention. They *cannot* count on being able to pay attention when they want to or need to. Having the stimulus of a deadline or a test helps sometimes, but not always. Attention "dysfunction" is a more accurate name than attention "deficit" for this disorder.

Another problem with the ADHD diagnosis is that not everyone who bears it is hyperactive. Some patients are truly hyperactive, like the out-of-control little boys many people think of when they hear the acronym "ADHD." However, there are, in fact, three subtypes of patients with ADHD: those with hyperactivity alone, those with a combination of inattention and hyperactivity, and those with inattention alone. As people mature, the symptom pattern of ADHD changes. Symptoms of hyperactivity tend to wane, while inattention persists. For many adults with the syndrome, hyperactivity and its consequences are not part of the clinical picture. Some adults were never hyperactive, and no one realized that they were inattentive as children. This pattern particularly affects women, whose problems as children and as adults tend to be unrecognized and overlooked.

A third problem with the diagnosis of ADHD in adults is, paradoxically, its popularity. We clinicians like to think that our minds are clear, our motives pure, and our diagnoses valid. Some people, however, use psychiatric diagnoses as excuses for bad behavior or for secondary gain. In some settings, our diagnoses can shield the guilty from the consequences of their actions. As any expert witness knows, this possibility is a particular tension in forensic work. People may use our diagnoses to get special treatment or accommodations they do not deserve. Although such behavior is off-putting, it should not keep us from making the diagnosis when it fits and from treating patients fully. The best approach is that of careful clinical work. First, get a full history. Whenever possible, have the patient provide outside documentation of problems with school and work and relationships. Finally, supplement information with material from those who know the patient well and are close to him or her. Chapter 10 ("ADHD Issues: Work, Women, and Family") further discusses the legal issues in diagnosing and treating patients with ADHD.

As with many psychiatric conditions, ADHD involves a range of symptoms and a range of severities. To qualify for the diagnosis, patients must demonstrate that symptoms affect their function in at least two settings. Naturally some patients will have more severe symptoms than others. Adults who come to outpatient-oriented clinicians in private practice for treatment of ADHD are likely to be some of the healthier of those affected. Such people, typically, have considerable resources.

> Bart, age 54, graduated from a fine college and had a "gilt-edged" M.B.A. He said, "You look as if you are thinking, 'What the hell are you doing here?'" That was exactly what I was thinking, and I told him so. He said, "In grad school I only scraped by because we did all our work in small groups. I'm an idea man. I got the others to put the paper together. Once I graduated, I surrounded myself with people who dotted the i's and crossed the t's for me. Yes, I have a fancy M.B.A., but I never made the big time. My wife loves me a lot, but she has complained for years that I never listen to what she says. Now she has threatened me with divorce if I don't do my part of the 'emotional work' of the family, whatever that is." On investigation, Bart proved to have ADHD not otherwise specified. He responded well to a combination of CNS stimulant medication and behavioral suggestions. He and his wife are in couples therapy. Feeling they are on more solid ground emotionally, they are more hopeful about the future. He's happy in his marriage and thriving in his entrepreneurial ventures.

For every Bart, with his resources and achievements, there are many adults who do not know that they have ADHD, do not know that treatment helps, and do not have access to affordable treatment. People with marginal financial resources struggle to survive. Looking for treatment for ADHD may seem unrealistic and unaffordable. Although our jails and our welfare rolls likely have substantial numbers of adults with unrecognized and untreated ADHD, there is virtually no formal study of the disorder in such populations. The reasons for this absence are unclear. The concept of adult ADHD is still relatively new. In such groups, there are scant treatment resources, and those that exist may focus on the psychotic disorders or on substance abuse or addiction. Looking for ADHD under such circumstances may seem unwarranted.

Many persons with the disorder cannot get treatment because they are unaware that the disorder affects them. Those with severe ADHD often have multiple psychiatric conditions, which combine to threaten their livelihood. They may see psychiatric care as beyond their reach. Racial, ethnic, cultural, and financial issues keep them from treatment. For a greater discussion of these factors, see Chapter 4 ("Allies in Treatment").

DIAGNOSTIC CRITERIA FOR ADHD IN CHILDREN

ADHD was first described in children. The diagnostic standards for adults evolved from their original use in evaluating children. The criteria for ADHD are in DSM-IV-TR (American Psychiatric Association 2000, pp. 92–93; see also Chapter 2, "Diagnosing ADHD in Adults," Table 2–1). To warrant the diagnosis, a child has to be symptomatic before age 7, and he or she has to show symptoms of hyperactivity or inattention, or both. These primary symptoms can cause a wide variety of symptoms in children. Affected youngsters cannot sustain their attention unless they have strong, immediate reinforcers (Douglas 1983). In ADHD, normal reinforcers fail to hold children who have defective processes of attention and poor impulse control. The DSM-IV-TR descriptors of hyperactivity include being on the go continually, being unable to sit still, being unable to study or do another intellectual task, speaking out impulsively, and shifting from task to task without completing any. Symptoms of inattention include failing to attend, drifting and dreaming, procrastinating, and being unresponsive. To merit the diagnosis, in addition to being hyperactive or inattentive (or both), a youngster must have problems in two or more of five categories: mood, temper, emotional overreactivity, disorganization, and the inability to complete tasks. Finally, the child's symptoms must interfere with more than one area of his or her life, for example, both at school and at home.

The clinician trying to diagnose a youngster with ADHD has to do more than talk with the child in the office. Other important people in the child's life, such as parents and teachers, furnish crucial information. School evaluations and report cards are often revealing. Anecdotal information can fill out the diagnostic picture. At times formal tests are helpful, but no one test is diagnostic.

Subtypes of Childhood ADHD

There are three subtypes of childhood ADHD: hyperactive, inattentive, and combined subtypes. It is only natural that the diagnosis of ADHD started with hyperactive little boys, because they were the ones who regularly drove their teachers and parents up the wall. Curious, restless, and relentless, these children would try the patience of a saint. They are distractible as well as hyperactive. Keep quiet in class? Sit quietly and do homework? One may as well tell them to stop breathing. They bound through life, leaving chaos in their wake. Some lucky ones are engaging, and it is hard to stay angry at them for long. Others are infuriating. They hear early in life that they are losers: "You're never going to get anywhere, young man. If you'd only settle down and try harder...." The dismal lecture goes on and on.

Although wild boys are the poster children for ADHD, many girls are hyperactive as well. While in the past teachers, parents, and physicians were less likely to think of the diagnosis for girls, this mind-set is changing. More girls and women are being evaluated and treated.

> Faith, age 55, reported, "In grade school, I was always in trouble with the nuns for disrupting class. On every report card I flunked deportment: 'Faith speaks out of turn.' 'Faith interrupts others when they are speaking.' 'Faith does not stay in her seat.' I was the oldest of six, supposed to be setting a good example. My poor mother, the perfect lady, with this out-of-control daughter! It was worse when I was a teenager. No one even thought of ADHD: I was just a bad child."

Hyperactivity is the first symptom many people link with ADHD. Inattentiveness is the other important one. Inattentive children tune out, and others may see them as daydreamers or "space cadets."

> As an adult in his early 40s, Jack remembered, "I never paid attention in school. Once in third grade, I suddenly realized that the teacher and all my classmates were looking at me and laughing. The teacher had written on the blackboard, 'Let's all stare at Jack until he comes to.'"

Some children who are hyperactive and inattentive qualify for the combined type of ADHD. Although the focus with children who have ADHD is typically on their learning problems at school and their behavior problems at home, they also have a wide range of social problems. They miss social cues, and other children find their behavior off-putting. It is harder for them to make and maintain friendships. Other children can be rejecting or teasing. The ADHD children complain that they do not have friends, that nobody invites them over to play, and that they cannot get onto sports teams. Adolescents with ADHD have fewer close friendships and experience more peer rejection than those without the disorder (Bagwell et al. 2001).

It is not just the hyperactive, impulsive youngsters who have social difficulties. The inattentive ones are also hampered because they are often withdrawn and shy. Their peers tend to ignore the inattentive children rather than tease or reject them outright. The results are social isolation and poor self-esteem (Maedgen and Carlson 2000). Children with ADHD appear to experience greater rejection than do youths with any other type of behavioral or emotional disorder (Asarnow 1988). As negative experiences accumulate, young people with ADHD can become severely impaired socially. One study comparing 48 adolescents with ADHD and 38 with learning disorders found the youngsters with ADHD had significantly more impaired socialization (Wilson and Marcotte 1996).

Issues in the Diagnosis of ADHD in Children

Although up to 10% of American children qualify for the diagnosis of ADHD, not all are properly diagnosed or treated. One estimate is that 2%–4% of the children in U.S. schools are receiving psychostimulant medication. Recent trends indicate a rise in the number of prescriptions each year, both here (Safer et al. 1996) and as far away as Australia (Valentine et al. 1997). Some people assert that too many children receive this diagnosis. Some assert that boys who are simply lively get labeled as having ADHD and that too many children take stimulants and other medications. However, according to a sizable study, "There is little evidence of widespread overdiagnosis of ADHD or of widespread overprescription of medication" (Goldman et al. 1998, p. 106). Some claim that ADHD is an American construct. The prevalence here has traditionally been higher than in other countries. In the past in Great Britain, for example, about 2% of child psychiatric outpatients had a diagnosis of ADHD, compared with up to 40% in the United States (Popper et al. 2003). Numerous studies confirm that hyperactive, impulsive, and inattentive symptoms co-occur as a coherent syndrome in other countries as well. Allowing for cultural differences and other factors, the symptoms of ADHD show high internal consistency and factor-analytic results across the world. Observations and reports of the syndrome in the United States resemble those from countries such as Italy, New Zealand, China, Germany, Puerto Rico, Brazil, and Japan (Bird 2002). Prevalence rates have become more uniform as different international diagnostic systems have come into greater concordance.

Current estimates are that 8%–10% of American school-age children have ADHD; an estimated 6% of adolescents have the disorder. Boys are diagnosed with the disorder three to four times as often as girls (Barbaresi et al. 2002). Recent studies, however, indicate far more similarities than differences between boys and girls in core ADHD symptoms (Rucklidge and Tannock 2001). Girls are at higher risk for more psychological impairment. They have more fear, depression, mood swings, cognitive difficulties, and language problems than do boys with ADHD. Their outcome is often worse than that of the boys. The idea that girls suffer silently, with minimal symptoms, is mistaken (Faraone et al. 2000).

FREQUENTLY ASKED QUESTIONS IN ADULT ADHD

Do Adults Have ADHD?

There are three hypotheses for what happens when children with ADHD grow up. The first, which long dominated clinical thinking, was that children outgrew their symptoms (Cantwell 1985). That hypothesis was appealingly simple. We did not look for ADHD in adults.

The second hypothesis was that ADHD symptoms in children evolve into disturbed behavior in adults. Many ADHD children, mischievous and impulsive, have conduct problems that cause trouble with parents and teachers. The unruly behavior of some ADHD adolescents can bring them to the notice of the police. Some adults with conduct problems have a history of childhood ADHD. Severe behavior problems in adults are labeled as antisocial or criminal. In our diagnostic system, adults with a pattern of antisocial behavior have a personality disorder: an Axis II diagnosis, not an Axis I clinical syndrome. A sizable proportion of persons currently in jail may have undiagnosed and untreated ADHD. However, not all children with ADHD have disturbed or disruptive behavior, and not all adult criminals are ADHD children grown up.

The third hypothesis about adult ADHD comes from the clinicians who treated affected children. Even when clinicians diagnosed ADHD early and treated it vigorously, many of their patients had symptoms that persisted into adult life. These patients had grown-up versions of childhood woes: problems finding stable and satisfying work, and difficulties making sustaining, happy, intimate relationships. In this third hypothesis, ADHD symptoms evolve as children mature into adulthood. Even though many patients learn to compensate for their difficulties and make the most of their strengths, some still have symptoms. Problems in social competence and rejection by peers, along with difficulties making and keeping friends, are major areas of impairment (Whalen and Henker 1992).

Careful follow-up studies of children support all three hypotheses. Some children do mature out of ADHD. Even without intervention, symptoms may wane over time. Maturation and increased coping skills may account for the improvement. Second, some ADHD children do show disturbed behavior as adults. ADHD significantly increases the risk of antisocial behavior and substance abuse in adults (Mannuzza et al. 1991; Weiss et al. 1985). Evidence supports the third hypothesis as well. ADHD children grown up often have difficulties with adult development: school failure, poor work histories, poor social interactions, and low self-esteem (Cantwell and Hanna 1989). They are at risk for psychiatric symptoms, especially anxiety, depression, and abuse of alcohol and other substances. Considering what they struggle with, what is impressive is how well many patients do.

What Percentage of Children With ADHD Have It as Adults?

The percentage of ADHD children who continue to have it as adults is controversial. Some think only 10% of children with ADHD have it as adults, whereas others claim the percentage is as high as 75%. An estimate of persistence into adulthood is likely 50%–68% of children with ADHD (Barkley et al. 2002a; Spencer et al. 1998). Children with ADHD are more likely to have the disorder persisting into adulthood if they have a family history of ADHD, comorbid psychiatric conditions, or psychosocial adversity. Having two or three of those risk factors multiplies the likelihood that ADHD will persist (Biederman et al. 1996). In two retrospective studies of young adults with a history of childhood ADHD, 31%–44% had the full syndrome and 9%–25% had a partial syndrome, with at least one bothersome symptom (Mannuzza et al. 1989; Weiss et al. 1985). Researchers in one prospective study followed 85 children with ADHD into young adulthood (average age, 24 years), comparing them with age peers who never had that diagnosis. In this study, only 4% of the children who had ADHD qualified for that diagnosis as young adults. However, compared with the "normal" control subjects, the young adults who had ADHD as children showed significantly more substance abuse (12% vs. 3%) and antisocial behavior (12% vs. 3%) (Mannuzza et al. 1998). The young adults with persisting ADHD had problems with inattention, disorganization, impulsivity, and distractibility that held them back in their academic and work lives (Weiss and Hechtman 1993). Young adults with ADHD more often had depression, anxiety, and abuse of alcohol and other substances than did their age peers who did not have the disorder (Fischer et al. 2002). In general, studies that follow ADHD children into adulthood show that those diagnostic criteria are reliable in adults (Greenfield et al. 1988).

In a recent meta-analysis of studies of children diagnosed with ADHD, 62% continued to be symptomatic in adulthood, although only 19% met full diagnostic criteria (Mick et al. 2004). For children, the good news is that when ADHD symptoms remit, the functioning of the child normalizes (Mannuzza et al. 1991). However, as the demands of adult life mount, patients do not need to meet full diagnostic criteria to feel the effects of ADHD. If symptoms persist even in attenuated form, they can have a significant impact. The functional outcome of ADHD is heterogeneous; thus, we need to assess patients specifically for both ADHD symptoms and functional impairments. Over a 4-year period, one study evaluated the course of children and adolescents who had persisting ADHD. At the end of that time, the authors found that 20% of participants had good emotional, educational, and social adjustment; 20% functioned poorly in all three domains; and 60% had intermediate outcomes (Biederman et al. 1998). The same researchers studied ADHD children as they matured past 20 years of age. Although 30% attained symptomatic remission, only 10% achieved functional remission, defined as a Global Assessment of Functioning score of 60 or more (Biederman et al. 2000). The natural history of ADHD seems to be to improve, somewhat, with age and maturation. Recent studies suggest, however, that improvement is partial and not total. Some adults who still have a partial syndrome suffer considerably because of it. What causes major problems for adults with ADHD are the comorbid conditions that come with the disorder (Biederman 2005).

How Many Adults Have ADHD?

ADHD is one of the most common psychiatric disorders of adulthood (Faraone and Biederman 2004a). Current estimates are that 4.1% of adults in the U.S. population have the disorder. However, this rate reflects only those adults who meet DSM-IV-TR criteria for active ADHD and who were diagnosed with the disorder as children or adolescents. The actual rate is likely to be higher (Kessler 2004). In the most recent data, ADHD is the fourth most common psychiatric disorder of English-speaking adults in the United States. Of the patients who had ADHD, the severity of the disorder was serious for 41.3%, moderate for 35.2%, and mild for 23.5% (Kessler et al. 2005). Table 1–1 summarizes the survey data.

In a recent telephone survey, researchers asked 1,019 randomly selected adults about symptoms of ADHD retrospectively (in grade school) and currently (in the past 6 months). In making diagnoses of ADHD, researchers used both narrow and broad criteria. By the narrow criteria, the participant required "strong" evidence of ADHD in both childhood and adulthood. According to these narrow criteria, 1.1% of participants received the diagnosis of ADHD hyperactive-impulsive subtype; 0.7% had the inattentive subtype; and 1.1% the combined subtype. The total was 2.9% with any diagnosis of ADHD. By the broad diagnostic criteria for ADHD, participants endorsed symptoms "sometimes" in both childhood and adulthood. According to the broad criteria, 3.7% of participating adults warranted a diagnosis of ADHD hyperactive-impulsive

TABLE 1–1.　ADHD in the spectrum of psychiatric disorders in adults[a]

Social phobia	6.8%
Major depressive disorder	6.7%
ADHD	4.1%
Posttraumatic stress disorder	3.5%
Alcohol abuse	3.1%
Panic disorder	2.7%
Bipolar disorder I or II	2.6%
Drug abuse	1.3%

[a]12-month prevalence data in 9,282 English-speaking subjects age 18 years and older.
Source.　Kessler RC, Chiu WT, Demler O, et al: "Prevalence, Severity, and Comorbidity of 12-Month DSM-IV Disorders in the National Comorbidity Survey Replication." *Archives of General Psychiatry* 62:617–627, 2005.

subtype, 5.8% the inattentive subtype, and 6.9% with the combined subtype. The total prevalence, using the broad criteria for diagnosis, was 16.4% (Faraone and Biederman 2004a). Although estimates of prevalence rate range from 2.9% to 16.9%, the most common is 4% (Faraone and Biederman 2004b). In adults, the ratio of men to women identified as having ADHD is approximately 1.5 to 1.0 (Biederman 1998b).

In 2001, adults accounted for 16% of the estimated 9.7 million visits to office-based clinicians for ADHD treatment (McDonnell et al. 2000). A retrospective cross-sectional analysis of managed care claims found the point prevalence of ADHD ranged from 0.3% to 1.1% in adults. Such adults use significantly more total medical resources than control subjects without the disorder ($P<0.0001$) (Davis et al. 2002). The worldwide prevalence of ADHD in adults is unclear, because disagreement lingers in other countries about how to diagnose the disorder. Epidemiologic studies of adults in the community who warrant a diagnosis of ADHD reveal that 40% were in treatment for psychiatric problems, including substance abuse. Only about 10% of the cases identified were receiving treatment for their ADHD. This is a much lower treatment rate than for anxiety, mood, or substance disorders (Kessler 2004).

What Symptoms Do Adults With ADHD Have?

Symptoms of ADHD in adults reflect poor control of their executive functions, which are a set of skills linked to the frontal regions of the brain (Barkley 1997). These executive functions include nonverbal working memory and the internalization of speech, also called verbal working memory; executive functions also include self-regulation of affect, motivation, arousal, and reconstitution. The final executive function, reconstitution involves two tasks: 1) *analysis,* in which sequences of events are broken down into parts; and 2) *synthesis,* in which these parts are used to construct, or reconstitute, new messages or responses.

The frontal brain contains a behavioral inhibition system that has three components. First, it inhibits an initial response to an event; next, it stops a response once begun; and, third, it protects a response from interference and distractions. When a person's behavioral inhibition system works properly, he or she performs executive functions well. Adults with ADHD may have difficulties in executive function if they have problems in any or all of the three areas of behavioral inhibition. Thinking about ADHD this way allows us to conceptualize how symptoms both of inattention and hyperactivity/impulsivity can arise from similar deficits (Adler and Cohen 2004).

The clinical picture of adult ADHD is often more complex than it is in children. People learn to cope with their symptoms, but as they mature, others demand more of them. They expect more of themselves. Although the natural history of ADHD symptoms is to improve, symptoms of inattention decline at a modest rate; hyperactivity/impulsivity symptoms lessen much more abruptly. Symptoms labeled "inattentive" in children dominate the clinical picture in adults (Biederman et al. 2000).

Patterns of hyperactivity and impulsivity can linger in adult behavior, although these patterns are less obvious than in children (Hart et al. 1995). Adults with the hyperactive subtypes of ADHD are less frenetic than affected children, but they are still restless. They may put their internal restlessness to good use, as a source of ambition and drive to accomplish. They may choose jobs, such as sales and marketing, where being active and energetic is important to their function. They may work very long hours or have two jobs (Adler and Cohen 2004).

Many have learned to suppress the urge to squirm in a meeting so they will not distract others. That effort, however, may keep them from attending fully to the purpose of the meeting (R. Doyle 2004). Adults with ADHD who outgrow the "whirling dervish" activity of some affected children may still have high energy levels. Without good executive function, that energy lacks a sustained focus, or it goes in unproductive directions. Many hyperactive ADHD children race around; few adults do. They may still frequently change their posture, tap their fingers, or swing their legs.

> "I can't work for more than 15 minutes at a time," said one patient. "Then I get up and run up and down the stairs for at least that long. After that I can pay attention to my work again, but people in my office think I'm an exercise nut."

The social dysfunction that is part of ADHD has its consequences in terms of impaired relationships. Adults with ADHD may not have ever learned to master the give-and-take of comfortable or intimate communication, a process that begins in childhood. They can be poor listeners. Many talk incessantly; they interrupt others without noticing the reactions they stir. Their moods are labile, and they have trouble maintaining adult friendships and social interaction. The marriages of adults with ADHD are more at risk. In one study, the divorce rate was twice that of control subjects (Biederman et al. 1993).

> "I don't 'get it' about relationships," said 38-year-old Sarah. She was divorced, and her current boyfriend was complaining about her unresponsiveness. "I miss the cues. I can't figure out what's going on between me and other people."

Patients with ADHD have problems related to higher education or vocational training. Fewer enter college than peers without ADHD. They have lower grade point averages and lower class rankings than those without the disorder, they drop out of higher education at a higher rate, and they have a much lower graduation rate as well (Barkley and Murphy 1998). Affected adults fail to develop age-appropriate executive skills: they cannot plan, focus, work steadily, and implement a series of related actions. Others often regard them as stubborn; they chronically have conflicts with authorities, difficulties in intimate relationships, frequent job changes, and poor frustration tolerance (Elliott 2002).

Problems with impulsivity appear in the way that many ADHD patients conduct their sexual life. Many start having sex at an earlier age than their age peers. They tend to have more sexual partners; in one study, the ADHD patients had had 19 partners, versus 7 for control subjects. Less likely to use contraceptives, individuals with ADHD have a higher teenage pregnancy rate. In that study, 38% of adolescents with ADHD became pregnant, as opposed to 4% of teenagers without the disorder. Young adults with ADHD are more likely to have children out of wedlock and to contract a sexually transmitted disease (17% vs. 4%) (Barkley and Gordon 2002).

> Talking about his vigorous sexual life, one patient said with a grin, "I've been a bad boy." At age 42 years, he was twice divorced. His most recent fiancée broke their engagement when she discovered he was cheating on her.

Impulsivity and hyperactivity (and inattention) cause problems when adults with ADHD drive automobiles. In tests using driving simulators, they steer more erratically and have more scrapes and crashes than peers without the disorder (Barkley et al. 2002b). Compared with age peers, young adults with ADHD have more speeding tickets and get into more accidents in which they total the car (49% vs. 16%) (Murphy and Barkley 1996b). They are less likely to use seat belts, and they are more likely to demonstrate excessive anger and aggression behind the wheel. They are more at risk of having their license suspended or revoked (24%–32% vs. 4% of control subjects; Cox et al. 2000). Teenagers and adults with ADHD are almost four times more likely to have an accident while driving. Male ADHD teens and adults with conduct disorder, especially those with increased alcohol use or abuse, have the highest risk of adverse driving records (Barkley 2004). Similar studies in New Zealand show a similar association of ADHD with increased risk of driving accidents and injuries (Woodward et al. 2000).

The research shows that the greater risks for driving are not because of comorbid disorders associated with ADHD, such as oppositional defiant disorder, conduct disorder, depression, or anxiety. Drivers with ADHD have less ability to operate an automobile and less skill at maneuvering it in traffic. They also often overestimate their driving abilities relative to normal adults (Barkley 2004).

Problems with impulsivity may contribute to the increased incidence of substance abuse in ADHD adults. There is a clear bidirectional overlap between ADHD and substance use disorders (Wilens et al. 1996). Adults with ADHD more often smoke cigarettes than other adults without the disorder. They have a harder time quitting than other smokers do (Pomerleau et al. 1995). Compared with age peers without the disorder, young adults with ADHD consume more alcohol, get drunk more often, and are told more often that they drink too much (Barkley et al. 1996). Whether they continue to drink more later in adulthood and have more alcohol-related problems than other people is unsettled. Young adults with ADHD tend to try to use other substances, especially marijuana. Their susceptibility to drug abuse complicates treatment (Wilens 2004).

Adults with ADHD still hyperfocus, as they did as children. They become absorbed in activities that interest them and have trouble disengaging from these activities. The challenge is to get that hyperfocus to work for their benefit.

Evan's immersion in the stock market paid off. His computer was in the kitchen at home. If needed, he could be online at 3 A.M. to check on a stock. He was still there, however, when his wife was trying to get their three children up, fed, and out to school. She was grateful that he made a lot of money but, as she said, "He's underfoot. He's always there!"

Certainly the hyperactivity and impulsivity of ADHD adults—and what they do as a result—cause problems. However, what adults with ADHD do *not* do, out of inattention and distractibility, causes even more trouble.

"I'm always tuned out," admitted Mick. "I put things off, wait until the last minute, miss deadlines. I find myself in a room and forget why I am there, or start one task and then do another, and then another. Nothing gets finished, and I wonder where the day went."

Parenting, with its demands for consistency and steady performance, is problematic for women and men with ADHD. Daily life is full of children's many assignments, appointments, teachers, and books. There is so much "stuff" to keep track of: clothing and pens and other articles of everyday life. It is even harder when, as is often the case, one or more of the children have ADHD as well.

In her first interview, Betty jumped up, saying, "I forgot to put Timmy's ADHD medicine out for him this morning. Can I call him? If he doesn't take it, I'll be getting a phone call from school about him." Once she had talked to Timmy, she said, "I can't take care of myself, and I'm supposed to be looking out for my children?" She shook her head, exasperated.

Being impulsive and inattentive also causes problems in the workplace. ADHD adults report more work problems, lower occupational status, and higher rates of self-employment than do their non-ADHD peers. They are more likely to be fired (53% vs. 31% of control subjects). They quit jobs more frequently (48% vs. 16%) and acknowledge more chronic employment difficulties (77% vs. 57%) (Murphy and Barkley 1996a).

The final common pathway for symptoms in adults who have ADHD is that they cannot manage their responsibilities. They have trouble with the mundane tasks of everyday life: paying bills, taking laundry to the dry cleaner, filing tax returns, or keeping appointments. They have problems looking ahead, organizing themselves, and implementing life goals. They lack the skills to manage life effectively, skills summarized by the phrase "executive function."

One wife said, "Nothing gets done, unless Ben wants to do it himself. Actually I have to be organized for four of us, because his two teenagers have ADD too."

Although inattention and hyperactivity/impulsivity are currently the two defining dimensions of ADHD in DSM-IV-TR, other clinical features are important. Organizational deficits, problems with motivation, and impaired time sense wreak havoc in the lives of adults as well as children. These problems may constitute additional dimensions of ADHD. Although the current concept of ADHD is useful and valid, the construct of the disorder is likely to become more differentiated and multidimensional (Popper et al. 2003).

What Features Are Associated With Adult ADHD?

In adults with ADHD, often one or more other psychiatric diagnoses also apply. For many persons, especially those who have not been able to get treatment, life is a series of painful setbacks. Patients with ADHD are vulnerable to depression, anxiety, and substance abuse. Adults with ADHD have average to above-average intellectual abilities, but cognitive deficits are common (Biederman et al. 1993). Although they are as smart as anyone else, they are less successful at work or in school than expected (Barkley and Gordon 2002).

A recent large study of 434 adults found that men and women with ADHD have symptom patterns that are like those of children and that their symptoms can be as severe as those of children. Women in the study demonstrated a lower incidence of conduct disorder and substance abuse disorder than did the men. The ADHD adults, both men and women, had significant rates of mood and anxiety disorders and similar patterns of impairment in psychosocial, cognitive, and academic development. Comorbid disorders emerged early, in childhood and adolescence. What was striking in the study was the continuity of symptoms from childhood and the persistent symptom severity in adulthood (Biederman et al. 2004). Finally, these patients may have a personality disorder as well as additional Axis I diagnoses.

What Are the Challenges in Recognizing and Treating Adult ADHD?

Like many members of the general public, some clinicians are skeptical that adult ADHD exists (Biederman 1998a). With that skepticism, many do not look for the clinical picture or make the diagnosis. The adults who have ADHD but are unaware of it do not seek treatment. They tend to see their difficulties as problems with other people. They think they are distracted because other people frequently interrupt them. They regard their lack of attention to details as simply a bad habit (Schwartz 2003).

Early in the evaluation process, clinicians typically ask questions and gather information as they try to make diagnoses and start treatment. That clinical process provides structure for the ADHD adult. Without intending to, our standard evaluation process may keep key patient characteristics such as poor organization, memory difficulties, distractibility, and impulsivity from surfacing. These may be far more disruptive at work or at home than in our offices. However, they may make themselves felt later in treatment. When that happens, the clinician needs to consider the possibility that the patient has ADHD. Otherwise, he or she may assume that the patient has little motivation to change, is irresponsible, or is resisting treatment. Forgetting or missing appointments, leaving medication refills until the last moment, and losing or misplacing prescriptions are all typical of adult ADHD patients (Schwartz 2003).

The diagnosis of adult ADHD has remained understandably controversial (Shaffer 1994). To make the diagnosis, clinicians rely on the patient's memories of distant childhood events. How accurate are these memories? Many people have problems remembering accurately what has just happened, much less events from their childhood. Second, patients with adult ADHD often have symptoms found in other disorders. Are the symptoms those of the other disorders or those of ADHD, or both? A further source of skepticism is that patients often self-diagnose. Clinicians have reason to be wary, especially of diagnoses with intense media coverage.

Many people resist the idea that adult ADHD is a real entity, saying, "Some people are just smarter than others." True enough, but many people with ADHD have a high IQ. Highly intelligent patients have come to me for treatment after they have earned advanced degrees, such as M.B.A.s, L.L.B.s, and Ph.D.s. Another dismissive argument is that "everyone has strong points and weak points, and some people are just weaker." Adults with ADHD are usually painfully aware of their weaknesses, because they struggle with them every day. Many have outstanding strengths—originality, creativity, and persistence—that others lack. Another view is simply that "these people are lazy." Of this view, an educator at Boston University says, "Some students have clinically valid ADHD. These high achievers really put a nail in the coffin of this argument. Anyone who has watched a highly successful adult with ADHD knows that he has worked many times harder than his peers without ADHD" (B.B. Doyle et al. 2000).

Why Do Adults Seek Treatment for ADHD?

Many adult patients come for treatment after one or more of their children are diagnosed with ADHD, are treated, and then improve. They see themselves in their child and they think, "Why shouldn't I get treatment, too?" Often a spouse points out the resemblance between the patient and the child (or children) and urges the adult partner to get evaluation and treatment. Sometimes the spouse will not put up any longer with dysfunctional behavior in the adult with ADHD. The spouse insists that the affected mate get treatment or the marriage will end.

> "I'm here because of my wife," said Tyrone, a 34-year-old African American electrician. "I've learned to work around my problems, but they sure bug her."

Other adults get discouraged after struggling for years. As adults, they want to use their resources and enjoy them, not limp along in life. They want more education, and they want to do well at it. They want to succeed at work; they want to be happy in an intimate relationship.

> "I'm just so tired of *being* this way," said one woman. "I just want a decent job with decent pay. Someone to come home to who loves and respects me. Is that too much to ask?"

Some highly intelligent children with ADHD, in schools that do not challenge them, do fine academically. It is only in higher education that problems become apparent.

> Noah came for treatment after earning his Ph.D. "I was a well-behaved kid. In college, I got decent grades only because my professors forgave my lateness. I finally passed in my graduate school thesis more than 2 years after it was due. I was lucky they even looked at it."

Spouses or significant others often help make the diagnosis. They have day-to-day, continuous contact that provides detailed information.

> Said one wife, "He forgets his keys, he's doing 10 things at once, and he never listens to what I say. We were at a party recently with his coworkers. After they had a drink or two, they asked me, 'How do you live with him? He drives us nuts, he's so disorganized.'"

To qualify for a diagnosis of ADHD as an adult, the patient needs to have a history of symptoms since childhood plus current symptoms of impulsivity and hyperactivity. The symptoms must occur in two different settings and adversely impact at least two aspects of the patient's life. Central to the diagnosis are problems in executive function: problems managing everyday life successfully. No single measure specifies ADHD in adults. Making the diagnosis is an empathic process that relies on data, ideally from multiple sources (Weiss and Murray 2003).

When the process of information gathering is complete, from the patient and significant others, then a discussion about the diagnosis follows. Does this diagnosis fit? Many patients have already read about ADHD and talked with other key persons in their lives about the disorder. Some patients profit by additional information in books or at pertinent Web sites (see Appendix).

ADHD AND COMORBID DISORDERS: DIFFERENTIAL DIAGNOSIS

Using the five-axis system in DSM-IV-TR encourages thinking fully about the patient. That includes due regard for coexisting psychiatric syndromes, personality disorders, general medical illnesses, stress level, and overall functioning. ADHD may be the first or primary psychiatric diagnosis, but often there are other disorders to diagnose in the patient. As many as 70% of patients with ADHD have comorbid conditions during their lifetime, such as mood or anxiety disorders, learning disabilities, behavior and personality disorders, and substance abuse (Pliszka 1998). These conditions receive a full discussion in Chapter 9 ("Comorbid and Treatment-Refractory ADHD"). Because many psychiatrists are more familiar with the comorbid disorders, we may do better at identifying and treating them than we do with identifying and treating adult ADHD. Thus the ADHD may stay hidden behind the comorbid conditions. Patients improve if treatment of the comorbid problems succeeds, but areas of impairment can linger.

It is easier to make a diagnosis of ADHD than to untangle it from comorbid conditions. Is the patient having symptoms other than those of ADHD now or in the past? Was the ADHD present before the other problems? If there are comorbid symptoms, what symptom needs treatment first? Managing these disorders may be as important as treating the ADHD. In fact, we may not be able to address the ADHD until we treat comorbid conditions adequately.

Sorting out the differential diagnosis takes time. Other psychiatric disorders are not the only ones to consider. Inattention, hyperactivity, and impulsivity can be present in many metabolic and neurological disorders, such as seizures and organic brain syndromes (Weiss et al. 1999).

SETTING AND MONITORING TREATMENT GOALS

Making a diagnosis and differential diagnosis (or diagnoses) is a start. Multiple diagnoses are the rule rather than the exception. Whatever is most debilitating gets treated first.

Only recently has it become apparent that the medications used for ADHD in childhood are also effective for adults. Often patients will require complex regimens, with combinations of medications and other interventions. Because most treatments for depression are not effective for ADHD, and vice versa, we may have to treat each separately (Spencer et al. 1999). Many patients think of ADHD just in the context of specific tasks, such as doing a job or studying, but ADHD symptoms occur 24 hours a day, 7 days a week. Do patients need medication continuously or just at certain parts of the day? What factors may improve treatment outcome and what may hinder it? Once clinicians have answers to these questions, a full treatment plan is possible.

Factors Influencing Patient Outcome

Some patients do better, especially those who have only ADHD. Patients most likely to thrive are those who have already accomplished something with their life and those who have a supportive social network. ADHD symptoms tend gradually to improve over time if they are not complicated by other comorbidities. Unfortunately, most adults with ADHD have additional psychiatric problems. Patients with a darker prognosis include those who have major mood fluctuations, severe impulsivity, and disorders such as substance abuse. The demoralized patient who has a history of many failures is also at risk. Our efforts may fail when persons important to the patient oppose the diagnosis of ADHD or object to its treatment (Biederman 1998b).

ADHD: PROBLEM OR ADVANTAGE IN LIFE?

Clinicians helping patients naturally focus on the problems that bring their patients to treatment. However, in focusing on helping people do better, we may overlook or forget that many adults with ADHD have impressive personality traits and achievements. Often these strengths come from decades of contending with the constraints of the disorder.

> Talking in an interview about his life with ADHD, the prominent political consultant James Carville said, "I've been struggling with growing up for 58 years, and I'm winning."

Some patients insist that their ADHD provides them with special qualities and abilities.

> Jesse, a wealthy real-estate entrepreneur, said, "My mind is like a jumping jack. Most people think linearly. I see situations in 3-D, and it works. Check out my bank account."

Rather than being a burden, for some people having ADHD is the key to their success.

> David Neeleman, the founder of JetBlue Airways, said, "On balance, ADD has been a positive. People with it tend to be more creative, to think outside the box more. They take more risks. I was at a conference of educators at Harvard, talking about ADD in my life, and one asked why I had never taken any medication for it. I said, 'I'm afraid I'll take it once, blow a circuit, and then I'd be like the rest of you'" (Neeleman and Lawlor 2003).

SUMMARY

- ADHD is still a controversial diagnosis, even more so in adults than it is in children. Affected individuals can focus and attend, but they cannot count on being able to do that in situations where they want to and know that they should. Central to the disorder is a lack of effective executive function (i.e., frontal lobe skills). The symptom picture in adults is complex, affected by maturation and coping skills. Symptoms of impulsivity and hyperactivity tend to wane, and symptoms of inattention tend to persist.
- The current estimate is that more than half of children who have ADHD will have symptoms as adults. Patients who are adults do not need to meet the full criteria for ADHD to have it impact their life. An estimated 4% of American adults, or more than 7 million people, warrant the diagnosis.
- The symptoms of ADHD in adults complicate daily life, interfere with academic progress, and contribute to workplace difficulties. Lingering impulsivity contributes to problems in patients' sexual life. Driving an automobile is often problematic. Social aspects of the disorder keep patients from finding and sustaining intimate relationships. They are more likely to divorce. ADHD patients are more likely to abuse substances such as alcohol and other drugs.
- Once alert to the possibility that the patient has the disorder, clinicians may find the diagnosis relatively easy to make. Disentangling the comorbid conditions is harder, because the patient rarely presents with symptoms of ADHD alone. The clinician has to treat the most impairing condition first; the treatment of ADHD may need to wait.
- Some adults with ADHD thrive because of the special way their brain works, but they are unusual. Most need full treatment to make the most of their resources.

REFERENCES

Adler LA, Cohen J: Diagnosis and evaluation of adults with attention-deficit hyperactivity disorder. Psychiatr Clin North Am 27:184–201, 2004

Amen DG, Goldberg B: Attention deficit hyperactivity disorder: a guide for primary care physicians. Primary Psychiatry 7:76–80, 1998

American Psychiatric Association: Diagnostic and Statistical Manual of Mental Disorders, 4th Edition, Text Revision. Washington, DC, American Psychiatric Association, 2000

Asarnow JR: Peer status and social competence in child psychiatric inpatients: a comparison of children with depressive, externalizing, and concurrent depressive and externalizing disorders. J Abnorm Child Psychol 16:151–162, 1988

Bagwell CL, Molina BS, Pelham WE Jr, et al: Attention-deficit/hyperactivity disorder and problems in peer relations: predictions from childhood to adolescence. J Am Acad Child Adolesc Psychiatry 40:1285–1292, 2001

Barbaresi WJ, Katusic SK, Colligan RC, et al: How common is attention-deficit/hyperactivity disorder? Arch Pediatr Adolesc Med 156:217–224, 2002

Barkley RA: ADHD and the Nature of Self-Control. New York, Guilford, 1997

Barkley RA: Developmental course, adult outcome, and clinic-referred ADHD adults, in Attention-Deficit Hyperactivity Disorder: A Handbook for Diagnosis and Treatment, 2nd Edition. Edited by Barkley RA. New York, Guilford, 1998, pp 139–163

Barkley RA: Driving impairments in teens and adults with attention-deficit/hyperactivity disorder. Psychiatr Clin North Am 27:233–260, 2004

Barkley RA, Gordon M: Research on comorbidity, adaptive functioning, and cognitive impairment in adults with ADHD: implications for a clinical practice, in Clinical Interventions for Adult ADHD: A Comprehensive Approach. Edited by Goldstein S, Teeter Ellison A. San Diego, CA, Academic Press, 2002, pp 46–71

Barkley RA, Murphy KR: Attention-Deficit/Hyperactivity Disorder: A Clinical Workbook, 2nd Edition. New York, Guilford, 1998

Barkley RA, Murphy KR, Kasich D: Psychological adjustment and adaptive impairment in young adults with ADHD. J Atten Disord 1:41–54, 1996

Barkley RA, Fischer M, Smallish L, et al: The persistence of attention-deficit hyperactivity disorder into young adulthood as a function of reporting source and definition of disorder. J Abnorm Psychol 111:279–289, 2002a

Barkley RA, Murphy KR, Dupaul GI, et al: Driving in young adults with attention deficit hyperactivity disorder: performance, adverse outcomes, and the role of executive functioning. J Int Neuropsychol Soc 8:655–672, 2002b

Biederman J: A 55-year-old man with attention-deficit/hyperactivity disorder. JAMA 280:1086–1092, 1998a

Biederman J: Attention-deficit hyperactivity disorder: a life-span perspective. J Clin Psychiatry 59 (suppl 7):4–16, 1998b

Biederman J: Course and outcome of ADHD. Paper presented at ADHD Across the Life Span, Boston, MA, March 2005

Biederman J, Faraone SV, Spencer T, et al: Patterns of psychiatric comorbidity, cognition, and psychosocial function in adults with ADHD. Am J Psychiatry 150:1792–1798, 1993

Biederman J, Faraone SV, Milberger S, et al: Predictors of persistence and remission of ADHD: results from a four-year prospective study of ADHD children. J Am Acad Child Adolesc Psychiatry 35:343–351, 1996

Biederman J, Mick E, Faraone SV: Normalized functioning in youths with persistent ADHD. J Pediatr 133:544–549, 1998

Biederman J, Mick E, Faraone SV: Age-dependent decline of symptoms of attention deficit hyperactivity disorder: impact of remission definition and symptom type. Am J Psychiatry 157:816–818, 2000

Biederman J, Faraone SV, Monuteaux MC, et al: Gender effects on attention-deficit/hyperactivity disorder in adults, revisited. Biol Psychiatry 55:692–700, 2004

Bird H: The diagnostic classification, epidemiology, and cross-cultural validity of ADHD, in Attention Deficit Hyperactivity Disorder: State of the Science, Best Practices. Edited by Jensen PS, Cooper JR. Kingston, NJ, Civic Research Institute, 2002, pp 2-1–2-16

Bradley W: The behavior of children receiving Benzedrine. Am J Psychiatry 94:577–585, 1937

Cantwell DP: Hyperactive children have grown up: what have we learned from what happens to them? Arch Gen Psychiatry 42:1026–1028, 1985

Cantwell DP, Hanna G: Attention deficit disorder, in American Psychiatric Press Review of Psychiatry, Vol 8. Edited by Tasman A, Hales RE, Frances AJ. Washington, DC, American Psychiatric Press, 1989, pp 134–161

Chess S: Diagnosis and treatment of the hyperactive child. N Y State J Med 60:2379–2385, 1960

Cox DJ, Merkel L, Kovatchev B, et al: Effect of stimulant medication on driving performance of young adults with attention-deficit hyperactivity disorder: a preliminary double-blind placebo controlled trial. J Nerv Ment Dis 188:230–234, 2000

Davis K, Chang LL, Horrigan J: Prevalence and economic burden of adult ADHD in managed care. Poster presented at the annual meeting of the American Academy of Child and Adolescent Psychiatry, San Francisco, CA, October 2002

Denhoff E, Laufer MW, Solomons G: Hyperkinetic impulse disorder in children's behavior problems. Psychosom Med 19:38–49, 1957

Douglas VI: Attentional and cognitive problems, in Developmental Neuropsychiatry. Edited by Rutter M. New York, Guilford, 1983, pp 280–329

Doyle BB, Montauk SL, Wender PH, et al: ADHD in adults: valid diagnosis and treatment strategies. Medical Crossfire 4:30–40, 2000

Doyle R: The history of adult attention-deficit hyperactivity disorder. Psychiatr Clin N Am 27:203–214, 2004

Elliott H: Attention-deficit/hyperactivity disorder in adults: a guide for the primary care physician. South Med J 95:736–742, 2002

Faraone SV, Biederman J: Prevalence of adult ADHD in the U.S. Presented at the annual meeting of the American Psychiatric Association, New York, May 2004a

Faraone SV, Biederman J: Prevalence of adult ADHD in the United States. Poster presentation at the 17th annual U.S. Psychiatric and Mental Health Congress, San Diego, CA, November 19, 2004b

Faraone SV, Biederman J, Mick E, et al: Family study of girls with attention deficit hyperactivity disorder. Am J Psychiatry 157:1077–1083, 2000

Fischer M, Barkley RA, Smallish L, et al: Young adult follow up of hyperactive children: self-reported psychiatric disorders, comorbidity, and the role of childhood conduct problems. J Abnorm Child Psychol 30:463–475, 2002

Goldman LS, Genel M, Bezman RJ, et al: Diagnosis and treatment of ADHD in children and adolescents. JAMA 279:100–107, 1998

Greenfield B, Hechtman L, Weiss G: Two subgroups of hyperactives as adults: correlations of outcome. Can J Psychiatry 33:505–508, 1988

Hart EL, Lahey BB, Loeber R, et al: Developmental change in attention-deficit hyperactivity disorder in boys: a four-year longitudinal study. J Abnorm Child Psychol 23:729–749, 1995

Johnston C, Freeman W: Parents' beliefs about ADHD: implications for assessment and treatment. ADHD Report 10:6–9, 2000

Johnston C, Patenaud R: Parent attributions for inattentive-overactive and oppositional-defiant behaviors. Cognit Ther Res 18:261–275, 1994

Kessler RC: Prevalence of Adult ADHD in the United States: results from the National Comorbidity Survey (NCS-R). Paper presented at the annual meeting of the American Psychiatric Association, New York, May 2004

Kessler RC, Chiu WT, Demler O, et al: Prevalence, severity, and comorbidity of 12-month DSM-IV disorders in the National Comorbidity Survey Replication. Arch Gen Psychiatry 62:617–627, 2005

Maedgen JW, Carlson CL: Social functioning and emotional regulation in the attention deficit hyperactivity disorder subtypes. J Clin Child Psychol 29:30–42, 2000

Mannuzza S, Klein RG, Konig PH, et al: Hyperactive boys almost grown up, IV: criminality and its relationship to psychiatric status. Arch Gen Psychiatry 46:1073–1079, 1989

Mannuzza S, Klein RG, Bonagura N, et al: Hyperactive boys almost grown up, V: replication of psychiatric status. Arch Gen Psychiatry 48:77–83, 1991

Mannuzza S, Klein RG, Bessler A, et al: Adult psychiatric status of hyperactive boys grown up. Am J Psychiatry 155:493–498, 1998

McDonnell MA, Doyle R, Surman C: Current approaches to the management of ADHD. Clinician Reviews 13:110–118, 2000

Menkes M, Rowe J, Menkes J: A five-year follow-up study of the hyperactive child with minimal brain dysfunction. Pediatrics 39:393–399, 1967

Mick E, Faraone SV, Biederman J: Age-dependent expression of attention-deficit hyperactivity disorder symptoms. Psychiatr Clin North Am 27:215–224, 2004

Murphy K, Barkley RA: ADHD adults: comorbidities and adaptive impairments. Compr Psychiatry 37:393–401, 1996a

Murphy K, Barkley RA: Prevalence of DSM-IV symptoms of ADHD in adult licensed drivers: implications for clinical diagnosis. J Atten Disord 1:147–161, 1996b

Neeleman D, Lawlor J: Rewards in restlessness. The New York Times, June 1, 2003, sec 3, p 12

Pliszka SR: Comorbidity of attention-deficit/hyperactivity disorder with psychiatric disorder: an overview. J Clin Psychiatry 59 (suppl 7):50–58, 1998

Pomerleau OF, Downey KK, Stelson FW, et al: Cigarette smoking in adult patients diagnosed with attention deficit hyperactivity disorder. J Subst Abuse 7:373–378, 1995

Popper CW, Gammon GD, West SA, et al: Disorders usually first diagnosed in infancy, childhood, or adolescence, in The American Psychiatric Publishing Textbook of Psychiatry, 4th Edition. Edited by Hales RE, Yudofsky SC. Washington, DC, American Psychiatric Publishing, 2003, pp 833–974

Rie HE, Rie ED (eds): Handbook of Minimal Brain Dysfunction: A Critical Review. New York, Wiley, 1980

Rucklidge JJ, Tannock R: Psychiatric, psychosocial and cognitive functioning of female adolescents with ADHD. J Am Acad Child Adolesc Psychiatry 40:530–540, 2001

Safer DJ, Zito JM, Fine EM: Increased methylphenidate usage for attention deficit disorder in the 1990s. Pediatrics 98:1084–1088, 1996

Schwartz MD: Recognizing and managing the treatment-disruptive effects of attention deficit disorder. Primary Psychiatry 10:59–62, 2003

Shaffer D: Attention deficit hyperactivity disorder in adults. Am J Psychiatry 151:633–638, 1994

Spencer T, Biederman J, Wilens TE, et al: Adults with attention-deficit/hyperactivity disorder: a controversial diagnosis. J Clin Psychiatry 59 (suppl 7):59–68, 1998

Spencer T, Biederman J, Wilens T: Attention-deficit/hyperactivity disorder and comorbidity. Pediatr Clin North Am 46:915–927, 1999

Still GF: Some abnormal physical conditions in children. Lancet 1:1008–1012, 1077–1082, 1163–1168, 1902

Strauss AA, Lehtinen LE: Psychopathology and Education of the Brain-Injured Child. New York, Grune & Stratton, 1947

Stryker S: Encephalitis lethargica: the behavior residuals. Training School Bulletin 22:152–157, 1925

Valentine J, Rossi E, O'Leary P, et al: Thyroid function in a population of children with attention deficit hyperactivity disorder. J Paediatr Child Health 33:117–120, 1997

Weiss G, Hechtman LT: Hyperactive Children Grown Up: Empirical Findings and Theoretical Considerations. New York, Guilford, 1986

Weiss G, Hechtman LT: Hyperactive Children Grown Up: ADHD in Children, Adolescents, and Adults, 2nd Edition. New York, Guilford, 1993

Weiss G, Hechtman L, Milroy T, et al: Psychiatric status of hyperactives as adults: a controlled prospective 15-year follow-up of 63 hyperactive children. J Am Acad Child Psychiatry 24:211–220, 1985

Weiss M, Murray C: Assessment and management of attention-deficit /hyperactivity disorder in adults. CMAJ 168:715–722, 2003

Weiss M, Hechtman LT, Weiss G: ADHD and other disorders, in ADHD in Adulthood. Baltimore, MD, Johns Hopkins University Press, 1999, pp 73–108

Wender P: Attention-Deficit Hyperactivity Disorder in Adults. New York, Oxford University Press, 1995

Whalen CK, Henker B: The social profiles of attention-deficit hyperactivity disorder: five fundamental facets. Child Adolesc Psychiatr Clin N Am 1:395–410, 1992

Wilens TE: Attention-deficit/hyperactivity disorder and the substance abuse disorders: the nature of the relationship, subtypes at risk, and treatment issues. Psychiatr Clin North Am 27:283–301, 2004

Wilens TE, Spencer T, Biederman J: Attention deficit disorder with substance abuse, in Subtypes of Attention-Deficit Disorders in Children, Adolescents, and Adults. Washington, DC, American Psychiatric Press, 1996, pp 319–339

Wilson JM, Marcotte AC: Psychosocial adjustment and educational outcome in adolescents with a childhood diagnosis of attention deficit disorder. J Am Acad Child Adolesc Psychiatry 35:579–587, 1996

Woodward LJ, Fergusson DM, Horwood LJ: Driving outcomes of young people with attentional difficulties in adolescence. J Am Acad Child Adolesc Psychiatry 39:627–634, 2000

CHAPTER 2

DIAGNOSING ADHD IN ADULTS

TO DIAGNOSE ADHD IN AN ADULT, the clinician has to document the presence of inattentive or hyperactive/impulsive symptoms, or both. The onset of symptoms should have been in childhood, before the age of 7. The patient must show impairment in at least two realms of current life, such as work and family, and the impairment must be manifest in at least two settings, such as at the office and at home. Finally, the clinician must determine that the symptoms are those of ADHD and not of another mental health disorder. Diagnosing ADHD in adults is a clinical process. Other sources of information such as questionnaires, neuropsychological tests, and laboratory examinations are helpful but not diagnostic. They are no substitute for clinical interviews.

Although ADHD is one diagnostic category in DSM-IV-TR (American Psychiatric Association 2000), the disorder likely comprises a cluster of syndromes we cannot yet specify well. In the future, we will likely split off more specific disorders. Improved neuroimaging or other techniques may clarify a different genetic transmission or different pathophysiology. For now, however, clinicians need to find evidence for problems in the area under the ADHD rubric.

DIAGNOSING ADHD IN CHILDREN

Many issues in diagnosing ADHD in children are important in working with affected adults. When diagnosing ADHD in a child, the clinician gathers information from interviews with the child; from parents, teachers, and other physicians; and from written records from school and elsewhere. Then the clinician confirms whether the child meets criteria in DSM-IV-TR.

At the start, the clinician should request reports of all prior psychiatric, psychological, developmental, and medical evaluations and treatments. Reviewing prior records gives important history and suggests more information that may be needed now.

The evaluator assesses the youngster's developmental level and temperament. Typically, a youngster with ADHD has developmental delays that show up in how well the child collaborates with the clinician and participates in treatment. The child's temperament counts as well. Youngsters with an "easy" temperament typically have a positive mood. They are adaptable and have regular biological rhythms. Children with a "difficult" temperament have intense, negative moods and irregular biological rhythms. Third are children with a "slow to warm up" temperament (Thomas and Chess 1986). How well a youngster fits his or her parents' temperaments, expectations, and child-raising skills significantly affects his or her life.

To formulate a diagnosis in children, clinicians interview the child and significant others. Ideally, that means interviewing both parents, even if they are divorced or live separately. A disproportionate number of adopted children have ADHD. Is the patient the biological child of these parents, or adopted? Have the parents or other children received a diagnosis and been treated with ADHD? Is there a family history of ADHD? Are there potential risks of medication abuse by the patient or family members, either parents or siblings?

What is the child's medical history, including seizures, head trauma, thyroid disorder, and medication use? Were there problems in the obstetrical history, such as maternal substance abuse or prenatal or perinatal injury? Does the child have sleep difficulties? Is there a history of trauma such as neglect or abuse? Are there environmental problems, such as exposure to lead?

Documentation from school about the child's behavior is essential. Report card comments are classic sources; for example, "cannot sit still," "erratic," "disruptive in class," and "inattentive." Documentation on how the youngster behaves in the cafeteria and on the bus may be as revealing as reports from class.

In addition to history from the child and supportive information from others, the clinician uses normed rating scales. Some scales the clinician fills out; others are for parents, teachers, and other observers. The child should have a full physical examination. Laboratory testing can identify thyroid disorders, among other problems. Questions about neurological status require specialized evaluation. Youngsters need tests such as an electroencephalogram or a brain scan only if they show focal neurological signs, indications of a seizure disorder, or a decline in neurological function.

Psychological test results are useful but not diagnostic. These tests can assess intellectual ability, academic achievement, and possible specific learning disorders. A normal performance on individual testing, however, does *not* rule out the diagnosis of ADHD (Dulcan et al. 2003). If a child has specific deficits, neuropsychological evaluation may be useful.

Subtypes of ADHD

To qualify for the diagnosis of ADHD the child must be either inattentive or hyperactive/impulsive or both. The DSM-IV-TR criteria describe symptoms of inattention and of hyperactivity/impulsivity (see Table 2–1).

By these diagnostic criteria, there are three main types of ADHD: inattentive, hyperactive-impulsive, and combined. Each appears to have a distinct prognosis and response to treatment. Therefore, it is necessary to assess patients separately for inattention and for hyperactivity/impulsivity (Popper et al. 2003). A fourth diagnosis, ADHD not otherwise specified (ADHD-NOS), covers ADHD syndromes that do not meet criteria for one of the other three. These diagnostic criteria are described below:

> **314.00 Attention-deficit/hyperactivity disorder, predominantly inattentive type (ADHD-PI):** The patient meets Criterion A1 but not A2 for the past 6 months, to a degree that is maladaptive and not suited to the developmental level.
>
> **314.01 Attention-deficit/hyperactivity disorder, predominantly hyperactive-impulsive type:** The patient meets Criterion A2 but not A1 for the past 6 months, to a degree that is maladaptive and not suited to the developmental level.
>
> **314.01 Attention-deficit/hyperactivity disorder, combined type:** The patient meets both Criteria A1 and A2 for the past 6 months, to a degree that is maladaptive and not suited to the developmental level.
>
> **314.9 Attention-deficit/hyperactivity disorder not otherwise specified (ADHD-NOS):** This diagnosis applies to patients with prominent symptoms of inattention or of hyperactivity/impulsivity who do not meet full criteria for ADHD. This category is important in diagnosing some adults. Examples include individuals whose symptoms and impairment meet the criteria for ADHD-PI, but whose age at onset is 7 years or later. This diagnosis also applies to "individuals with clinically significant impairment who present with inattention and whose symptom pattern does not meet the full

TABLE 2–1.   DSM-IV-TR diagnostic criteria for attention-deficit/hyperactivity disorder

A.   Either (1) or (2):

   (1)   six (or more) of the following symptoms of **inattention** have persisted
         for at least 6 months to a degree that is maladaptive and inconsistent
         with developmental level:

   Inattention
   (a)   often fails to give close attention to details or makes careless
         mistakes in schoolwork, work, or other activities
   (b)   often has difficulty sustaining attention in tasks or play activities
   (c)   often does not seem to listen when spoken to directly
   (d)   often does not follow through on instructions and fails to finish
         schoolwork, chores, or duties in the workplace (not due to
         oppositional behavior or failure to understand instructions)
   (e)   often has difficulty organizing tasks and activities
   (f)   often avoids, dislikes, or is reluctant to engage in tasks that
         require sustained mental effort (such as schoolwork or
         homework)
   (g)   often loses things necessary for tasks or activities (e.g., toys,
         school assignments, pencils, books, or tools)
   (h)   is often easily distracted by extraneous stimuli
   (i)   is often forgetful in daily activities

   (2)   six (or more) of the following symptoms of **hyperactivity-
         impulsivity** have persisted for at least 6 months to a degree that is
         maladaptive and inconsistent with developmental level:

   Hyperactivity
   (a)   often fidgets with hands or feet or squirms in seat
   (b)   often leaves seat in classroom or in other situations in which
         remaining seated is expected
   (c)   often runs about or climbs excessively in situations in which it is
         inappropriate (in adolescents or adults, may be limited to
         subjective feelings of restlessness)
   (d)   often has difficulty playing or engaging in leisure activities
         quietly
   (e)   is often "on the go" or often acts as if "driven by a motor"
   (f)   often talks excessively

   Impulsivity
   (g)   often blurts out answers before questions have been completed
   (h)   often has difficulty awaiting turn
   (i)   often interrupts or intrudes on others (e.g., butts into
         conversations or games)

TABLE 2–1. DSM-IV-TR diagnostic criteria for attention-deficit/hyperactivity disorder *(continued)*

B. Some hyperactive-impulsive or inattentive symptoms that caused impairment were present before age 7 years.
C. Some impairment from the symptoms is present in two or more settings (e.g., at school [or work] and at home).
D. There must be clear evidence of clinically significant impairment in social, academic, or occupational functioning.
E. The symptoms do not occur exclusively during the course of a pervasive developmental disorder, schizophrenia, or other psychotic disorder and are not better accounted for by another mental disorder (e.g., mood disorder, anxiety disorder, dissociative disorder, or a personality disorder).

Code based on type:

314.01 Attention-Deficit/Hyperactivity Disorder, Combined Type: if both Criteria A1 and A2 are met for the past 6 months

314.00 Attention-Deficit/Hyperactivity Disorder, Predominantly Inattentive Type: if Criterion A1 is met but Criterion A2 is not met for the past 6 months

314.01 Attention-Deficit/Hyperactivity Disorder, Predominantly Hyperactive-Impulsive Type: if Criterion A2 is met but Criterion A1 is not met for the past 6 months

Coding note: For individuals (especially adolescents and adults) who currently have symptoms that no longer meet full criteria, "In Partial Remission" should be specified.

Source. Reprinted from American Psychiatric Association: *Diagnostic and Statistical Manual of Mental Disorders,* 4th Edition, Text Revision. Washington, DC, American Psychiatric Association, 2000. Used with permission.

criteria for the disorder but have a behavioral pattern marked by sluggishness, daydreaming, and hypoactivity" (American Psychiatric Association 2000, p. 93).

The diagnostic category of ADHD-NOS might appear to be one of convenience rather than one that is biologically distinct. However, researchers using quantitative electroencephalography and evoked response potentials have found electrophysiological characteristics that distinguish it from the three main subtypes of the disorder (Kuperman et al. 1996). This suggests that ADHD-NOS is an additional subtype of ADHD.

The diagnostic criteria of DSM-IV-TR allow specifying whether symptoms are mild, moderate, or severe. For individuals who once warranted an ADHD diagnosis but who no longer meet full criteria, the proper specifier is "in partial remission."

Despite apparent differences between the inattentive and combined subtypes of ADHD in demographics, disruptive behavior, and cognitive tempo, research has failed to find differences between the subtypes in key neuropsychological functions. The deficit in ADHD-PI seems to be associated with stimulus processing and related to the "arousal system," which is mainly noradrenergic. Combined-type ADHD, in contrast, appears to be associated with response processing and related to the "activation system." This system involves motor preparedness and output functions that are primarily dopaminergic (Solanto 2004).

The predominance of an ADHD subtype may shift over time within the same person. One study followed children who received a diagnosis of ADHD at 4–6 years of age. Of the youngsters who initially received a diagnosis of the hyperactive-impulsive form of ADHD, just over 40% improved within 5 years. Of the remaining 60%, a large proportion appeared to shift into the combined type of ADHD. Few children become hyperactive/impulsive who were not from the start. The symptoms of hyperactivity and impulsivity wane faster than those of inattention (Lahey et al. 2004).

Differential Diagnosis of Childhood ADHD

The clinician needs to be alert for explanations other than ADHD for the child's problems. If the symptoms are new and short-lived, the child may have an adjustment disorder. Medical illnesses and environmental problems, such as inadequate nutrition and sleep, can interfere with attention and concentration. Thyroid disturbances, as well as medications such as theophylline, benzodiazepines, or phenobarbital, may also cause attentional problems. Abused, neglected, or undernourished children can be impulsive, scattered, and inefficient. Among teenagers, abuse of substances such as marijuana and alcohol can wreak havoc on study habits and life achievement.

Like adults with ADHD, children rarely present with only that disorder. The clinician may need systematic observation of the child before deciding whether the child's symptoms are those of ADHD, another disorder, or both. Many common, co-occurring conditions have symptoms that overlap those of ADHD, especially affective and anxiety disorders. Some children have learning disabilities, such as in reading or in doing mathematics, which result from localized decrements in brain function. Children who have more global central nervous system (CNS) deficiencies are mentally retarded. They may be referred for ADHD evaluation because they have trouble staying on task and following directions in school or at home.

Children with behavior disorders, either oppositional defiant disorder or the more severe conduct disorder, usually provoke and misbehave deliberately. The youngster with ADHD may fail to comply more out of inattention and disorganization. Many children, unfortunately, have both ADHD and a behavior disorder.

The clinician needs particularly to rule out the possibility of a psychotic disorder. CNS stimulants can worsen psychotic symptoms and disorganization. Many children with ADHD are distractible and talkative. They can display loose thinking, but they do not have hallucinations, delusions, or a formal thought disorder (Dulcan et al. 2003).

DIAGNOSING ADHD IN ADULTS

Evaluating adults for ADHD is a clinical process, as it is for children. DSM-IV-TR does not provide specific diagnostic criteria for adults.

Diagnosing an adult with ADHD can have legal and career ramifications. In recent years, adults with ADHD have sought special accommodation in higher education and in the workplace. The diagnosis has received considerable attention in the popular press. Some persons have used the diagnosis as an excuse for failure to perform. (Chapter 10, "ADHD Issues: Work, Women, and Family," contains a fuller description of the legal issues involved in working with adults with ADHD.)

Most patients require multiple evaluative interviews. Making a diagnosis of ADHD is a first step; next is assessing the patient for comorbidity. The evaluation is complete when a full treatment plan prioritizes the patient's problems and provides a suitable range of interventions. Recommendations for organizing the office evaluation of ADHD are in Table 2–2.

Before the first scheduled interview, it is useful to ask the identified patient to confirm the time and date. That initial phone contact helps the patient to connect with the clinician. It also counteracts any ADHD-related tendency to forget or mislay information.

At the start of the assessment, obtain and review the results of prior testing, treatment, or both. This includes materials from nonpsychiatric physicians such as past pediatricians, prior psychiatrists or other mental health professionals, and educational or other evaluators.

When assessing adults, the clinician must translate into suitable terms the childhood criteria for ADHD. Adult manifestations of problems with inattention and hyperactivity/impulsivity are different. Inat-

TABLE 2–2.   Office evaluation of ADHD in adults

History of attentional complaints

> Duration, primary symptoms
>
> Are symptoms diffuse or specific to modality or to setting?
>
> Is there evidence of hyperactivity? Can the patient sit to study, or through dinner or a movie?
>
> Can the patient read effectively (decode, comprehend)? How long can he or she read at one time? Can the patient recall what was read? Does he or she read for pleasure?
>
> Can the patient take effective notes from an oral presentation and follow the presentation?
>
> Does he or she have problems from being disorganized or misplacing things?
>
> Does the patient keep his or her belongings in good order?
>
> Does the patient daydream? Do his or her thoughts jump around?
>
> Is the patient frequently forgetful? Does he or she often feel overwhelmed?
>
> Does the patient have problems completing tasks?
>
> Does he or she lose interest quickly and shift from one task to another?
>
> Can the patient listen to others and keep track of a conversation?
>
> Is he or she easily distracted, impulsive, or impatient? Can he or she wait in line? Is he or she short-tempered, irritable?
>
> Does the patient blurt out answers and interrupt others?
>
> Does his or her mood change frequently?

History from patient and other informants

> Developmental history: history of brain injury, tics, conduct disturbance
>
> Academic history: highest educational level, grades at each level, best and worst subjects, resource help, special education, repetition of a grade, history of hyperactivity in school
>
> Work history: nature and number of jobs, work satisfaction, status of career goals
>
> Psychiatric history: in particular, anxiety and affective disorders, especially bipolar spectrum disorders
>
> Social history: relationships past and present with spouses, partners, family members, children
>
> Sexual history: age at initiation, number of partners, sexually transmitted diseases, unplanned or unexpected pregnancies, current status
>
> Driving history: tickets for speeding or other infractions; accidents or wrecks
>
> Legal history: misdemeanors, felonies, or convictions

TABLE 2–2. Office evaluation of ADHD in adults *(continued)*

Office tests (adapted to developmental level)

Recitation of the months of the year backward or a digit span

Repetition of a short story

Test-free articulation of ideas: describe a paragraph he or she read or answer open-ended questions

Arithmetic problems: addition, multiplication, subtraction, division

Reading: fluency, comprehension, educational level

Brief writing sample

Verbal fluency

Abstraction

Figure copying

Memory

General information

Estimate of general intelligence

Observation of problem-solving strategy: carefulness, consistency, frustration and anxiety levels

Source. Adapted from Cohen RA, Salloway S, Zawacki T: "Neuropsychiatric Aspects of Disorders of Attention," in *The American Psychiatric Publishing Textbook of Neuropsychiatry and Clinical Neurosciences,* 4th Edition. Edited by Yudofsky SC, Hales RE. Washington, DC, American Psychiatric Publishing, 2002, p. 516. Used with permission.

tentive ADHD adults often have problems sustaining attention while in meetings, reading, or doing paperwork. They may procrastinate extensively; they are slow, disorganized, and inefficient, with poor time management. Hyperactive ADHD adults often have an inner restlessness, staying overscheduled and often overworking. Their constant activity, and their propensity for talking and not listening, can cause family friction. Impulsivity in ADHD adults can have serious consequences when it results in rapid changes of jobs and relationships or in driving too aggressively.

It is harder to assess adult patients' developmental level than that of children. An important developmental marker is autonomy, the patient's ability to sustain himself or herself in the world. Has the patient made suitable work choices and shown work achievement? Does he or she have sustained, intimate relationships? What are the patient's coping mechanisms? Resourceful adults can minimize their symptoms, but often at hidden, high emotional costs. Adulthood makes larger demands on the person's executive functions than childhood does.

Many psychiatrists who treat adults lack the developmental perspective that colleagues trained in child psychiatry bring to their work with children. Focused on the patient's current life, we may neglect to ask questions that trace problems with inattention, hyperactivity, and impulsivity over time (Adler and Cohen 2004). Thus, we may overlook the diagnosis. Persons with ADHD who are biologically adults often have developmental delays. Because these adults typically have problems learning, they may have less formal education or take longer to graduate than their age peers. They may have fewer formal qualifications and often launch their adult work life later. Their work record may be uneven. Many adults with ADHD are personable, but they may also have frustrated spouses and disgruntled bosses.

When evaluating patients, clinicians must recognize and support the patients' strengths as well as help them remedy weaknesses. This task is particularly important in assessing adults who come with questions about ADHD. They often do not know the answer to the question, "Who are you, at your best?" They have always been struggling, only having access to their full resources from time to time. Many are resilient, resourceful, and tenacious, but some get overwhelmed. To help patients succeed, encourage them to look for their natural inclinations, interests, and strengths and build on them.

PRACTICE PARAMETERS FOR THE ASSESSMENT OF ADULT ADHD

Comprehensive practice parameters for assessing adults for ADHD are available from the American Academy of Child and Adolescent Psychiatry (AACAP; 1997). A summary of the recommended initial evaluation appears in Table 2–3.

Clinicians develop their own process for evaluating patients. Some choose a different sequence of elements or emphasize some elements more than others. The AACAP recommendations are a fine framework for the evaluation. They can serve as a guide to information that may be overlooked. The next discussion follows the framework of elements proposed by AACAP.

1. Clinical Interviews

As it is with children, the clinical interaction is at the heart of the matter in diagnosing adults. Usually an evaluation requires several interviews, which respects the complexity of the adult's situation. In a few instances, the clinician can reach a diagnosis of ADHD and start treatment on the basis of one interview. Although this may be possible with an adult who has severe symptoms and a long, well-documented history, such patients are rare. Most ADHD adults do not display their symp-

TABLE 2–3. Initial evaluation of adults for ADHD

1. Clinical interviews
    Developmental history
    Past and present DSM-IV-TR symptoms of ADHD
    How symptoms have developed to produce impairments
    History of other psychiatric diagnoses and treatment
    Symptoms of possible alternative and comorbid psychiatric
        disorders, especially mood disorders (depression, mania), anxiety
        disorders, substance use disorders, learning disorders, and
        personality disorder
    Strengths: talents and abilities
    Mental status examination
2. Standardized rating scales
    Adult ADHD Self-Report Scale
    Barkley System of Diagnostic Scales
    Brown Attention-Deficit Disorder Scales
    Conners' Adult ADHD Rating Scale
    Other applicable scales
3. Medical history and evaluations
4. Family history
    ADHD
    Other psychiatric disorders, including developmental/learning
    Family coping style, organization, resources
    Family stresses
    Abuse or neglect (as victim or perpetrator)
5. Interview with significant other or parent, if available
6. School and work evaluations
7. Further evaluations as indicated
    Educational evaluation
    Psychological testing
    Neuropsychological testing
    Neuroimaging
    Vocational evaluation

Source. Adapted from the American Academy of Child and Adolescent Psychiatry: "Practice Parameters for the Assessment and Treatment of Children, Adolescents and Adults With Attention-Deficit/Hyperactivity Disorder." *Journal of the American Academy of Child and Adolescent Psychiatry* 36(suppl):85S–121S, 1997.

toms in the office interview; they report problems in their current life and in their past. Their performance on cognitive tasks in a structured setting may be normal (Cohen et al. 2002). They have a "sophisticated chief complaint": they say that they "are not fulfilling their potential" or that they "are having issues in their marriage or close relationships"

(Biederman 2005). It takes time and documentation to fill out their clinical picture, with corroborating information from other persons.

More important, adults who have ADHD usually have comorbid psychiatric conditions. These conditions complicate the treatment of the ADHD and require thoughtful planning about the sequence and nature of interventions. The clinician needs full information, for example, on the presence or history of affective disorder, especially bipolar spectrum disorders, before prescribing for ADHD. The clinician also needs to determine past or present substance abuse, which may make it unsafe to use some medications that can improve the symptoms of ADHD.

Developmental History

The developmental history provides a framework for the entire evaluation. Review the patient's life, including details of his or her mother's pregnancy, labor, and delivery. A developmental history is useful, with a timeline for when the patient reached major milestones. An educational history is essential; school is so often where ADHD symptoms first come to outside attention. The work history often shows turbulence and underachievement, especially in conventional job settings. Patients may be able to succeed when they are their own boss, setting their own hours and doing work they like. Many smart, resourceful ADHD adults succeed that way. Others struggle through their education, even completing graduate school. They tire of their extra burdens as life's challenges continue to mount.

For the strict DSM-IV-TR diagnostic criteria to be met, there must be evidence of childhood underachievement as well as failure to meet the normal milestones of adult development. The problems in adulthood are versions of childhood difficulties. These problems occur in the adult's work or career, in establishing personal autonomy, and in finding and maintaining intimate relationships. The clinician wants a full understanding of where the patient is in adult life. What are the discrepancies between the patient's potential and his or her actual function?

Past and Present DSM-IV-TR Symptoms of ADHD

What difficulties bring the patient into the evaluation? What bothers the patient most? Open-ended inquiry is always a good place to start. More than acute symptoms, what bothers most adults with ADHD are long-standing patterns of impaired function. ADHD is a continuous problem, not acute and sporadic. Difficulties are likely to persist over many years.

Patterns of distractibility can be apparent even in the patient's first few sentences. If the patient is presenting for an ADHD evaluation, how and when did that diagnostic possibility come up? Is it the patient's idea? Have others suggested it—perhaps a spouse, coworkers, friends, or relatives? If the patient is a parent, did the diagnosis of ADHD come up because one or more children received the diagnosis or have been treated for the disorder? What has suggested the diagnosis to the patient or to others close to him or her? Once the patient has explained the difficulties in his or her own words, the clinician can ask specific questions or use standard rating instruments, such as a diagnostic criterion checklist or a self-report form, as an aid to complete the history.

How Symptoms Have Developed to Produce Impairment

Typically, many people experience or complain of the behaviors associated with ADHD: they forget, procrastinate, make careless mistakes, daydream, fidget, and resist taking on sustained, unappealing work. The clinical task is seeing if and how these symptoms impair the patient more often and more intensely than most persons of the same age or life stage (Brown 1995). Sometimes impairment is obvious. Sometimes it is subtler, such as chronic unhappiness because a spouse resents his or her ADHD partner's inefficiency or unresponsiveness (Brown 1995). Impairment is situation dependent. Patients with ADHD can organize and pay attention when something really interests them, but not when the task does not appeal. Even when they know jobs are desirable or even necessary, they cannot force themselves to perform (Denckla 1993). Many affected adults function "well enough," but they feel that they could be, and should be, doing better. Impairment is relative to the patient's capacity. Record the patient's failure to perform at expected skill levels, both to establish impairment and to have markers to document progress (Biederman 2005).

Most adults give a true account of their childhood and adult symptoms (Biederman et al. 2000). Contrary to claims that patients exaggerate or make up symptoms for secondary gain, adults tend to underreport difficulties (Barkley et al. 2002). Some patients may have had symptoms for a long time but never labeled them as ADHD. They regard themselves as immature, spacey, or just lazy. Evidence that symptoms have lasted many years supports the possibility of ADHD, regardless of whether anyone considered the diagnosis when the patient was young (Brown 1995).

An estimated 70%–85% of adult ADHD patients have a history of symptoms in childhood (Ingram et al. 1999). Some remember little about their childhood. Some do not have others who can verify their story or fill out their clinical picture. If symptoms must be documented before the age of 7, some patients who would profit by treatment may be missed (Cuffe et al. 2001). Some clinical researchers suggest using less stringent criteria for diagnosing ADHD in patients age 17 years or older (Barkley and Murphy 1998).

Some patients who were treated for ADHD as children assumed they would outgrow their ADHD symptoms. They stopped taking medication or other treatment as teenagers. Now although the pattern of their symptoms has changed, they are still having difficulties. Many who were hyperactive have settled down, but they still cannot pay attention consistently or work steadily. What treatment has the patient tried? What helped and what didn't?

The adult who warrants a diagnosis of ADHD should have a history, since childhood, of problems related to inattention, hyperactivity, or both. The patient should have had impairing symptoms by age 7. There must be clear evidence of impairment in two or more areas of function: social (family and peer relationships), academic, and occupational. Symptoms must cause demonstrable past and present impairment in two or more settings, such as at work and at home.

Regarding the patient's work life, has the patient completed the education he or she wanted? If not, why not? What is his or her work history? How is the patient doing in his or her work now? If it is not going well, why? Does the patient have new performance demands that exceed his or her coping skills? If the patient has succeeded without formal education, how? What personal qualities account for his or her success?

In the social domain, consider the patient's family, intimate, and peer relationships. What is the nature of the patient's relationships with members of his or her family of origin? If the patient has a life partner or spouse, are both partners happy in the relationship? What is the other person's view of the patient? If the patient is divorced, what did he or she contribute to the problems—did he or she seem not to listen when spoken to? Did the patient fail to follow through with the mundane tasks of domestic life? Was he or she unfaithful? Did he or she lose jobs repeatedly? If the couple is an effective team, what keeps them together? Are they allies who foster each other's strong points and selectively ignore differences? Does the patient have special qualities that enhance his or her desirability as a mate, qualities such as resourcefulness, spontaneity, and vitality?

If the patient has children, assess his or her performance as a parent. ADHD can be a benefit to a parent, if he or she has the creativity and zest that many children prize. How are the children doing? Have any been diagnosed or treated for ADHD and, if so, what was their response? Knowing whether an affected child responded to treatment, and in which modalities, can directly impact work with the adult with ADHD.

Supplement the usual inquiry about education/work life and social life with questions about key other areas. Hyperactivity, impulsivity, and inattention in adolescents and adults often have legal and sexual consequences. Persons with ADHD often begin sexual activity earlier than their age peers and have more sexual partners. They are more susceptible to contracting sexually transmitted diseases and to having unplanned pregnancies. Questions about sexual development and current practices, including birth control, are often illuminating. Also ask about the patient's driving record. Automobile driving is the kind of complex task, requiring sustained attention, that is hard for persons with ADHD. They commonly have a history of accidents, whether fender benders or crashes, and of speeding, with or without multiple tickets (Murphy and Barkley 1996). Arrests for these or other legal infractions, and any history of antisocial or criminal behavior, are important information.

History of Other Psychiatric Diagnoses and Treatment

Persons with ADHD are susceptible to having a full range of other psychiatric disorders. Often they have been treated for these disorders for years, without ADHD being considered. To help the patient best, it is important to know what other disorders have been diagnosed and treated.

Symptoms of Possible Alternative and Comorbid Psychiatric Disorders

When assessing the adult who may have ADHD, consider alternate etiologies for the current symptoms and alternate diagnoses that fit the patient in addition to ADHD. Later chapters in this book address the challenges of differential diagnosis and comorbidity. Essential to the initial evaluation is that the clinician be aware of other confounding symptoms and disorders. Prominent among these are the unipolar and bipolar mood disorders and the anxiety disorders. Inquire about substance use and abuse, especially of alcohol, marijuana, and cocaine. What substances does the patient use, how much, and how often? Has the patient's health or work or social relationships suffered? Also ask about the use or abuse of legal substances such as caffeine and nicotine. What functions does the substance abuse have in the patient's life? Does he or she want an occasional "high" with friends? Does using drugs help the patient focus, concentrate, and work effectively? Or is the drug use a driven, true dependence?

Comorbid learning disorders often go unsuspected and unrecognized in adults. Personality disorder in the ADHD patient complicates treatment and darkens prognosis, as it does in any other patient with any Axis I disorder. What caregivers has the patient seen for which problems, and what was the outcome? Especially if the patient had unrecognized and untreated ADHD, treatment results for other conditions may be poorer than expected.

Strengths: Talents and Abilities

Searching for problems and difficulties, although necessary, should not keep the clinician from looking for, acknowledging, and encouraging strengths and abilities. There is no one ADHD "personality." Interpersonal style can vary markedly, from the lively and engaging to the quiet and withdrawn. ADHD patients often feel they have to work harder than their peers to make their way successfully in life. For some, their personality and their unconventional ways of thinking are precious: they worry that treatment will dampen their prospects, not enhance them. Thus it is important, from the start of treatment, that the patient and clinician have the shared goal of supporting and developing the patient's strengths.

Patients such as the ones who seek out my metropolitan private practice are likelier to be among the healthier adults who have ADHD. Not only do they have to be aware of their disorder, but they have to find a suitable psychiatrist, make and keep appointments, and pay for treatment, including medicine. All these tasks require resources. Many adults with ADHD who are trapped in ignorance and poverty or in jail may not be able to get treatment.

Mental Status Examination

Although there are no standard or diagnostic symptoms in the mental status examination of ADHD patients, some findings are suggestive. One is the failure of the patient to show up for appointments. When adults with ADHD are late or miss appointments, they may be resisting treatment or they may be showing their symptoms: they forget.

Appearance and behavior.   While there are rarely diagnostic clues in the patient's appearance, his or her behavior may be instructive. Hyperactive/impulsive patients can be "all over the place," literally and figuratively, from the time they enter the room.

Speech.   Although most patients have normal speech, others talk rapidly, darting off onto tangents and then wondering aloud, "Where was

I?" or "Where was I going with this?" as if you know better than they do. Some interrupt, repetitively answering questions before hearing them out to the end. They may speak with some urgency.

Mood. Although changeable mood is characteristic, the fluctuations typically last hours to days, not the course of an interview. Patients with ADHD may be deeply depressed, in the classical sense, or they may have a gray mood due to their chronic frustrations and disappointments. They may have an irritable or resentful, edgy quality. Some have affect that belies their mood.

> One woman said, "My friends call me Little Mary Sunshine, but when I get home at night I just crash. I'm exhausted from giving the impression that I'm happy all day."

Mental content. Many patients review their difficulties in work and in their social life and their struggles with always feeling different and not knowing why. Even seasoned patients, well aware of their ADHD, are self-critical when they forget appointments, mislay objects, miss deadlines, or otherwise fail to measure up. Patients often have disappointments and setbacks. They may acknowledge ongoing problems with depression and with anxiety. With patients who are helpless or despairing, investigate suicidality.

Mental function. In their conversation, patients show readily if they are alert and oriented to time, place, and person. The patient may be spacey in the interview, his or her attention drifting elsewhere. You may lose the patient in the middle of a set of questions because he or she is off on another thought path. Traditional simple clinical tasks can be revealing, such as reciting the months of the year backward or doing a digit span. Doing arithmetic problems with addition, multiplication, subtraction, and division gives a rapid view of skill level. Similarly, having the patient read shows fluency, comprehension, and educational level. Asking patients to describe a paragraph that they read or to answer open-ended questions about it allows them to articulate ideas in a test-free situation. Having them give a brief writing sample shows the level of expression and the state of their handwriting. Such simple tasks can provide a sense of their general information, memory, and capacity to abstract. The clinician listens to the history to understand the patient's problem-solving strategy: How careful and consistent is the patient? How easily frustrated? How high is his or her anxiety (Chang et al. 1995)?

Memory.   Persons with ADHD regularly complain that they "can't remember anything," but their memory loss is selective. The same student who cannot remember that her term paper in modern European history is due on Monday can name every movie that the Coen brothers ever made, when the movies were released, and who starred in them. The person with ADHD remembers what is personally meaningful. Everyday matters may not register. ADHD patients have memory problems because they do not attend in the first place, not because they cannot retrieve information already stored in the brain.

Insight.   Many adults with ADHD are painfully aware that something is wrong and that their symptoms affect other people. When offered treatment, such patients welcome it. Others, unaware of the impact of their symptoms, may need repeated confrontations before they can get help. Although some have good reason to assert that their ADHD is the key to their success in life, many more regard it as a burden.

Judgment.   Most ADHD adults have "good enough" judgment to get by in everyday life. Many, however, show poor judgment by repeating behaviors that get them into trouble. They seem not to learn from their mistakes.

2. Standardized Rating Scales

Current rating scales make diagnosing ADHD more standardized. They show how prevalent symptoms are in the normal population and what level of a specific dimension is statistically abnormal. Many scales exist in multiple formats that can be used by the clinician, the patient, and significant others. Cost-effective and efficient, scales allow raters to compare the patient's responses with those of many other age- and gender-matched peers. Going through the questionnaire is often instructive and therapeutic for the patient. It is obvious from the questionnaire that others suffer as he or she does. Symptoms that seemed isolated suddenly make patterns. Difficulties that seemed vague take on greater solidity as data because of the quantitative rating scales. Using the instruments, the clinician can measure the severity of the patient's symptoms initially and later can document and quantify change.

Adult ADHD Self-Report Scale

The Adult ADHD Self-Report Scale Symptom Checklist–v1.1 is an 18-item instrument that asks about the diagnostic symptoms in DSM-IV-TR (Adler et al. 2003). The questions are about adult behavior and activities rather than those of children. Patients rate their responses with a four-point Likert severity scale, where 0=none, 1=mild, 2=moderate, and 3=severe. Scoring guidelines assess the total score and the inattentive and hyperactive/impulsive subsets. This well-validated instrument is often a useful starting point for talking more in depth about the patient's history.

Barkley System of Diagnostic Scales

The Barkley System of Diagnostic Scales contains different rating scales that together provide a comprehensive picture of the patient (Barkley and Murphy 1998). On the Current Symptoms Scale Self-Report Form, patients assess themselves on 18 items that correspond to the DSM-IV-TR diagnostic criteria. The rating is a Likert frequency scale, where 0=never or rarely, 1=sometimes, 2=often, and 3=very often. Odd-numbered questions assess the frequency of inattentive symptoms, while even-numbered items assess hyperactivity/impulsivity. Patients report the age at onset of their symptoms and also how much the symptoms interfere with school, relationships, home, and work. Significant others can fill out a similar form, the Current Symptoms Scale–Other Report. Prospective patients can fill out other instruments as well: a Childhood Symptoms Scale Self-Report Form; Developmental Employment, Health, and Social History Form; and a Work Performance Rating Scale Self-Report Form. Versions of these forms are available for observers for both current and childhood symptoms.

Brown Attention-Deficit Disorder Scales

The Brown ADD Diagnostic Form is filled out by the clinician. It covers clinical history, including the impact of symptoms on the important major domains of the patient's life (Brown 1999). It includes questions about family history and the patient's general medical health, sleep habits, and substance use. The 40-item diagnostic scale covers five areas of executive function: activating and organizing for work; focusing and sustaining attention; sustaining alertness, energy, and effort; managing frustration and modulating feelings; and using working memory and accessing recall. Using the Brown ADD Scales for adults (Brown 1996), the clinician asks the patient to give a numerical, Likert response (from 0 to 3) to each of 40 questions. The scale allows for adding the total score and specifying subscores for the five executive function areas. Patients, parents, or significant others can also fill out other versions of the Brown ADD Scales. The form is standardized and validated for both clinician and self-reporting.

Conners' Adult ADHD Rating Scale and Diagnostic Interview

The Conners' Adult ADHD Rating Scale assesses the 18 DSM-IV-TR symptoms of ADHD (Conners et al. 1999). The first question is: "What is going on in your life that leads you to believe you have attention deficit hyperactivity disorder, or ADHD?" The scale provides questions about history and current status in the domains of education, work, and social relationships. The 30-question instrument grades the patient for both frequency and severity of symptoms. The scale uses a four-point Likert scale, where 0=not at all, 1=rarely; 2=often; and 3=very frequently. Clinicians, patients, and significant others can complete these validated, normed scales.

Wender Utah Rating Scale

For persons who cannot document symptoms from the past, the Wender Utah Rating Scale (WURS) is useful (Ward et al. 1993). The patient fills out the questionnaire. A score over 60 means that he or she likely had ADHD as a child.

Summary

Patients and others can fill out these scales outside of the office, efficiently expanding on the clinician's database. In clinical practice, combining the results of the Adult ADHD Self-Report Scale and one other rating scale such as the Brown ADD Scales is usually sufficient. This combination gives the clinician normed information to supplement the clinical evaluation. Naturally, different clinicians prefer different scales. Table 2–4 gives information about obtaining scales.

3. Medical History and Evaluation

Is the patient in good health? Does he or she have illnesses that contribute to problems with attention, such as disorders of the thyroid? Has sexual impulsivity had consequences in sexually transmitted diseases, unplanned pregnancies, or both? Is the patient taking medications that can interfere with sustained attention and focus?

The patient should provide the results of a full recent physical examination and laboratory tests. If no such examinations or testing has been done in the past year, the patient should be referred for a medical evaluation. Suspicion that the patient has medical components to his or her symptoms should trigger referral for further medical assessment and laboratory testing, including for thyroid disorders and neurological illnesses. In the absence of specific indicators or suggestive symptoms,

TABLE 2–4. Obtaining scales

Scale	Available from
Adult ADHD Self-Report Scale Symptom Checklist–v1.1	World Health Organization Web site and http://www.med.nyu.edu/ Psych/training/adhd.html
Barkley Current Symptoms Scale and other forms	Barkley RA, Murphy KR: *Attention Deficit Hyperactivity Disorder: A Clinical Workbook*, 2nd Edition, New York, Guilford, 1998
Brown Attention-Deficit Disorder Scales and Diagnostic Form	The Psychological Corporation
Conners' Adult ADHD Rating Scale and Diagnostic Interview	Multi-Health Systems, Inc. P.O. Box 950, North Tonawanda, NY 14120-0950
Utah Criteria (Wender-Reimherr Adult Attention-Deficit Disorder Scale)	c/o F. W. Reimherr, M.D. Mood Disorders Clinic, Department of Psychiatry, University of Utah Health Science Center, Salt Lake City, UT 84132

Source. Adapted from Adler LA, Cohen J: "Diagnosis and Evaluation of Adults With Attention-Deficit/Hyperactivity Disorder." *Psychiatric Clinics of North America* 27:196, 2004.

however, a baseline electroencephalogram, electrocardiogram, and thyroid evaluation are neither essential nor cost-effective (Popper et al. 2003).

4. Family History

Do any of the patient's blood relatives have a history of ADHD? Have they been treated, and if so, how have they responded? Alternatively, is information about family history unavailable because the patient is adopted? That alone raises the likelihood that the patient has ADHD.

Relevant family history includes inquiry about other psychiatric disorders, including developmental and learning disorders. What are the family's coping style, level of organization, and resources? What are significant family stressors? Is there abuse or neglect, with family members as perpetrators or victims?

5. Interviews With Significant Others

Conjoint interviews with other family members are helpful. Parents have unique information, and siblings often have stories to tell. Older siblings may remember better than the patient what he or she was like as a child. Younger siblings may recall contending with a disorganized or inattentive older brother or sister. Did the patient have a nickname that reflected ADHD symptoms, like "space cadet" for boys or "ditz" for girls? Whenever possible, have relatives provide written documentation such as school report cards or other evaluations.

Typically, the spouse of an adult ADHD patient has long known about the symptoms and is eager to talk. Family attitudes toward the patient and toward ADHD can determine whether treatment succeeds or fails. Although the clinician's relationship with the patient is primary, the alliance with family members is crucial for the success of treatment.

6. School and Work Evaluations

The results of standardized rating scales and narrative reports from childhood about learning, academic productivity, and behavior are helpful. Grades, transcripts, and records from schools, colleges, and universities are useful, especially ones that provide written comments as well as grades. They are particularly helpful in documenting symptoms at an earlier age, especially if the patient had no formal testing or treatment for ADHD as a child. If adult patients do not have such academic records—and many do not—inquire about their availability from parents or other family members.

Similarly, records of written evaluations at work can shed light on the patient's status, including information about strengths as well as problem areas.

7. Additional Evaluations, as Indicated

Educational Testing

Educational testing instruments help assess academic achievement and intelligence, including cortical functioning. IQ testing can be instructive. The patient may need formal testing to assess learning disabilities, often overlooked in the adult with ADHD who was not evaluated as a child.

Psychological Tests

Psychological tests compare the individual's responses with those of many other persons. However, the tests fail to differentiate persons with ADHD from those who do not have the disorder. They are not a standard instrument necessary to diagnose ADHD in adults, but they can provide useful supplemental information.

Continuous performance tests are specialized psychological instruments that assess a person's capacity to pay ongoing attention. They measure the speed and accuracy of the patient's information processing. The person watches a monitor or listens to the auditory output from a computer program. He or she responds when a specific target signal appears, ignoring nontargets. The computer records the patient's responses and compares the results with those of control subjects. However, being in the test situation itself stimulates patients to pay attention and to stick to the task. The Test of Variables of Attention is one of the many available. The results are unreliable, and the tests can miss up to 50% of ADHD cases (Greenberg and Kindschi 1996).

Neuropsychological Testing

The relationship of psychological symptoms to their biological bases is the domain of neuropsychology. Although neuropsychological tests are used in clinical research about ADHD, they do not produce a classical or instant diagnostic picture. On such tests, the profile of adults with ADHD resembles that of patients with frontal lobe brain damage. Both groups of patients show problems paying attention, holding memories, and organizing material. However, the neuropsychological tests have low sensitivity and specificity, and they miss many diagnoses. Many patients with ADHD do not show abnormal findings on these tests (Biederman 2005). Although not necessary or specific in diagnosing ADHD, they may provide useful information about the person who clearly has the diagnosis but is not responding well to treatment.

Neuroimaging Techniques

Neuroimaging techniques are finding increasing applications throughout psychiatry. Researchers using a radiolabeled compound that binds to dopamine transporters found that adults with ADHD showed twofold more binding to the transporter than did other persons. The clinical significance of this striking finding is unclear. Before neuroimaging can be used as a diagnostic test, researchers must replicate studies and test more individuals (Wilens 2001). Experts currently agree that although neuroimaging has no formal or standard role for diagnosing ADHD now, the technique may be useful later, when we have more information (Biederman 2005).

Vocational Evaluation

Formal evaluation of the patient's work history, strengths, and weaknesses can help make the diagnosis of ADHD. The evaluation is often more useful once the diagnosis is made and efforts turn to providing a full treatment program.

FINAL STEPS IN THE DIAGNOSTIC PROCESS

DSM-IV-TR Criteria

The clinician accumulates information from interviews, other documentation, and medical, psychological, and other tests. Rating scales provide useful diagnostic indicators. The next task is determining whether the patient meets the DSM-IV-TR criteria for ADHD (see Table 2–1). This requires adapting diagnostic criteria originally developed for children (Table 2–5).

The three subtypes of ADHD used in the diagnosis of children also apply to the diagnosis of adults with ADHD. Because the symptoms of hyperactivity tend to decline with age, most often adults present with the predominantly inattentive subtypes of ADHD. If the patient's symptoms meet the criteria for inattention but not hyperactivity for the past 6 months, the patient warrants the diagnosis of ADHD-PI (coded in DSM-IV-TR as 314.00). Such patients who have "silent" symptoms are as likely to have academic or social impairment, or both, as those who are hyperactive (Solanto 2000). Inattentive patients may respond to lower dosages of stimulant medication than those with the hyperactivity subtypes (Barkley 1997).

Patients with the hyperactive subtype (314.01) have met criteria for hyperactivity, but not for inattention, for the past 6 months. Impulsive irritability and hyperactivity occur in adults but often in more socially acceptable ways than in childhood. This is the rarest subtype in adults.

A combined inattentive and hyperactive subtype of ADHD (also 314.01) is the third diagnostic category. Adults with the combined type of ADHD usually have a strong history of both types of symptoms in childhood, and the symptoms have persisted.

Current estimates are that 5% of adults have the predominantly inattentive form of ADHD, 5% have the predominantly hyperactive form, and 70% have the combined form of the disorder (Michelson et al. 2003). In another recent clinical trial, however, the prevalence of ADHD-PI was the same as for the combined form of the disorder (Spencer et al. 2001). Both studies reflect the natural trend of ADHD patients to display fewer symptoms of hyperactivity/impulsivity as they mature (Adler and Cohen 2004).

Some clinical researchers assert that the number of symptoms to diagnose ADHD with a 93% confidence level declines over time. In one study of 467 adults with ADHD, 17- to 29-year-olds required only four of the nine inattentive or five of the nine hyperactive-impulsive symptoms. Accurate diagnosis was possible for adults ages 30–49 years with only four of nine symptoms, and adults 50 and over only required three of nine symptoms (Murphy and Barkley 1995). Clinicians making formal diagnoses with medicolegal or research consequences may still prefer to adhere to the strict requirements of DSM-IV-TR.

The diagnosis of ADHD-NOS (314.9) applies to patients whose symptoms of inattentiveness or hyperactivity-impulsivity do not meet criteria for the other types of the disorder. This diagnosis is useful for patients who have symptoms in adulthood but who may not remember or cannot document symptoms before the age of 7. The diagnosis of ADHD "in partial remission" applies to adults who had the full syndrome as children and now have a partial syndrome.

The diagnostic criteria require patients to show clinically significant impairment in two different settings. For the impaired adult these might include school or work, home, or community. The patient must show clinically significant impairment in social, academic, or occupational functioning. An example of educational impairment could be repeated academic failure. Occupational impairment could show as a string of lost jobs that seemed to fit the person's skills and interests.

The DSM-IV-TR criteria emphasize the three core symptoms of inattention, hyperactivity, and impulsivity. Other symptoms are important as well, including mood variability, unpredictability, difficulty sustaining interest and completing projects, and simple frustration and discouragement. These associated features of ADHD, which contribute to poor motivation and self-organization, may interfere more with adult life than do the core features of the disorder (Popper et al. 2003).

The primary diagnostic challenge is not differentiating ADHD from normal behavior but from other disorders. The difficult diagnostic criterion to meet is that "the symptoms do not occur exclusively during the course of other disorders and are not better accounted for by another mental disorder" (Biederman et al. 1991, p. 574). For information on the substantial problems of comorbidity, see Chapter 9 ("Comorbid and Treatment-Refractory ADHD").

The European diagnostic criteria for ADHD in the *International Statistical Classification of Diseases and Related Health Problems*, 10th Revision (ICD-10; World Health Organization 1992), resemble the diagnostic

---

TABLE 2–5.   DSM-IV-TR criteria for the diagnosis of ADHD, adapted for adults

---

Criterion A.   At least six of nine symptoms of inattention, or six of nine symptoms of hyperactivity/impulsivity, or both, have persisted for at least 6 months to a degree that is maladaptive and inconsistent with developmental level. (Specific examples of adult complaints are in parentheses.)

Inattention: the nine symptoms include the following:
- (a) often fails to give close attention to details; makes careless mistakes in school, work, or other activities (fails to proofread, edit, or otherwise polish written work)
- (b) often has difficulty sustaining attention in work or leisure activities (cannot complete a long-term or complex project, gets lost following conversations)
- (c) often does not seem to listen when spoken to directly (others complain he/she is "tuned out" or "not there," have to repeat his/her name to get attention)
- (d) often does not follow through on instructions; fails to finish jobs, household tasks, or other projects (misses deadlines, cannot multitask. Failure is not due to oppositional or passive-aggressive behavior or inability to understand the directions)
- (e) has difficulty organizing tasks and activities (does not plan ahead, depends on others to keep on track, is late and inefficient)
- (f) often avoids, dislikes, and is reluctant to engage in tasks that require sustained mental effort (shirks sizable work projects or reports; avoids tracking household expenses; is late to file tax reports or fails to file them at all)
- (g) often loses things necessary for tasks or activities (lists, pens, keys, wallet, or tools)
- (h) is often easily distracted by extraneous stimuli (deflected from task by noise from the corridor or by nearby conversation)
- (i) is often forgetful in daily activities (neglects to use personal digital assistant [PDA] or other organizer, misses appointments. Frequently scrambles for prescription medication because of forgetting to contact the clinician in a timely manner)

Hyperactivity-impulsivity: the nine symptoms include the following:
Hyperactivity
- (a) fidgets or moves, is unable to sit quietly (taps fingers, swings leg, chews nails)
- (b) often cannot stay still or seated when expected (cannot sit and watch a movie or even the evening news on television)
- (c) often moves about excessively; has subjective restlessness (cannot sit still)

TABLE 2–5. DSM-IV-TR criteria for the diagnosis of ADHD, adapted for adults *(continued)*

Hyperactivity-impulsivity (continued):
Hyperactivity (continued)
- (d) has difficulty engaging in leisure activities quietly (talks loudly on cell phone or in movies or restaurants)
- (e) is often "on the go" or "driven" (cannot relax)
- (f) often talks excessively (talks over others, others cannot interject)

Impulsivity
- (a) blurts out answers before another person completes a question (speaks without thinking)
- (b) often has difficulty waiting his/her turn (in traffic or in stores)
- (c) often interrupts or intrudes into the conversation or activities of others (others find behavior intrusive or obnoxious)

Criterion B.   Some hyperactive-impulsive or inattentive symptoms that caused impairment were present before age 7 years.

Criterion C.   Some impairment from the symptoms is present in two or more settings (e.g., work, home).

Criterion D.   There must be clear evidence of clinically significant impairment in social, academic, or occupational functioning.

Criterion E.   These symptoms do not occur during the course of schizophrenia or another psychotic disorder, and they are not better accounted for by another mental disorder (e.g., mood disorder, anxiety disorder, or personality disorder).

Source.   Adapted from American Psychiatric Association: *Diagnostic and Statistical Manual of Mental Disorders,* 4th Edition, Text Revision. Washington, DC, American Psychiatric Association, 2000. Used with permission.

criteria for ADHD in DSM-IV-TR. This diagnostic similarity helps in the response to critics who assert that ADHD, especially the adult version, is an exclusively American phenomenon.

Case Example

The following clinical example, drawn from experience with several patients, shows how history, supplemental information, and rating scales combine to indicate the diagnosis of ADHD in an adult.

Micah, a 34-year-old salesman, complained, "I have to be a grown-up now, and I can't manage it. My customers love me, but they get pissed because I'm late and disorganized. My sales area has expanded fast, but more travel means more screwups. At least automated ticketing gives me one less piece of paper to lose. I have to check in with my secretary every morning, because otherwise I would miss appointments, even with my BlackBerry. Reports, filing expenses, and getting reimbursed— I can't manage these details! I drink six to eight diet colas a day on top of two 20-ounce coffees, and I still can't stay focused.

"I'm an only child. I was going to get the family car dealerships eventually, so who cared about grades? I grew up in L.A., smoking cigarettes and drinking at 13. Weed never did much for me, but cocaine— ah, cocaine! I totaled my first car 3 months after I was 16. I banged up two other cars and finally totaled one of them racing at night with my friends.

"My parents suspected that I was drinking and drugging. They didn't know about me and sex. I was jerking off at 9, before I could even come. Got laid for the first time when I was 13. Always desperate for women.

"I barely got into one college, and then I drank, snorted cocaine, and chased girls. I couldn't study for more than 10 minutes at a time, but somehow I always crammed and passed. Cocaine actually helped me study; isn't that weird? My friends called me the 'crazy druggie.'

"It took me 6 years to graduate, and then I ticked off my parents by not going into the business. Instead, I stayed East and married Shirley. She said, 'It's me or drugs, and that includes booze and coke.' So I chose her. I've hopped from job to job. I made money and split before they could catch up with me. I was doing OK, until this damn job and three kids."

In a conjoint interview, Shirley said, "I've been telling him since college that he has ADD. His parents deny it: their son, the god-prince, with ADD? Ridiculous! Of course they never saved any school reports. He's only here because I told him I'd divorce him otherwise. Micah is a great guy. He adores me and the kids, but he never listens. If I make any demands, I am 'a controlling bitch,' like his mother. The one thing I ask him to do is keep his fish tank clean—they're his tropical fish—and the algae are suffocating them!"

Micah had seven symptoms of inattention and six of hyperactivity/ impulsivity. His difficulties, which dated back to grammar school, caused problems at home and at work and threatened his career and his marriage. His wife corroborated his story. On the Adult ADHD Self-Report Scale he scored 26/36 on measures of inattention and 25/36 on measures of hyperactivity/impulsivity, for a total score of 51/72. On the Brown Adult ADD Scales he scored 83, well into the diagnostic range. He had ADHD, combined type. He also had adjustment disorder with anxious and depressed mood. Although discouraged at times, he had no episodes of clinical depression. He was energetic but never manic. Aside from his caffeine, he had stopped his extensive substance abuse. Impulsive and immature, he was also warm, loving, and generous. At his best, he was a super salesman. The Clinical Global Impression Severity (CGI-S) rating was 4, moderately ill.

Utah Criteria

Most clinicians find the standard DSM-IV-TR diagnostic criteria sufficient for adults. However, Wender's Utah criteria, although not standard, can fill out the clinician's picture. In addition to hyperactivity and inattention, the patient must show at least two of five other symptoms: affective lability, hot temper and emotional overreactivity, disorganization, inability to complete tasks, and impulsivity (Wender 1995).

Presenting the Diagnosis of ADHD to Adults

The clinician gathers the information and reviews it to make the diagnosis, when applicable. It is important to gauge the patient's response to the diagnosis. Many patients have read about the disorder and talked about it with key persons in their life, and they are already expecting the diagnosis. Others are surprised. In addition to discussion, they may profit by direction to reading materials or, increasingly, to Web sites (see Appendix). A more difficult clinical task is dealing with the responses of patients who expect the diagnosis but do not qualify for it.

Differential Diagnosis of ADHD in Adults

The task of differential diagnosis of the adult with ADHD can be much harder than making the diagnosis itself. Does an alternate disorder account better for the patient's symptoms? Is the ADHD one of several psychiatric disorders? Many etiological factors produce ADHD or conditions that look like it. Some look-alike conditions will be more suitable diagnoses than ADHD, and some are best regarded as comorbid with ADHD. Because conditions that resemble ADHD are so common, and because ADHD is so often comorbid with other disorders, the clinician needs to consider these disorders and the etiological factors involved. Table 2–6 lists the range of differential diagnoses in adults.

ADHD may be unique in psychiatry in being highly prevalent but often *not* diagnosed in a large proportion of cases. Although misdiagnosis can impair the proper understanding and treatment of any medical condition, ADHD is a special example because of the high frequency of diagnostic error (Popper et al. 2003). More than 50% of patients with ADHD have comorbid conditions, with mood and anxiety disorders high on the list (Pliszka 1998). Unfortunately, often the comorbid diagnoses are the only ones made. ADHD may stay hidden behind the comorbid conditions. Treating co-occurring symptoms helps the patient, but ADHD impairments linger. ADHD may not rank high on the clinician's list of suspected diagnoses in adults.

TABLE 2–6.   Differential diagnosis of ADHD in adults

Psychiatric

> Affective disorders: dysthymic disorder, major depression, or
>   bipolar disorder
> Anxiety disorders: adult separation, panic, phobic, or posttraumatic
>   stress disorder
> Dissociative disorders
> Schizophrenia
> Substance use disorders (intoxication or withdrawal)
> Personality disorder
> Attention-seeking or manipulative behavior

Psychosocial

> Physical or sexual abuse
> Neglect
> Boredom
> Overstimulation
> Sociocultural deprivation

Medical

> Thyroid disorders
> Medicine-induced agitation (e.g., carbamazepine, theophylline,
>   pseudoephedrine)
> Recreational stimulant use
> Barbiturate or benzodiazepine use

Extreme prenatal or perinatal (rare)

> Brain damage (following trauma or infection)
> Lead poisoning (postnatal toxicity)
> Teratogenic effect of exposure to alcohol, cocaine, lead, or nicotine and
>   other substances in cigarette smoke

Dietary

> Excessive caffeine

Hunger

Normal behavior

Source.   Adapted from Popper CW, Gammon GD, West SA, et al: "Disorders Usually First Diagnosed in Infancy, Childhood, or Adolescence," in *The American Psychiatric Publishing Textbook of Clinical Psychiatry,* 4th Edition. Edited by Hales RE, Yudofsky SC. Washington, DC, American Psychiatric Publishing, 2003, p 848. Used with permission.

Determining which symptoms are due to ADHD and which to other psychiatric disorders is a challenge. Often symptoms overlap. Hypomania, substance intoxication and withdrawal, intermittent explosive disorder, posttraumatic stress disorder, mental retardation, Tourette's

TABLE 2–7. Psychiatric disorders associated with ADHD

Anxiety disorders, including posttraumatic stress disorder and obsessive-compulsive disorder

Affective disorders, including unipolar and bipolar disorders

Learning disorders

Motor skills disorder

Substance use disorders

Communication disorders

Tourette's disorder

Schizophrenia

Mental retardation

Pervasive developmental disorders

Antisocial, borderline, and other personality disorders

Source. Adapted from Popper CW, Gammon GD, West SA, et al: "Disorders Usually First Diagnosed in Infancy, Childhood, or Adolescence," in *The American Psychiatric Publishing Textbook of Clinical Psychiatry,* 4th Edition. Edited by Hales RE, Yudofsky SC. Washington, DC, American Psychiatric Publishing, 2003, p. 848. Used with permission.

disorder, and adjustment disorder present in adults with symptoms that look like ADHD.

Several general medical conditions also suggest ADHD. A partial list includes head injury, hyperthyroidism or hypothyroidism, epilepsy, stroke, dementia, vitamin deficiencies, drug side effects, and CNS tumors (Waid et al. 1997).

If comorbid disorders are identified, what symptoms need treatment first? Comorbid symptoms may be more pressing. For more information about the challenges of comorbid and refractory ADHD, please see Chapter 10 ("ADHD Issues: Work, Women, and Family"). Table 2–7 lists the psychiatric disorders more commonly associated with ADHD.

Sometimes when clinicians cannot be definitive about a diagnosis, we use a preliminary one as a basis for treatment. When considering ADHD as a possibility, some clinicians do an empirical trial with CNS stimulant medication. The patient who responds positively to the stimulant still may *not* have ADHD; many people without ADHD or with another psychiatric diagnosis can respond favorably to those medications. Conversely, a negative response to a stimulant does *not* rule out ADHD. Many patients with the disorder respond to certain stimulants and not to others or to another class of medication altogether. At times we have to keep the diagnostic process open-ended, relying on clinical data as they emerge to confirm or refute our initial impressions (Popper et al. 2003).

IS ADULT ADHD A VALID DIAGNOSIS?

Adult ADHD is still a new diagnosis, not yet in the standard diagnostic system. Is adult ADHD a valid diagnosis?

There are three aspects of validity: descriptive, predictive, and concurrent (Spencer et al. 1994). These are discussed below.

Does It Have Descriptive Validity?

For a diagnosis to have descriptive validity, affected individuals must have a syndrome with characteristic symptoms. In a survey of 720 healthy community adults, 4.7% reported past or present symptoms consistent with ADHD. Persons in the study with ADHD symptoms did not go as far in school or do as well at work as those individuals without ADHD symptoms (Murphy and Barkley 1996).

In one study, 50% of adults with a childhood history of ADHD had a full or partial syndrome as adults. In contrast, only 5% of these patients' adult siblings did. Although the adults with persistent ADHD were as intelligent and as highly educated as their siblings without the disorder, they had less successful careers and made less money (Borland and Heckman 1976).

Does It Have Predictive Validity?

For a diagnosis to have predictive validity, the disorder must have a characteristic clinical course and outcome, with an expectable response to standard treatment. In many studies of ADHD adults, researchers note childhood onset and the persistence of expectable symptoms. Reports by parents or other adults confirm the patients' self-reports. Patients show poor academic performance despite adequate intelligence. They frequently conflict with peers, spouses and authorities. They have turbulent work histories, with high rates of absenteeism and frequent job changes. Their co-occurring psychiatric symptoms resemble those of children and adolescents with ADHD (Biederman et al. 1993).

One difference between childhood and adult ADHD is in the sex ratio. Until recently, far more boys than girls were diagnosed with ADHD in childhood; the percentage is more equal in adult men and women. It may be as close as 1.5 men to every 1 adult woman (Biederman et al. 1994). Girls, because they are less hyperactive and disruptive than boys, are less often referred in childhood (Shaywitz and Shaywitz 1987).

Does It Have Concurrent Validity?

For a diagnosis to have concurrent validity, its proposed etiology must agree with its proposed pathophysiology. Central to ADHD are problems in brain function, especially impairments in attention and in executive function: organizing, planning, carrying through with plans, and doing more than one thing at a time. These impairments appear as characteristic patterns in neuropsychological tests in many patients, even though the tests themselves are not necessarily diagnostic (Shue and Douglas 1992). More information about the concurrence of symptoms and brain structure and function is in Chapter 3 ("Biological Basis of ADHD").

Summary: Adult ADHD Is a Valid Diagnostic Entity

ADHD in adults is a controversial diagnosis. However, many clinical studies report on adults who are impulsive, inattentive, and restless and who "look like" children who have ADHD. Children with documented ADHD often continue to express the same syndrome in adulthood. In addition, adults with the disorder do well by treatments that help children with ADHD: medication (CNS stimulants and others) plus varied structuring interventions. Like children with ADHD, adults with ADHD have more than their share of problems: they have a greater tendency to abuse alcohol and other substances, experience more anxiety and depression, and exhibit more dysfunctional personality patterns than adults without the disorder. They do worse academically and in their work life than adults without the syndrome.

The clinical and cognitive characteristics of adults retrospectively diagnosed with ADHD show demographic, psychiatric, psychosocial, and cognitive patterns identical to those of children with the disorder (Biederman et al. 1993). Prospective studies are more valid, however. The few studies that followed ADHD children as they matured support the findings of retrospective studies (Borland and Heckman 1976).

Another measure of validity is whether the disorder is an independent entity or a subset of other psychiatric illnesses. If ADHD were simply a subset of another disorder, then it would occur only in the presence of those disorders, such as anxiety, depression, substance abuse, and antisocial personality disorder. ADHD does occur in the context of other disorders, but in reported studies, approximately 40% of adults with ADHD do not have another psychiatric disorder (Spencer et al. 1998).

There is growing international consensus about the rates of ADHD prevalence (Goldman et al. 1998). Cultural differences impact whether individuals see their ADHD symptoms as problematic, whether they need treatment, and what treatment they will seek. More information on cultural, racial, and ethnic factors is in Chapter 4 ("Allies in Treatment").

WHEN THE DIAGNOSIS IS *NOT* ADHD

Despite efforts to make diagnosing ADHD in adults more specific and reliable, there are good reasons to be cautious. The diagnostic criteria are inexact, and some patients use the diagnosis for secondary gain. There is concern about inappropriate diagnosis of ADHD in adults. In one retrospective sample, 50% of the patients referred for evaluation of ADHD did not meet the diagnostic criteria (Chang et al. 1995).

Parents who seek an evaluation for themselves after their child is diagnosed and treated for ADHD do not necessarily have the disorder. Procrastination and underachievement, by themselves, do not mean that someone warrants a diagnosis of ADHD. Other diagnostic possibilities can cause those and other life difficulties.

> Savannah, age 53, reported, "At my recent review my boss criticized my 'disorganization, excessive talkativeness, and intruding on others.' I'm worried about losing my job. I'm single, this is my sole income, and I've been with the same company for over 20 years. My office is a mess, but I know where everything is. I do miss deadlines, but my clients never complain about quality. Just because some of my colleagues have a professional degree doesn't make them smarter than me. What it boils down to is that I don't know when to keep my mouth shut. A friend told me that if I have ADD, it could save my job.
>
> "My apartment is cluttered. Too many magazine subscriptions, and too little time to read. I don't like to sleep; there's too much I want to do! Besides, I never did like housework.
>
> "Growing up, I was 'the social one.' I never paid attention in school, and none was required. My college grades were bad because I cared more about my beaus than my courses."
>
> Savannah did not have ADHD. Her distress came from resenting her colleagues and feeling entitled to do things her way. Over time, her dramatic manner annoyed her coworkers. Her past poor academic record reflected her social priorities, not problems focusing or concentrating. She had an adjustment disorder with anxious and depressed mood. Her high energy, little sleep, and omnivorous reading suggested hypomania, but her symptoms never met full criteria for that as a formal diagnosis. Her histrionic and narcissistic personality traits interfered with her effectiveness. Her unfavorable work review was painful, but she resolved to behave better, and she did. Able to accept that she did not have ADHD, Savannah made good use of the psychiatric evaluation process.

Some patients, emotionally invested in what the diagnosis of ADHD may provide, are indignant if the outcome of the evaluation is not what they expect. Such patients need a clear rationale for alternate diagnoses, if others exist, and specific recommendations for treating what does burden them.

WHEN THE DIAGNOSIS *IS* ADULT ADHD

The evaluation process for an adult who warrants the diagnosis of ADHD can itself be therapeutic. Patients often come for help after struggling for years, sensing they are different and having had repeated setbacks and disappointments. No matter how energetic and resourceful they are, they tire of fighting uphill. Especially for adults who were not diagnosed in childhood, learning that they have the disorder can be a relief. They are not lazy or stupid, and they are not alone; many other people have the same or similar problems. Although they still have to work hard on their ADHD and its comorbidities, for many patients accurate and specific diagnosis is the first step forward.

Making a diagnosis of ADHD in adults is more complicated than it once was, because clinicians now recognize the importance of assessing the patient for the presence or absence of many other disorders (see Table 2–8). Making the diagnosis usually requires more than one office visit, because acquiring sufficient clinical data requires time.

The diagnosis of ADHD in adults, as in children, relies heavily on clinical judgment. Using behavioral rating scales helps solidify the diagnosis. Teasing apart cognitive, anxiety, and affective symptoms is complex as we try to differentiate ADHD from look-alike disorders. Still needed are objective methods that reliably assess both inattention and impulsivity/hyperactivity. Identifying specific, sensitive diagnostic criteria will help differentiate ADHD from normalcy and from other psychiatric disorders.

SUMMARY

- Diagnosing ADHD in adults is a clinical process adapted from the one used for diagnosing ADHD in children. Document the patient's symptoms of inattention, hyperactivity, or both that have occurred since childhood. Show that these symptoms significantly impact the patient's function in at least two domains, in at least two settings. Supplement clinical interviews of the adult with documents or with information from significant others, or both. Record the patient's strengths and resources as well as his or her difficulties and vulnerabilities.

- In adults, while ADHD can present alone, it usually does not. In the majority of cases, one or more comorbid conditions are present. Look especially for affective or anxiety disorders, substance abuse, learning disabilities, and personality disorder.
- The diagnosis of adult ADHD is a valid diagnosis. Abundant evidence supports its descriptive, concurrent, and predictive validity. Making the diagnosis of ADHD in an adult may itself be therapeutic. However, it may be difficult for patients who do *not* have ADHD to accept other diagnoses.

REFERENCES

Adler LA, Cohen J: Diagnosis and evaluation of adults with attention-deficit/hyperactivity disorder. Psychiatr Clin North Am 27:187–201, 2004

Adler LA, Kessler RC, Spencer T: Adult ADHD Self-Report Scale-v1.1 (ASRS-v1.1) Symptom Checklist. New York, World Health Organization, 2003

American Academy of Child and Adolescent Psychiatry: Practice parameters for the assessment and treatment of children, adolescents and adults with attention-deficit/hyperactivity disorder. J Am Acad Child Adolesc Psychiatry 36(suppl):85S–121S, 1997

American Psychiatric Association: Diagnostic and Statistical Manual of Mental Disorders, 4th Edition, Text Revision. Washington, DC, American Psychiatric Association, 2000

Barkley RA: ADHD and the Nature of Self-Control. New York, Guilford, 1997

Barkley RA, Murphy KR: Attention Deficit Hyperactivity Disorder: A Handbook for Diagnosis and Treatment, 2nd Edition. New York, Guilford, 1998

Barkley RA, Fischer M, Smallish L, et al: The persistence of attention-deficit/hyperactivity disorder into young adulthood as a function of reporting source and definition of disorder. J Abnorm Psychol 111:279–289, 2002

Biederman J: Course and outcome of ADHD. Paper presented at ADHD Across the Life Span, Boston, MA, March 2005

Biederman J, Newcorn J, Sprich S: Comorbidity of attention-deficit hyperactivity disorder with conduct, depression, anxiety and other disorders. Am J Psychiatry 148:564–577, 1991

Biederman J, Faraone SV, Spencer T, et al: Patterns of psychiatric comorbidity, cognition and psychosocial functioning in adults with ADHD. Am J Psychiatry 150:1792–1798, 1993

Biederman J, Faraone SV, Spencer T, et al: Gender differences in a sample of adults with ADHD. Psychiatry Res 53:13–29, 1994

Biederman J, Faraone SV, Spencer T, et al: Use of self-ratings in the assessment of symptoms of ADHD in adults. Am J Psychiatry 157:1156–1159, 2000

Borland BL, Heckman HK: Hyperactive boys and their brothers: a 25-year follow up study. Arch Gen Psychiatry 33:669–675, 1976

Brown TE: Differential diagnosis of ADD versus ADHD in adults, in A Comprehensive Guide to ADD in Adults. Edited by Nadeau KG. New York, Brunner-Mazel, 1995, pp 93–108

Brown TE: The Brown Attention-Deficit Disorder Scales—Adults. San Antonio, TX, Psychological Corporation/Harcourt Brace Jovanovich, 1996

Brown TE (ed): Attention-Deficit Disorders and Comorbidities in Children, Adolescents, and Adults. Washington, DC, American Psychiatric Press, 1999

Chang K, Neeper R, Jenkins M, et al: Clinical profile of patients referred for evaluation of adult attention deficit disorder. J Neuropsychiatry Clin Neurosci 7:400–401, 1995

Cohen RA, Salloway S, Zawacki T: Neuropsychiatric aspects of disorders of attention, in The American Psychiatric Publishing Textbook of Neuropsychiatry and Clinical Neurosciences, 4th Edition. Edited by Yudofsky SC, Hales RE. Washington, DC, American Psychiatric Publishing, 2002, pp 489–524

Conners CK, Erhardt D, Sparrow EP: Conners' Adult ADHD Rating Scales. North Tonawanda, NY, Multi-Health Systems, 1999

Cuffe SP, McKeown R, Jackson K, et al: Prevalence of attention-deficit/hyperactivity disorder in a community of older adolescents. J Am Acad Child Adolesc Psychiatry 40:1037–1044, 2001

Denckla M: The child with developmental disabilities grown up: adult residua of childhood disorders. Neurol Clin 11:105–125, 1993

Dulcan M, Martini DR, Lake MB: Concise Guide to Child and Adolescent Psychiatry. Washington, DC, American Psychiatric Publishing, 2003, pp 23–63

Goldman LS, Genel M, Bezman RJ, et al: Diagnosis and treatment of attention-deficit/hyperactivity disorder in children and adolescents. Council on Scientific Affairs, American Medical Association. JAMA 279:1100–1107, 1998

Greenberg LM, Kindschi CL: Test of Variables of Attention: A Clinical Guide. St. Paul, MN, TOVA Research Foundation, 1996

Ingram S, Hechtman L, Morgenstern G: Outcome issues in ADHD: adolescent and adult long-term outcome. Ment Retard Dev Disabil Res Rev 5:243–250, 1999

Kuperman S, Johnson B, Arndt S, et al: Quantitative EEG differences in a nonclinical sample of children with ADHD and undifferentiated ADD. J Am Acad Child Adolesc Psychiatry 35:1009–1017, 1996

Lahey BB, Pelham WE, Schaughency EA, et al: Subtypes of ADHD change over time. Current ADHD Insights 3:2–3, 2004

Michelson D, Adler L, Spencer T, et al: Atomoxetine in adults with ADHD: two randomized, placebo-controlled studies. Biol Psychiatry 53:112–120, 2003

Murphy K, Barkley RA: Preliminary normative data on DSM-IV criteria for adults. ADHD Report 8:6–7, 1995

Murphy K, Barkley RA: Prevalence of DSM-IV syndromes of ADHD in adult licensed drivers: implications for clinical diagnosis. J Atten Disord 1:147–161, 1996

Pliszka SR: Comorbidity of ADHD with psychiatric disorders: an overview. J Clin Psychiatry 59(suppl):50–58, 1998

Popper CW, Gammon GD, West SA, et al: Disorders usually first diagnosed in infancy, childhood, or adolescence, in The American Psychiatric Publishing Textbook of Clinical Psychiatry, 4th Edition. Edited by Hales RE, Yudofsky SC. Washington, DC, American Psychiatric Publishing, 2003, pp 833–974

Shaywitz SE, Shaywitz BA: Attention deficit disorder, current perspectives. Pediatric Neurol 3:129–135, 1987

Shue KL, Douglas VI: Attention deficit hyperactivity disorder and the frontal lobe syndrome. Brain Cogn 20:104–124, 1992

Solanto MV: The predominantly inattentive subtype of attention deficit hyperactivity disorder. CNS Spectr 5:45–51, 2000

Solanto MV: Neuropsychological findings in the predominantly inattentive and the combined forms of ADHD. Current ADHD Insights 3:1–2, 2004

Spencer T, Biederman J, Wilens T, et al: Is attention deficit disorder in adults a valid disorder? Harv Rev Psychiatry 1:326–335, 1994

Spencer T, Biederman J, Wilens TE, et al: Adults with attention-deficit/hyperactivity disorder: a controversial diagnosis. J Clin Psychiatry 59 (suppl 7):59–68, 1998

Spencer T, Biederman J, Wilens T, et al: Efficacy of a mixed amphetamine salts compound in adults with attention deficit/hyperactivity disorder. Arch Gen Psychiatry 58:775–782, 2001

Thomas A, Chess S: Temperament in Clinical Practice. New York, Guilford, 1986

Waid LR, Johnson DE, Anton RF: Attention-deficit hyperactivity disorder and substance abuse, in Dual Diagnosis and Treatment: Substance Abuse and Comorbid Medical and Psychiatric Disorders. Edited by Kranzler HR, Rounsaville BJ. New York, Marcel Dekker, 1997, pp 393–425

Ward MF, Wender PH, Reimherr FW: The Wender Utah Rating Scale: an aid in the retrospective diagnosis of ADHD. Am J Psychiatry 150:885–890, 1993

Wender PH: Attention-Deficit Hyperactivity Disorder in Adults. New York, Oxford University Press, 1995, pp 245–247

Wender PH: Attention deficit hyperactivity disorder in adults: a wide view of a widespread condition. Psychiatr Ann 27:556–562, 1997

Wilens T: Update on diagnosis and treatment of attention deficit hyperactivity disorder. Currents in Affective Illness 20:5–12, 2001

World Health Organization: International Statistical Classification of Diseases and Related Health Problems, 10th Revision. Geneva, World Health Organization, 1992

C H A P T E R   3

THE BIOLOGICAL BASIS OF ADHD

PSYCHIATRIC SYNDROMES ARISE FROM the interplay of biological, psychological, and social forces. Cultural, ethnic, and spiritual or religious factors affect the expression of these syndromes. More than ever, clinical researchers look for a biological basis for psychiatric disorders. The biological rubric covers many possibilities, from structure to chemical functions to the genetic coding material within cells.

What is the biology of ADHD? How does the brain of a person with ADHD differ from the brain of a person who does not have the disorder? We have some theories, and some evidence, but no definitive answers yet. Advances in technology both support older theories and make new ones possible.

BIOLOGY OF ATTENTION

According to William James: "Everyone knows what attention is. It is the taking possession by the mind, in clear and vivid form, of one of what seem several simultaneous possible objects or trains of thought. Focalization, concentration of consciousness, is of its essence. It implies withdrawal from some things in order to deal effectively with others" (James 1890, p. 138).

Our minds cannot process at any one time all the stimuli that bombard us. We need processes that select, filter, and organize information into manageable and meaningful units. Attention is the cognitive apparatus for that dissemination. Attention has four components: 1) attentional capacity, 2) selective attention, 3) response selection and executive control, and 4) sustained attention (Cohen et al. 2002).

65

Attentional Capacity and Focus

We each have only so much capacity to attend and to focus. Many factors influence the capacity to attend. Some are extrinsic, such as how pressing a stimulus is and how many other stimuli clamor for attention. Others are intrinsic, such as energetic or structural factors. The energetic factors include arousal, affective state, and drive and motivation. They vary greatly among individuals. Structural factors, which are more stable among individuals, include processing speed, memory capacity, and the spatial and temporal dynamics of the system. Of these factors, processing speed varies the most. In general, the faster we process, the more we can master in a given time.

Focused attention requires that we actively invest resources in a particular task. As the number of stimuli rises, or as tasks get harder, our attentional performance declines.

Selective Attention

Selectivity is the most fundamental quality of attention. Selective attention means we process and respond to task-relevant information so we perform at our best. As we select certain stimuli we suppress others, keeping the total amount manageable. It is somewhat like the workings of a camera. Changing the depth of field and the focal point, our selective attention allows us to concentrate on the most important external events and internal operations (Cohen et al. 2002).

Response Selection and Executive Control

Usually we link our attention to a goal-directed course of action. When we respond to a stimulus, we choose among possibilities. Our intentions shape our behavior. A girl racing down a field in a soccer game may well focus her attention and guide her behavior toward making a goal.

The attentional processes in response selection relate to the executive functions. These executive functions, a broader class of cognitive functions, include intention, selection, initiation, inhibition, facilitation, and switching. The executive functions in turn underlie complex processes such as categorizing, organizing, and abstracting, all of which we need to function at our best. Neural mechanisms can either enhance (increase) responsiveness to target stimuli or suppress (decrease) responsiveness to nontarget stimuli. For best executive function, we have to switch from enhancing to inhibiting, as needed.

Sustained Attention

Although many sensory processes, such as primary perception and memory, are stable over time, this quality is less true for attention. Whether we detect a particular stimulus, or process it further, depends on our disposition and on what else is happening in our environment. Sustaining attention is hard work that requires us to continually reprocess positive and negative feedback from our prior actions. We have limited capacity to sustain attention. Most of us can listen attentively to a half-hour talk. The 3-hour lecturer, however, loses us.

Vigilance is attention sustained toward specific targets. Being vigilant makes us detect and respond to small changes in the environment that occur randomly (Colquhoun and Baddeley 1967). As any nighttime sentry will attest, that sustainability is hard to do. Information flows through the four major components of attention: sensory selection, attentional capacity, response selection control, and sustained attention. Motivation, boredom, and fatigue affect our ability to stay vigilant.

A NEUROLOGICAL MODEL OF ATTENTION

By definition, attention is not a single process. It spans multiple domains and includes many neural systems. What we call "attention" intersects with many other constructs: memory, consciousness, vigilance, motivation, and alertness. Building conceptual models of the constructs and systems in attention is complex. To do that, clinical researchers have used information from neuroanatomy, from basic neuroscience, and from patients with neurological lesions. Clearly, neural networks interact to mediate attention (Mesulam 1981). The key structures are the reticular activating system, the thalamus and striatum, the nondominant posterior parietal cortex, the prefrontal cortex, and the anterior cingulate gyrus and the limbic system.

Mesulam (1985) subdivided attention into two major categories: 1) a matrix, or state, function and 2) a vector, or channel, function. The matrix function is primarily the domain of the reticular activating system. It regulates overall information-processing capacity, focus, and vigilance. The vector function, which regulates the direction or target of attention, is analogous to selective attention. Neocortical systems govern these aspects of attention. In the normal brain, the two systems function well together.

BRAIN STRUCTURE AND ADULT ADHD

Interrelated brain areas contribute to attentional/executive function and to behavioral regulation. The dorsolateral prefrontal cortex supports planning and executive control, including shifts of attentional focus and working memory. The basal ganglia participate in circuits essential for executive function. The cingulate cortex plays an important role in motivation and in selecting and inhibiting responses. The lateral prefrontal and parietal cortices activate during sustained and directed attention. The parietal lobule and the superior temporal sulcus are polymodal areas that help target stimuli. The brain stem reticular activating system, especially involving thalamic nuclei, regulates attentional tone and filters interference. Thus many brain regions are likely sites for the dysfunction in ADHD (Seidman et al. 2004b).

Central to ADHD are abnormalities in the connections between the frontal cortex and the striatum (Zametkin et al. 1987). The disorder also involves neural circuits between the frontal lobes and the cerebellum; the latter helps coordinate higher-order cognitive processes (Mega and Cummings 1994). In Biederman's (2004) description:

> The disorder is associated with dysregulation of inhibitory influences of fronto-cortical activity, which are predominantly noradrenergic, and of lower striatal structures, which are predominantly dopaminergic. Striatal structures driven by dopaminergic agonists controlled or modulated by higher initiatory structures are sensitive to adrenergic agents. This has practical consequences in treatment: medications for ADHD either work upstream (noradrenergic) or downstream (dopaminergic).

Frontal Lobe Function

Our executive center is in the frontal lobes of the cerebral cortex. These overlie the brain stem, our center for primitive functions and reflexes. Problems with frontal lobe function are central to the symptoms of ADHD. The frontal lobes regulate functions such as abstract thought, sequencing ability, drive, and executive control.

Sequencing ability is our working memory: our capacity to handle information in a logical set of steps, despite distractions. *Drive* refers to our capacity to do what we want or need to get done.

Executive control is the term for a skill set that determines our success in the real world. One metaphor for executive function might be the conductor of a symphony orchestra. Although the conductor does not play an individual instrument, he or she organizes, focuses, integrates, and directs all the players so that beautiful music results (Brown 2000).

Persons with poor executive control may be impulsive and distractible and have difficulty completing tasks. They may be smart, but they may be prone to behave thoughtlessly or recklessly. They may not fulfill their academic and other kinds of potential. In short, they may be like someone who has ADHD, especially the hyperactive type.

Frontal Lobe Damage

Someone who has damage to the frontal lobes may lose cognitive ability, but sometimes his or her executive function suffers even more.

> In the nineteenth century Phineas Gage was accidentally felled by a spike into the frontal lobes of his brain. After his accident, Mr. Gage was described as "fitful, irreverent, indulging at times in gross profanity (not previously his custom), manifesting little deference for his fellows, impatient with advice when it conflicts with his desires, at times pertinaciously obstinate, yet capricious and vacillating, devising many plans of future operations which are no sooner ranged than they are abandoned, in turn, for others appearing more feasible. A child in his intellectual capacity and manifestations, he has the animal passions of a strong man. Previous to his injury, he was looked upon as a shrewd, smart businessman, energetic and persistent. In this regard his mind was radically changed, so decidedly that his friends and acquaintances said that he was 'no longer Gage.'" (Sacks 1995)

This case report illustrates another useful clinical point. Frontal lobe patients such as the unfortunate Mr. Gage have cognitive abilities that developed normally before any brain damage. With ADHD, the dysfunctional neural networks are probably present from conception. They evolve during pregnancy and after birth, with ongoing impact on cognitive development.

Neurologists have pointed out similarities between adult patients with frontal lobe damage and children with ADHD (Mattes 1980). Persons with ADHD share cognitive features of people with traumatic frontal lobe damage. However, persons with ADHD have no such gross pathology. To understand what is happening in their brain, we need modern high-tech studies. Neurological exams, magnetic resonance imaging (MRI), and computed tomography (CT) scans show that individuals with ADHD typically have frontal lobe malfunction (Sudderth and Kandel 1997). Without good executive function, disinhibition of the frontal lobes occurs. Instead of a grown-up, a risk-taking adolescent is at the controls. The ride may be exhilarating but reckless, and the patient may crash—literally as well as figuratively.

Neuroanatomic Studies

Nearly all the brain imaging studies of ADHD children, adolescents, and adults show evidence of structural abnormalities, especially of the frontal lobe. CT scans and MRI consistently show smaller volumes in the frontal cortex, cerebellum, and subcortical structures (Faraone 2004). The changes mean that patients with ADHD can complete tasks, but they do so inefficiently.

Most studies report on findings in children. One MRI study showed a decrease of 4%–6% of white matter in the brains of children with ADHD. Disturbances in white matter, the anatomical basis for brain connectivity, may be crucial to ADHD (Overmeyer et al. 2001). A new technology, diffusion tensor imaging (DTI), can safely assess white matter development in children. In studies to come, DTI may shed more light on postnatal brain development and the role of white matter in ADHD (Schmithorst et al. 2002).

Another MRI study of children with ADHD showed subtle but real decrements in both gray and white matter of the entire brain, with a reduction of 4%–5% of total brain volume. The developmental curves of these youngsters, although lower, paralleled those of healthy children. Whatever produced the volumetric deficits occurred early in life. The clinical symptoms of ADHD may reflect the expression of early neurobiological insults. In this study, a small subgroup of ADHD children who never had been medicated had much less white brain matter than comparison normal control subjects or ADHD children who had received stimulant medication. This study suggests that some brain abnormalities in ADHD are independent of psychiatric comorbidity and medication. Stimulants may enhance the normalization of white matter growth and development in children with ADHD (Castellanos et al. 2002).

In a study using high-resolution MRI, the brains of children with ADHD showed consistent reductions bilaterally in the dorsal prefrontal cortex as compared with control subjects. These ADHD children also had reduced brain size bilaterally in the temporal cortex. The children with ADHD also had substantially increased gray matter in the posterior temporal and inferior parietal cortices. There were no significant differences in findings between boys and girls. Children with lesser volumes of gray matter tended to be more inattentive; children with significantly larger frontal lobes showed more hyperactivity (Sowell and Peterson 2003).

Some studies have reported a smaller right frontal cortex in children with ADHD. This finding is consistent with decreased blood flow in the frontal regions of ADHD children compared with control subjects, and with a defect in cortical-striatal-thalamic-cortical circuits in the right hemisphere (Lou et al. 1998).

Another MRI study of ADHD boys and their siblings suggests that common genetic factors, not the disorder itself, causes ADHD changes in brain morphology. Compared with control subjects, the ADHD boys and their siblings showed reductions in volume of up to 9.1% in the right prefrontal cortex and the left occipital region. Overall the ADHD boys had a volume reduction of 4.0%, with a similar trend in unaffected siblings. The boys with ADHD also had a reduction in right cerebellar volume of 4.9%, which their siblings did not share. Something characteristic about ADHD may impact the cerebellum of affected children. Alternatively, unshared genetic characteristics may explain this finding (Durston et al. 2004).

Other studies of ADHD girls and boys show reduced cerebellar volume, particularly the posterior inferior lobe of the vermis. As well as regulating motor control and inhibition, the cerebellum may factor in cognitive processes, including executive function. A prefrontal-thalamic-cerebellar network may operate in the core symptoms of ADHD. Some researchers consider that this network, not frontal or striatal change, is the key regional anatomical abnormality in patients with ADHD (Castellanos et al. 2001).

The caudate region shows abnormal structural asymmetry on MRI examination of ADHD children. This finding fits with the idea that ADHD involves a disruption of the normal developmental transfer of functions from the basal ganglia to the frontal cortex (Pueyo et al. 2000). The putamen helps regulate motor behavior. It may be involved in ADHD as well (Teicher et al. 2000).

Clinical researchers theorize that the corpus callosum is important in the transfer of information between the hemispheres. In one MRI study, anterior portions of the corpus callosum were significantly smaller in children who had ADHD than in children who did not have ADHD. This finding is yet more evidence of frontal lobe problems (Giedd et al. 1994). Findings in other studies of the corpus callosum in children have been inconsistent (Overmeyer et al. 2000). Only one structural MRI study of adults with ADHD is currently available, in which researchers found that 8 men with ADHD had a significantly smaller left orbital-frontal cortex compared with 17 control subjects (Hesslinger et al. 2002).

Functional Neuroimaging Studies

Functional MRI studies of the dorsal anterior cingulate cortex in children and in adults with ADHD show functional deficits regardless of whether the subjects had learning disabilities (Seidman et al. 2004a).

A recent functional MRI study of 7- to 11-year-old children with and without ADHD showed distinct patterns of functional abnormalities. Researchers measured responses to two distinct cognitive tasks. On an interference suppression task, children with ADHD showed reduced frontal-striatal-temporal-parietal engagement compared with youngsters without ADHD. In doing another task that involved response inhibition, the children with ADHD relied more on superior temporal engagement, whereas the children without ADHD used more frontal-striatal circuits. The researchers implicated the ADHD children's inability to activate the caudate nucleus as a "core abnormality in the disorder" (Vaidya et al. 2005). Such research shows that the disorder is more complex than we previously supposed.

More support for the frontal lobe theory of ADHD comes from studies using positron emission tomography (PET). Intensely working brain areas have a high rate of glucose metabolism. PET scans read the differences between brain areas that are and are not metabolizing glucose rapidly. One PET scan study of adults showed decreased glucose utilization in the frontal lobes of ADHD patients compared with matched control subjects. This decrease was especially marked in the anterior sections, which regulate attention and carry out other executive functions. In ADHD patients doing attentional tasks, frontal lobe glucose metabolism may be as much as 10% lower than in control subjects. Other, deeper areas of the brain of the ADHD patients also showed diminished glucose metabolism; overall, there was a reduction of 8% (Zametkin et al. 1990). More recent PET scan evidence showed redistribution of blood flow after ADHD patients were treated with psychostimulants (Popper et al. 2003). These data support the view that there is relative hypofrontality in ADHD.

In one study, participants did an intellectual task in which they had to make decisions by weighing short-term rewards against long-term losses. The researchers compared which parts of the brain activated in 10 persons with ADHD versus 12 control subjects. When making decisions, all subjects activated the ventral and dorsolateral prefrontal cortex and insula. However, the ADHD patients activated fewer brain regions than the control group. They did not activate regions involved in emotion and memory, such as the hippocampus and anterior cingulate cortex. They did, however, recruit the caudal part of the right anterior cingulate more than the healthy subjects did. The anterior cingulate cortex, on the medial surface of the frontal lobe, is a paralimbic structure closely connected with the dorsolateral prefrontal cortex. It may have a critical role in complex, effortful cognition. It helps motivate attention; it selects and inhibits responses. ADHD patients also involved the hippocampus less. That structure monitors ongoing processes, continuously records new and uncertain conditions, and determines how reinforcing stimuli are. This comparative lack of hippocampal activity may explain why persons with ADHD respond less to reinforcements (Ernst et al. 2003).

The ADHD patients also showed less activation in the insula. This brain region integrates sensory events with emotional responses. This finding may explain why ADHD subjects respond less to certain stimuli. The result may be lower motivation: less willingness to push toward goals.

Thus adults with ADHD have different neural circuits for making decisions. They may rely less on brain structures involved in complex cognitive-emotional processes and more on structures involved in more primary processes, such as coding sensorimotor aspects of stimuli (Ernst et al. 2003).

A recent study of working memory showed that adults with ADHD have a relative lack of task-related activity in frontal regions and more extrastriate activity. This finding suggests that adults with ADHD struggle to engage frontal regions for difficult executive tasks and that they use more visual imagery to compensate (Schweitzer et al. 2000). The deficits in working memory typical of ADHD implicate an entire network of the brain, including the anterior hippocampus, portions of the thalamus, the anterior cingulate, the parietal cortex, and the dorsolateral prefrontal cortex (Faraone 2004).

Many other areas of the brain may be involved. Three subcortical structures—the caudate, the putamen, and the globus pallidus—are involved in motor control, executive function, inhibition of behavior, and the modulation of reward pathways. The right prefrontal and caudate areas may have specific cognitive functions. Studies of ADHD patients show correlations between anatomical changes in the right frontal-striatal neuronal circuits and changes in performance on neuropsychological tasks that require response inhibition (Teicher et al. 2000). Frontal-striatal-pallidal-thalamic circuits give feedback to the cortex for regulating behavior (Alexander et al. 1986). Some studies have suggested that damage to the striatum is part of the pathogenesis of ADHD (Lou 1996). The volume of the basal ganglia is 5%–10% smaller in patients with ADHD compared with control subjects (Biederman 2004).

The reticular activating system is crucial to a person's becoming and remaining alert. If this system is not intact and functioning, the cerebral cortex cannot maintain its awake and receptive state. Animals with a damaged reticular activating system are more distractible. The locus coeruleus is central to the brain's noradrenergic system. In persons with ADHD, the locus coeruleus is unusually active (Sudderth and Kandel 1997). The resulting "emergency/alert" status may contribute to the distractibility of persons with ADHD.

In summary, neuroimaging studies show widely distributed brain dysfunction in ADHD, not simply frontal-striatal pathology. Researchers cite involvement of the lateral prefrontal cortex, the dorsal anterior cingulate cortex, the basal ganglia (especially the caudate), the corpus callosum, and the cerebellum. These studies have deepened our understanding of ADHD. To date, however, the neuroimaging studies are not sensitive or specific enough to be valid diagnostic tools (Biederman 2004).

PSYCHOPHYSIOLOGY OF ATTENTION

Detecting physiological activity allows us to localize the brain regions involved in attention and to measure its intensity. The most common psychophysiologic methods use autonomic or central nervous system (CNS) indices: skin conductance, change in heart rate, pupil dilation, and electromyographic changes. CNS studies use electroencephalographic measurement. Most routine clinical electroencephalograms of patients with ADHD are read as normal. However, using quantitative electroencephalographic data, it is possible to categorize 93% of children with ADHD as showing either hyperarousal or hypoarousal compared with age peers without the disorder. These data suggest subtle abnormalities that are not specific or diagnostic (Chabot and Serfontein 1996).

In the brain, sensory or cognitive tasks produce evoked response potentials. Researchers average the electroencephalographic activations from a series of stimuli to produce an event-related potential (ERP) linked to specific brain regions. By measuring ERP changes as tasks change, we can see how different attentional tasks affect brain activity. Studies of ERPs in children with ADHD show abnormal arousal and attention (Popper et al. 2003). ERPs allow us to study normal attentional responses and to characterize disturbances of attention in patients. However, ERPs are not widely used in the standard clinical assessment of ADHD patients (Cohen et al. 2002).

NEUROPSYCHOLOGY OF ADULT ADHD

Neuropsychological tests measure human perception, cognition, and behavior and link them to specific brain functions. They help specify the clinical features of ADHD (Weiss and Seidman 1998). Evaluating attention requires data from multiple tasks that reflect the disorder's different and specific manifestations. Comprehensive assessment requires using a neuropsychological battery with several standardized paradigms. Neuropsychological measures, grouped by the domains of attention they assess, are listed in Table 3–1.

Neuropsychological testing of patients with ADHD demonstrates problems with response inhibition. This capacity to withhold or suppress an expected physical or mental response has the effect of keeping impulsive reactions in check. Delaying such responses, which are often semiautomatic, allows us to think before we act. ADHD patients typically display difficulty delaying responses (Schachar et al. 2000). Some researchers propose that this difficulty is central to the disorder. Affected individuals do not accurately appraise the moment-to-moment consequences of their actions and interactions with others; they are poor at self-monitoring. They have difficulty multitasking (Barkley et al. 2001).

ADHD is, by definition, a disorder of attention. Some neuropsychological researchers, however, assert that adults with ADHD have more problems with motor response and output than they do with attention. In one study, affected adults did as well as control subjects on measures of sustaining attention and encoding speed. They significantly lagged behind control subjects on performing tasks that required motor output and response organization (Himelstein and Halperin 2000).

The neuropsychological test results of adults with ADHD resemble those of children and teenagers who have the disorder (Seidman et al. 2004a). The many deficits experienced by adults with ADHD especially affect higher-level abilities. The neuropsychological impairments of ADHD in adults increase as the cognitive demands or complexity of the task increases. This may explain why many adults first seek treatment for ADHD when they contend with the escalating challenges of adult life (Johnson et al. 2001). The similarity of the neuropsychological deficits among children, adolescents, and adults with ADHD suggests that the disorder in adults is the same as in children (Faraone 2004).

Neuropsychological studies of ADHD individuals suggest that impaired executive dysfunction is associated with abnormal brain structures (Seidman et al. 2004b). The circuitry of the prefrontal cortex is complex, and we can only infer so much from these tests. Are the abnor-

---

TABLE 3–1.   Neuropsychological measures of attentional domains

---

Sensory selective attention
>   Double simultaneous stimulation
>   Letter or symbol cancellation
>   Line bisection
>   Spatial cueing paradigms
>   Dichotic listening
>   Wechsler Adult Intelligence Scale—Revised (WAIS-R):
>   picture completion
>   Orienting response
>   Event-related potential (ERP) tasks

Response selection and control (executive control)
>   Motor impersistence task
>   Go/no-go task
>   Reciprocal motor programs
>   Trail Making Test
>   Wisconsin Card Sorting Test
>   Porteus Maze Test
>   Controlled word generation
>   Design fluency
>   Spontaneous verbal generation

Attentional capacity—focus
>   Digit span forward, digit span backward
>   Corsi Blocks
>   Serial addition/subtraction
>   Consonant Trigrams
>   Symbol-digit tasks
>   Stroop Test
>   Reaction time paradigms
>   Paced Auditory Serial Addition Task (PASAT)
>   Dichotic Listening Test

Sustained performance and vigilance
>   Continuous Performance Test
>   Motor continuation
>   Cancellation tasks

Source.   Reprinted from Cohen RA, Salloway S, Zawacki T: "Neuropsychiatric Aspects of Disorders of Attention," in *The American Psychiatric Publishing Textbook of Neuropsychiatry and Clinical Neurosciences,* 4th Edition. Edited by Yudofsky SC, Hales RE. Washington, DC, American Psychiatric Publishing, 2002, p. 499. Used with permission.

malities in ADHD due to lesions of the prefrontal cortex or to brain areas with prefrontal projections? The best term to describe the involved brain regions may be *frontosubcortical*: that is, the behavioral or cognitive dysfunction looks frontal but may be influenced by subcortical projections (Faraone 2004).

We need additional research. Not all studies describe impairment of the same tasks or functions. Not all studies control for various confounders, such as comorbid psychiatric conditions (Hervey et al. 2004). Also note that a substantial proportion of ADHD children and adults do *not* show any abnormalities on neuropsychological tests (Doyle et al. 2000).

BRAIN CHEMISTRY IN ADHD

In the nervous system, electrical impulses move along the axons of neurons. The electrical nerve impulse, hitting the presynaptic neuron membrane, triggers the release of neurotransmitters into the synapse. These strike the postsynaptic neuron, signaling it to go (*activate*) or stop (*inhibit*). The chemical neurotransmitters have a natural cycle. Synthesized and stored in the presynaptic neuron, they move into the synapse when they are triggered. Some of the neurotransmitters strike the postsynaptic membrane, generating or stopping further nerve impulses. Some neurotransmitters are metabolized in the synapse. Alternatively, a reuptake process returns neurotransmitters to the presynaptic neuron. There they remain until another electrical impulse triggers their release.

More than 30 neurotransmitters are biologically active monoamines, the catecholamines. One, serotonin, clearly helps regulate mood. Among the other neurotransmitters, norepinephrine (adrenaline) and dopamine are important in the biological basis of ADHD. The interaction of both of these neurotransmitters is discussed in a later subsection, "Dopamine, Norepinephrine, and Inattention."

Role of Dopamine

The dopaminergic system may contribute to inattention symptoms. Dopamine directly activates the neuronal networks in attention, especially the anterior cortical system, which is home for the executive functions (Servan-Schreiber et al. 1998).

If the brains of ADHD patients work less efficiently than the brains of non-ADHD individuals, and if dopaminergic neurotransmission regulates or runs the parts involved, then ADHD patients may have a relative dopamine deficiency (Wender 1995). In one study, ADHD children tended to have lower levels of dopamine metabolic products in their cerebrospinal fluid (CSF) than did control subjects (Shaywitz et al. 1977). In another study, researchers tested the CSF level of dopamine metabolites in adults with ADHD both before and after they took methylphenidate at therapeutic doses. Eleven of 15 adults in the study who responded well to Ritalin had low CSF levels of dopamine metabolites homovanillic acid and 5-hydroxyindoleacetic acid. The four test subjects who responded poorly to methylphenidate had higher CSF levels of dopamine metabolites (Reimherr et al. 1984).

CSF studies suggest a relative dopamine deficiency in ADHD, but they do not indicate the basic problem. Where is the source of the relative deficiency? Is too little synthesized? Is too much metabolized before it can act? Or is too much transported back into the presynaptic neuron?

To answer these questions, researchers investigated several hypotheses. A person with ADHD may have too little of dopamine's metabolic precursors: the amino acids phenylalanine, tyrosine, and L-3,4-dihydroxyphenylalanine (L-dopa). However, giving increased amounts of these amino acid precursors has not proven a practical treatment for ADHD. Obviously, the disorder involves more than a deficiency of dopamine or its chemical precursors (Wender 1995). Another hypothesis is that adults with ADHD may have a problem with dopamine synthesis. DOPA decarboxylase is a key enzyme in that process, and there is lower activity of that enzyme in the prefrontal cortex of ADHD adults (Ernst et al. 2003). Last, the transporter system for dopamine that carries the transmitter back to the presynaptic neuron may be particularly active. A study using single proton emission computed tomography (SPECT) reported a 70% increased density of striatal dopamine transporters in ADHD adults compared with control subjects (Dougherty et al. 1999). Another researcher who used a different SPECT ligand, however, did not replicate this finding.

Dopamine, Norepinephrine, and Inattention

Along with dopamine, norepinephrine may be important in ADHD. Norepinephrine neuronal projections actively alert the posterior attention system of the cortex to receive incoming stimuli. The following findings support a norepinephrine/activity and dopamine/attention model of ADHD, especially if we define *activity* to include hyperactivity, impulsivity, and behavioral self-control (Pliszka et al. 1996):

1. Noradrenergic medications, such as tricyclic antidepressants, and alpha-agonist medications, such as clonidine, help relieve hyperactivity/impulsivity symptoms, more often seen in children (Spencer et al. 1996).
2. The CNS stimulants encourage the release of norepinephrine and dopamine into the synapse and tend to block their reuptake.

3. The tricyclic antidepressants and bupropion (Wellbutrin) block the reuptake of both norepinephrine and dopamine.
4. Clonidine (Catapres) and guanfacine (Tenex) increase the release of norepinephrine and dopamine into the synapse.
5. The monoamine oxidase inhibitor antidepressants reduce the degradation of norepinephrine and dopamine in the presynaptic neuron, keeping them active (Spencer et al. 1996).

The most complex biological systems regulate our highest mental functions. Even a dopamine/norepinephrine theory of ADHD may be simplistic. We may be observing the correlates of a process, not the cause. To date, biochemical studies of ADHD do not distinguish between primary and secondary abnormalities (Wender 1995). More sophisticated models now suggest that multiple neurotransmitter systems govern brain functions (Popper et al. 2003).

A NEUROBIOLOGICAL MODEL FOR ADHD CLINICAL SUBTYPES

One researcher proposed a theory that four clinical subtypes of ADHD result from neurotransmitters acting at specific brain sites. One subgroup of adults with ADHD who have increased norepinephrine activity show symptoms of cortical arousal, such as distractibility. Others have primary cognitive deficits due to less dopamine in the input pathways of the prefrontal cortex and the regulatory systems of the midbrain. Another subgroup has problems with impulsivity; their prefrontal cortex may not sufficiently inhibit behavior. Because they need increased serotonergic output to diminish impulsivity, they may respond best to a combination of serotonergic antidepressants and stimulants. In a fourth subtype, because of problems in a combination of neurotransmitters, the primary dysfunction may be in attachment and reward processes that regulate self-directed attention (Hunt 1997).

OTHER BIOLOGICAL POSSIBILITIES

The search continues for other biological factors in the development of ADHD. After a pandemic of the viral encephalitis lethargica (von Economo's encephalitis) in the 1920s, many children and adults developed a neurological syndrome much like ADHD (Wender 1995). Survivors sustained damage to the dopamine-rich substantia nigra. The virus that caused the encephalitis had long-lasting effects on behavior. After the epidemic, clinicians for the first time linked pathological restlessness to neurological deficits rather than to psychological difficulties (Adler and Cohen 2004).

Other biological factors associated with ADHD include other encephalitides, brain damage (especially frontal cortex), neurological disorders, low birth weight, prematurity, head trauma, and extreme perinatal anoxia. Intrauterine exposure to toxic substances including alcohol, lead, and probably cocaine can produce damaged behavior in offspring. Fetal alcohol syndrome, for example, produces hyperactivity, impulsivity, and inattention as well as physical abnormalities and diminished intelligence (Popper et al. 2003). There is a clear link between maternal smoking in pregnancy and ADHD in children. In one sample, 22% of 140 children with ADHD had mothers who smoked in pregnancy, versus 8% of 120 control subjects (Milberger et al. 1996). A rare form of thyroid disease has been linked to ADHD (Sudderth and Kandel 1997). Nonlocalizing neurological soft signs such as clumsiness, left-right confusion, perceptual-motor dyscoordination, and dysgraphia are common in children with ADHD (Popper et al. 2003).

Nutrition is crucial to the proper development of the CNS. Severe early malnutrition may be a common cause of ADHD worldwide. Of children who have severe malnutrition in the first year of life, 60% show inattention, impulsivity, and hyperactivity persisting at least into adolescence (Galler et al. 1983). Theories abound in the popular press about nutritional factors in causes of, or treatment for, ADHD. There has been recurrent enthusiasm for various nutritional theories, such as the idea that ADHD is related to "excessive sugar intake" in children. However, special diets, with specific attention to sugar and other nutrients, have not relieved the symptoms of ADHD (Spencer et al. 1996). To date, we do not know whether or how specific nutritional deficiencies contribute to the etiology of ADHD (Popper et al. 2003).

The onset of ADHD after childhood may indicate acquired neuropathological changes such as traumatic brain injury, encephalitis, or CNS infection. Preadolescents with pediatric autoimmune neuropsychiatric disorders associated with streptococcal infections (PANDAS), such as obsessive-compulsive disorder and Tourette's disorder, may present with ADHD symptoms. About half of preadolescents diagnosed with PANDAS have symptoms of ADHD (Peterson et al. 2000).

RIGHT HEMISPHERE SYNDROME

Right hemisphere syndrome comprises cortical deficits that appear as difficulties with learning, memory, concentration, and organization

(Garcia-Sanchez et al. 1997). Usually evident from birth, the syndrome is not a medical disorder resulting from injury or disease. It is not a learning disorder, in the sense of specific skill deficits in mathematics or reading. The entire right hemisphere appears to be involved.

Affected individuals have "social dyslexia." They miss or misread social cues; they fail to understand other people's sense of humor; they are socially awkward. Others regard them as odd. As a result, the affected persons can become angry and isolated, vulnerable to depression. Although the ADHD-like symptoms of right hemisphere syndrome respond poorly to medication, cognitive-behavioral treatment is often helpful. Affected individuals need structured treatment, such as that for patients with major traumatic brain damage. This type of treatment teaches step-by-step approaches to developmentally appropriate life tasks. Adolescents, for example, might need specific instructions about social interactions such as dating (Popper et al. 2003).

GENETICS OF ADHD

Genetics—the science of inheritance—provides information about the biological basis of ADHD. Data available now suggest that persistent or adult ADHD is more genetic than the childhood type. The solid evidence of cross-generational transmission of ADHD from adults to children makes the diagnosis of the adult form of the disorder even more valid. In family studies, twin studies, and adoption studies, there is clear evidence of a genetic basis for ADHD. Researchers may be close to finding a molecular basis for ADHD as well. When considered together, results of genetic investigations demonstrate a striking similarity. These findings suggest a polygenic inheritance that creates vulnerability but does not guarantee that the disorder will occur. Today's data require confirmation to increase the reliability of the findings on specific genetic contributions. In the future, molecular genetics will help us match the patient's genetic makeup with optimal treatment (Faraone 2004).

Family Studies

ADHD runs in families. The clearest association of ADHD is between fathers and sons ("he's his father's son"). Some researchers assert that parents of children with ADHD have a two- to eightfold increase in risk for the disorder (Frick et al. 1991; Schachar and Wachsmuth 1990). Other investigators do not agree. However, a dramatic finding is that 41% of siblings of adults with ADHD have the disorder, compared with 0% of siblings of control subjects (Manshadi et al. 1983). Grandparents of children with ADHD are at higher risk for the disorder (Faraone et al. 1994). A higher incidence of the disorder is among first-degree relatives (siblings, parents, and children) of patients with ADHD than in families without the disorder (Faraone 2004).

If ADHD is a valid disorder, children of affected adults should have a higher prevalence than children of parents without the disorder. The risk for children of ADHD adults is much higher than among siblings of children with the disorder. In one study, 57% of children with an ADHD parent had the disorder, whereas only 15% of siblings of ADHD children had it (Biederman et al. 1995).

The high familial loading of adult ADHD suggests that genes are more important for symptoms persisting into adulthood than for those that remit. Both prospective and retrospective studies support this finding. These results are somewhat surprising. If the diagnosis of adult ADHD is fragile, subject to faulty recollection and to claims made for secondary gain, we should find more false-positive cases among adults than among children. We should find less evidence for familial transmission in families sampled through adults than in those sampled through children. The opposite is true. From a familial perspective, not only is the adult ADHD diagnosis valid, but it may be more valid than the childhood one (Faraone 2004).

In a study investigating the validity of the adult ADHD diagnosis, researchers found that having a child with ADHD did not bias adults to overreport ADHD symptoms (Faraone et al. 1997b). Researchers analyzed structured interviews with members of 280 ADHD and 242 non-ADHD families. The ADHD families showed significantly more familial aggregation of ADHD symptoms for adult relatives than for nonadult relatives. This finding was true for both past and current symptoms, for inattentive and hyperactive symptoms, and for relatives with and without psychiatric comorbidity (Faraone et al. 2000a). Families of ADHD patients have significantly more psychiatric illness than do families without the disorder (Wender 1995). ADHD in children with bipolar disorder may be a distinct familial subtype (Faraone et al. 1997a). Although family studies suggest that genetic and nongenetic factors contribute substantially to ADHD, the genetic factors appear to predominate (Faraone and Doyle 2001).

Twin Studies

Some of the most convincing evidence for a genetic basis of ADHD comes from twin studies. Identical twins, who share 100% of their genetic endowment, are alike in appearance, intelligence, and personality.

In contrast, fraternal or dizygotic twins share only 50% of their genes; the two individuals are no more alike than any two brothers or sisters or any pair of brother and sister. Now, through DNA testing, we can rapidly and accurately determine whether twins are identical or fraternal. When we study twins, we look for greater concordance: that both more often share an attribute than expected by chance. We assume that higher concordance is due to genetic factors.

We expect identical twins to share more attributes than fraternal twins do. Their genetic material is identical, so a disorder with a genetic basis ought to occur more often in both. Study after study shows that identical twins have higher concordance for ADHD than do fraternal twins (Sudderth and Kandel 1997). In a study in which one twin had ADHD, 51% of identical twins had the disorder, but only 33% of fraternal twins did (Goodman and Stevenson 1989). To show a significant biological link, monozygotic twins do not need 100% concordance. The percentages for ADHD are similar to the figures for twins with diabetes mellitus (56% monozygotic, 11% dizygotic) and bipolar disorder (58% monozygotic, 11% dizygotic) (Wender 1995).

Twin studies allow the measurement of heritability, which is the degree to which genetic factors influence a disorder. Heritability ranges from zero to one; the higher the number, the greater the degree of genetic determination. Heritability estimates from 17 twin studies of ADHD indicate that approximately 80% of ADHD is due to genes and the interaction of genes with environmental risk factors (Faraone 2004). A study of ADHD children in Australia found that specific genetic and environmental influences were highly similar in boys and in girls (Rhee et al. 1999).

A recent study of twin pairs in the Netherlands showed robust additive genetic influences in the disorder while attesting to the importance of environmental factors. Data, using the Conners' Rating Scale for ADHD—Revised, came from the mothers of 1,595 7-year-old monozygotic and dizygotic twin pairs. The prevalence of ADHD was about 4%. Surprisingly, more girls (5.1%) than boys (3.4%) were scored as having clinically diagnostic ADHD. Genetic analyses of the data provided a model of the disorder that includes dominant genetic factors (48%), additive genetic factors (38%), and unique environmental factors (22%). As expected, the correlations between monozygotic twins were higher than those between dizygotic twins. Additive genetic variance reflects the cumulative additive effect of individual genes. The research study suggested that different genetic influences act at different ages in the development of ADHD (Hudziak et al. 2005).

Adoption Studies

Twin studies do not tell us what roles heredity (nature) and environment (nurture) play in how a condition appears. Biological parents providing genetic material (nature) differ from adoptive parents providing the psychological environment (nurture). Studying the adoptive and biological relatives of adopted probands allows us to tease out which sources of familial transmission are genetic and which are environmental.

Adoption studies demand careful documentation over time. Such studies show conclusively that ADHD very highly correlates with the genes of the biological parents. The presence of the disorder has little to do with who rears the child or the child's age when adopted (Sudderth and Kandel 1997).

Because adoptive parents are highly screened, they generally show less psychopathology than do biological parents. Adoptive parents, then, should do a better job of parenting. If quality of upbringing determines whether children develop ADHD, we would expect fewer adopted children to have the disorder. In fact, adopted children show ADHD independent of the quality of the parenting of their adoptive parents. The incidence of ADHD is higher among adopted children, whose biological parents often have ADHD. The pregnancy itself may reflect the poor impulse control of many adoptees' ADHD adolescent and young adult mothers. This evidence that ADHD is genetic counters arguments that the disorder is primarily one of parenting, that children with ADHD are "spoiled kids who need discipline" (Wender 1995).

Adoptive relatives of adopted ADHD probands had lower rates of ADHD and associated disorders than did the biological relatives. As expected, the adoptive relatives of adopted ADHD probands had ADHD and associated disorders at rates similar to those in relatives of control probands (Sprich et al. 2000).

Current opinion is that ADHD is strongly genetic. However, the specific subtype of ADHD—that is, whether predominantly hyperactive or predominantly inattentive—does not seem to be inherited. Most researchers consider ADHD a complex polygenic disorder (Malaspina et al. 2002).

Molecular Genetic Studies

Molecular genetic studies use two main approaches: genome scans and candidate gene studies. Genome scans examine *all* chromosomal locations without any prior guesses about which genes underlie susceptibility to a disorder. In contrast, candidate gene studies examine one or more genes that appear to be specifically linked to a disorder.

Genome Scans

Few genome scans exist for ADHD. Two such studies found some evidence of ADHD genes in chromosomes 16p13 and 17p11 (Smalley et al. 2002) and at chromosome locations 7p13 and 15q15 (Bakker et al. 2003). Analyses of candidate chromosomal regions from 308 affected sibling pairs of children with ADHD showed three genomic regions that yielded empirically significant linkage to ADHD: 6q12, 16p13, and 17p11. A fourth region, 5p13, contains suggestive evidence of linkage to ADHD (Ogdie et al. 2004).

Candidate Gene Studies

The more numerous candidate gene studies in ADHD focus on the likely genetic sources of problems. Very small stretches of DNA transmit together across generations. As a result, if a DNA marker is within a disease gene or close to it, a version of that marker will be more common among persons with the disorder.

ADHD is most likely a polygenic disorder involving dopamine, norepinephrine, serotonin, γ-aminobutyric acid (GABA), and other neurotransmitters (Comings et al. 2000a). The natural area of molecular genetic interest in ADHD, then, is the neurotransmitter systems, especially those using dopamine and norepinephrine (Faraone 2004). Genes for components of the dopamine neurotransmitter system have received the most attention. Association studies have implicated three dopaminergic system genes. One association is between ADHD and the gene that encodes the D_4 dopamine receptor (*DRD4*) on chromosome 11. Researchers also reported an association between novelty seeking and a polymorphic region of the DRD4 gene that encodes the third cytoplasmic loop of the protein (Benjamin et al. 1996). The behavioral construct, which the authors described as "excitement follows novel stimuli," might describe characteristic symptoms of ADHD. Some studies have replicated this association (Sullivan et al. 1998).

Studies have focused on a variant of *DRD4*, the seven-repeat allele, which mediates a *blunted* response to dopamine. Persons with this version of the DRD4 gene are approximately twice as likely to have ADHD as persons who do not carry that variant. People with ADHD are approximately 50% more likely to have a parent transmit the seven-repeat variant to them, compared with other variants (Faraone et al. 2001). Five other clinical studies implicate this variant of *DRD4* (Faraone 2004). In one, researchers evaluated 133 children with ADHD using neuropsychological tests associated with attention, impulse control, and response inhibition. Children who had the seven-repeat allele of the DRD4 receptor significantly more often made incorrect responses and clearly had an inaccurate, impulsive response style (Langley et al. 2004). About half of all studies of *DRD4* report a positive association between the seven-repeat allele and ADHD. A decreased response to postsynaptic dopamine may be a mechanism behind some forms of ADHD. This "gene polymorphism" might be a marker for nonresponse to stimulants (Seeger et al. 2001b). Other information about *DRD4* bolsters its role in ADHD: both dopamine and norepinephrine are potent agonists of *DRD4* (Lanau et al. 1997).

Molecular genetic studies of other aspects of the dopaminergic system implicate a variant of the dopamine transporter gene (*DAT1*) on chromosome 5 (Waldman 2001). The 10-repeat allelic variant of the DAT1 gene may relate to hyperefficient reuptake of dopamine from the synaptic cleft. Reduced intrasynaptic dopamine may be another potential mechanism for ADHD. Some PET scan studies have documented 30%–40% more dopamine transporter in adults with ADHD (Spencer et al. 2004). Most, but not all, studies have confirmed the links between the allelic variants of the DRD4 and DAT1 genes (Payton et al. 2001).

A version of the dopamine D_5 receptor (*DRD5*), the 148-bp allele, may be a risk factor for the inattentive and combined forms of ADHD (Lowe et al. 2004).

Molecular genetic studies also implicate the noradrenergic neurotransmitter system in ADHD. Postulated genes include those for the norepinephrine receptor α-1C, dopamine β-hydroxylase, the epinephrine-synthesizing enzyme phenylethanolamine N-methyltransferase, and the catecholamine breakdown enzymes catechol-O-methyltransferase and monoamine oxidase A (Comings et al. 2000b). This preliminary genetic evidence fits with the utility of noradrenergic reuptake inhibitors in ADHD (Michelson et al. 2001).

Other molecular genetic studies suggest that serotonergic systems, although not central to ADHD, also play a role (Callaway et al. 1992). There may be an association between ADHD and a polymorphism of the promoter region for the serotonin transporter gene (*5-HTTLPR*) (Seeger et al. 2001a). This polymorphism may interact with the dopamine DRD4 gene (Auerbach et al. 1999).

Current genetic research efforts are developing approaches for standardizing diagnosis (Curran et al. 2000) and optimizing pedigree composition for genetic studies by using ADHD populations with comorbid disorders (Faraone et al. 2000b). There are eight genes for which the same variant has been studied in three or more case-control or family-based studies. Of the eight genes, seven have a statistically significant association with ADHD, based on the pooled odds ratio across the studies: *DRD4, DRD5, DAT, DBH, 5-HTT, HTR1B,* and *SNAP25*. These genes of small effect may combine with each other and with environmental risk factors to cause ADHD (Faraone et al. 2005).

Up to 98% of children respond to the stimulants when both methylphenidate and dextroamphetamine are tried. However, about 80% of subjects have a preferential response to one or the other. This preference suggests that genes, such as *SNAP25*, may play a role in drug response (Elia et al. 1991). Already, genetic tracers suggest which children respond poorly to methylphenidate, for example (Roman et al. 2002).

THINKING BROADLY ABOUT THE BIOLOGY OF ADHD

The brain's multiple regions, each with specialized architecture, all interact. The attention system links information processing across the brain. The cognitive and sensory systems closely connect with areas that control feeling states. Information starts at the sensory organs and then goes to brain areas for pattern recognition, identification, interpretation, prioritization, analysis, and response selection. At each site, information selectively amplifies or diminishes. These complex operations all take place without conscious interruption of thoughts (Hunt 1997).

Information arriving at the eyes travels down the optic tracts to the occipital cortex. These pathways connect to the hippocampus, which transmits messages to other regions for further analysis. Norepinephrine is the crucial neurotransmitter for these tasks. The amygdala, the central alerting system, scans constantly to determine danger or opportunity. In the midbrain, the thalamus monitors and integrates the internal drives. Memory retrieval is complex. It involves pattern recognition and associations encoded by concept, event, sequence, and affect. The associative cortex builds the visual, auditory, tactile, and olfactory components of a stimulus into a multisensory construction. The prefrontal cortex judges what are suitable responses and behavior. These signals go to the speech generation system in the frontal cortex and to other sites for other responses.

Errors in information processing can occur anywhere on this path. Attention, which links all these centers, is central to perceiving and recognizing stimuli. It helps us form associations, tap into memory, and develop appropriate responses. An elaborate network of thought and abstraction connects to long-term memory. Our conscious thinking is processed at multiple neurophysiologic levels. Immediate memory stores stimuli that seem potentially significant. Short-term memory (immediate to several minutes) retains stimuli requiring conscious transformation or forethought. Because short-term memory has limited storage capacity, meaningful material is transferred into the active or working memory for further processing.

In considering a biological basis for ADHD, we have to think broadly about brain problems. One clinical researcher summarized ADHD as "a label for a heterogeneous group of dysfunctions related to each of several nodes along the attentional/intentional network…from the cerebellum, up to and including prefrontal cortex. [ADHD] includes neural substrates of activation, orientation, motivation and vigilance as these connect with and influence executive function" (Denckla 1993, p. 237). Conditions that are commonly comorbid with ADHD share a close anatomical, neurochemical, and functional locus in the basal forebrain and anteromedial frontal lobe (Cohen et al. 2002).

So far, we have many suspects for the biological basis of ADHD but no one model successfully discusses the underlying pathophysiology of the disorder (Spencer 2006). Clearly the disorder has a genetic basis. The frontal lobes of persons with ADHD behave differently than those of other people. On that basis alone, we can expect differences in symptom patterns, in penetrance, and in severity.

What we now call ADHD is likely more than one disorder. This type of realization is a common issue in psychiatry: a symptom or set of symptoms turns out to be multiple disorders. What lies under the umbrella term *ADHD*? We need precise measures of inhibitory capacity, working memory, and temporal processing to identify specific phenotypes of ADHD. Then we will be able to make more sense of the results of neuroimaging research.

FUTURE DIRECTIONS IN THE BIOLOGY OF ADHD

New and better technology, such as functional MRI, will make it possible to better visualize specific areas of the brain. Radioactively labeled medications and neurotransmitters will help specify which brain systems are involved and how and where medications work. A second element of understanding will come from molecular genetics. With these techniques, we will study individual genes, locate and specify genetic abnormalities, and begin to separate patients into genetically homogeneous groups. Another facet of knowledge will come from more precise cognitive-behavioral measures. With all these elements in place, we will be better able to separate ADHD into discrete clinical entities.

SUMMARY

- Genetic studies show that ADHD is strongly inherited. There is significantly increased incidence in the first-degree relatives of affected individuals. Identical twins show much higher concordance for the disorder than do fraternal twins. Adoption studies show that nature (genetic inheritance) is much more important than nurture (parenting style) in determining ADHD.
- Clinical observation and laboratory studies (MRI, PET scans) support the theory that ADHD is a syndrome of frontosubcortical dysfunction. Biochemically, ADHD is more than the result of too little brain dopamine. The central lesion in the disorder may be another process entirely. Clearly the disorder involves multiple neurotransmitter systems.
- In the future, molecular genetics will allow us to study groups of genetically homogeneous individuals. We will have enhanced neuroimaging techniques and more specific cognitive and behavioral measurements. This trio of molecular genetics, neuroimaging techniques, and cognitive-behavioral measures will enable us to better identify and treat what are probably multiple ADHDs.

REFERENCES

Adler L, Cohen J: Diagnosis and evaluation of adults with attention-deficit/ hyperactivity disorder. Psychiatr Clin North Am 27:187–201, 2004

Alexander GE, DeLong MR, Strick PL: Parallel organization of functionally segregated circuits linking basal ganglia and cortex. Annu Rev Neurosci 9: 357–381, 1986

Auerbach J, Geller V, Lezer S, et al: Dopamine D_4 receptor (DRD4) and serotonin transporter (5-HTTLPR) polymorphisms in the determination of temperament in 2-month-old infants. Mol Psychiatry 4:369–373, 1999

Bakker SC, van der Meulen EM, Buitelaar JK, et al: A whole-genome scan in 164 Dutch sib pairs with attention-deficit/hyperactivity disorder: suggestive evidence for linkage on chromosomes 7p and 15q. Am J Hum Genet 72:1251–1260, 2003

Barkley RA, Edwards G, Laneri M, et al: Executive functioning, temporal discounting, and sense of time in adolescents with attention deficit hyperactivity disorder (ADHD) and oppositional defiant disorder (ODD). J Abnorm Child Psychol 29:541–556, 2001

Benjamin J, Li L, Patterson C, et al: Population and familial association between the D_4 dopamine receptor gene and measures of novelty seeking. Nat Genet 12:81–84, 1996

Biederman J: Current concepts in the neurobiology of ADHD. Paper presented at the annual meeting of the American Psychiatric Association, New York, May 2004

Biederman J, Faraone SV, Mick E, et al: High risk for attention deficit hyperactivity disorder among children of parents with childhood onset of the disorder: a pilot study. Am J Psychiatry 152:431–435, 1995

Brown TE: Emerging understandings of attention-deficit disorders and comorbidities, in Attention-Deficit Disorders and Comorbidities in Children, Adolescents, and Adults. Edited by Brown TE. Washington, DC, American Psychiatric Press, 2000, pp 3–55

Callaway CW, Rempel N, Peng RY, et al: Serotonin 5-HT1-like receptors mediate hyperactivity in rats induced by 3, 4-methylenedioxymethamphetamine. Neuropsychopharmacology 7:113–127, 1992

Castellanos FX, Giedd JN, Berquin PC, et al: Quantitative brain magnetic resonance imaging in girls with attention-deficit/hyperactivity disorder. Arch Gen Psychiatry 58:289–295, 2001

Castellanos FX, Lee PP, Sharp W, et al: Developmental trajectories of brain volume abnormalities in children and adolescents with attention-deficit/hyperactivity disorder. JAMA 288:1740–1748, 2002

Chabot RJ, Serfontein G: Quantitative electroencephalographic profiles of children with attention deficit disorder. Biol Psychiatry 40:951–963, 1996

Cohen RA, Salloway S, Zawacki T: Neuropsychiatric aspects of disorders of attention, in The American Psychiatric Publishing Textbook of Neuropsychiatry and Clinical Neurosciences, 4th Edition. Edited by Yudofsky SC, Hales RE. Washington, DC, American Psychiatric Publishing, 2002, pp 489–524

Colquhoun WP, Baddeley AD: Influence of signal probability during pretraining on vigilance decrement. J Exp Psychol 73:153–155, 1967

Comings DE, Gade-Andavolu R, Gonzalez N, et al: Comparison of the role of dopamine, serotonin and noradrenaline genes in ADHD, ODD and conduct disorder: multivariate regression analysis of 20 genes. Clin Genet 57:178–196, 2000a

Comings DE, Gade-Andavolu R, Gonzalez N, et al: Multivariate analysis of associations of 42 genes in ADHD, ODD and conduct disorder. Clin Genet 58:31–40, 2000b

Curran S, Newman S, Taylor E, et al: Hypescheme: an operational criteria checklist and minimum data set for molecular genetic studies of attention deficit and hyperactivity disorders. Am J Med Genet 96:244–250, 2000

Denckla MD, Reader MJ: Education and psychosocial interventions: executive function and its consequences, in Handbook of Tourette's Syndrome and Related Tic and Behavioral Disorders. Edited by Kurlan R. New York, Marcel Dekker, 1993, pp 431–451

Dougherty DD, Bonab AA, Spencer TJ, et al: Dopamine transporter density in patients with attention deficit hyperactivity disorder. Lancet 354:2132–2133, 1999

Doyle A, Biederman J, Seidman LJ, et al: Diagnostic efficiency of neuropsychological test scores for discriminating boys with and without attention deficit-hyperactivity disorder. J Consult Clin Psychol 68:477–488, 2000

Durston S, Hulshoff Pol HE, Schnack HG, et al: Magnetic resonance imaging of boys with attention-deficit/hyperactivity disorder and their affected siblings. J Am Acad Child Adolesc Psychiatry 43:332–340, 2004

Elia J, Borcherding BG, Rapoport R, et al: Methylphenidate and dextroamphetamine treatments of hyperactivity: are there true nonresponders? Psychiatry Res 36:141–155, 1991

Ernst M, Kimes AS, London ED, et al: Neural substrates of decision making in adults with attention deficit hyperactivity disorder. Am J Psychiatry 160:1061–1070, 2003

Faraone SV: Genetics of adult attention-deficit/hyperactivity disorder. Psychiatr Clin North Am 27:303–321, 2004

Faraone SV, Doyle AE: The nature and heritability of attention-deficit/hyperactivity disorder. Child Adolesc Psychiatr Clin N Am 10:299–316, 2001

Faraone SV, Biederman J, Milberger S: An exploratory study of ADHD among second-degree relatives of ADHD children. Biol Psychiatry 35:398–402, 1994

Faraone SV, Biederman J, Mennin D, et al: Attention deficit hyperactivity disorder with bipolar disorder: a familial subtype? J Am Acad Child Adolesc Psychiatry 36:1378–1387, 1997a

Faraone SV, Biederman J, Mick E: Symptom reports by adults with attention-deficit/hyperactivity disorder: are they influenced by attention-deficit hyperactivity disorder in their children? J Nerv Ment Dis 185:583–584, 1997b

Faraone SV, Biederman J, Feighner JA, et al: Assessing symptoms of attention-deficit hyperactivity disorder in children and adults: which is more valid? J Consult Clin Psychol 68:830–842, 2000a

Faraone SV, Biederman J, Monuteaux MC: Toward guidelines for pedigree selection in genetic studies of attention deficit hyperactivity disorder. Genet Epidemiol 18:1–16, 2000b

Faraone SV, Doyle AE, Mick E, et al: Meta-analysis of the association between the 7-repeat allele of the dopamine D(4) receptor gene and attention deficit hyperactivity disorder. Am J Psychiatry 158:1052–1057, 2001

Faraone SV, Perlis RH, Doyle AE, et al: Molecular genetics of attention deficit hyperactivity disorder. Biol Psychiatry 57:1313–1323, 2005

Frick PJ, Lahey BB, Christ MG, et al: History of childhood behavior problems in biological relatives of boys with attention deficit hyperactivity disorder and conduct disorder. J Clin Child Psychol 20:445–451, 1991

Galler JR, Ramsey F, Solimano G, et al: The influence of early malnutrition on subsequent behavioral development, II: classroom behavior. J Am Acad Child Adolesc Psychiatry 22:16–22, 1983

Garcia-Sanchez C, Estevez-Gonzalez A, Suarez-Romero E, et al: Right hemisphere dysfunction in subjects with attention-deficit disorder with and without hyperactivity. J Child Neurol 12:107–115, 1997

Giedd JN, Castellanos FX, Casey BJ, et al: Quantitative morphology of the corpus callosum in attention deficit hyperactivity disorder. Am J Psychiatry 151:665–669, 1994

Goodman R, Stevenson J: A twin study of hyperactivity, I: an examination of hyperactivity scores and categories derived from Rutter teacher and parent questionnaires. J Child Psychol Psychiatry 30:671–689, 1989

Hervey AS, Epstein J, Curry JF: The neuropsychology of adults with attention deficit hyperactivity disorder: a meta-analytic review. Neuropsychology 18:485–503, 2004

Hesslinger B, Tebartz van Elst L, Thiel T, et al: Fronto-orbital volume reductions in adult patients with attention deficit hyperactivity disorder. Neurosci Lett 328:319–321, 2002

Himelstein J, Halperin JM: Neurocognitive functioning in adults with attention-deficit hyperactivity disorder. CNS Spectr 5:58–64, 2000

Hudziak JJ, Derks EM, Althoff RR, et al: The genetic and environmental contributions to attention deficit hyperactivity disorder as measured by the Conners' Rating Scales—Revised. Am J Psychiatry 162:1614–1620, 2005

Hunt RD: Nosology, neurobiology and clinical patterns of ADHD in adults. Psychiatr Ann 27:572–580, 1997

James W: Principles of Psychology. New York, Holt, 1890

Johnson DE, Epstein JN, Waid LR, et al: Neuropsychological performance deficits in adults with attention deficit/hyperactivity disorder. Arch Clin Neuropsychol 16:587–604, 2001

Lanau F, Zenner M, Civelli O, et al: Epinephrine and norepinephrine act as potent agonists at the recombinant human dopamine D_4 receptor. J Neurochem 68:804–812, 1997

Langley K, Marshall L, van den Bree M, et al: Association of the dopamine D_4 receptor gene 7-repeat allele with neuropsychological test performance of children with ADHD. Am J Psychiatry 161:133–138, 2004

Lou HC: Etiology and pathogenesis of ADHD: significance of prematurity and perinatal hypoxic-haemodynamic encephalopathy. Acta Paediatr 85:1266–1271, 1996

Lou HC, Andresen J, Steinberg B, et al: The striatum in a putative cerebral network activated by verbal awareness in normals and in ADHD children. Eur J Neurol 5:67–74, 1998

Lowe N, Kirley A, Hawi Z, et al: Joint analysis of the DRD5 marker concludes association with attention-deficit/hyperactivity disorder confined to the predominantly inattentive and combined subtypes. Am J Hum Genet 74:348–356, 2004

Manshadi M, Lippmann S, O'Daniel RG, et al: Alcohol abuse and attention deficit disorder. J Clin Psychiatry 44:379–380, 1983

Malaspina D, Corcoran C, Hamilton SP: Epidemiological and genetic aspects of neuropsychiatric disorders, in The American Psychiatric Publishing Textbook of Neuropsychiatry and Clinical Neurosciences, 4th Edition. Edited by Yúdofsky SC, Hales RE. Washington, DC, American Psychiatric Publishing, 2002, pp 323–415

Mattes JA: The role of frontal lobe dysfunction in childhood hyperkinesis. Compr Psychiatry 21:358–369, 1980

Mega MS, Cummings JL: Frontal-subcortical circuits and neuropsychiatric disorders. J Neuropsychiatry Clin Neurosci 6:358–370, 1994

Mesulam M-M: A cortical network for directed attention and unilateral neglect. Ann Neurol 10:309–325, 1981

Mesulam M-M: Principles of Behavioral Neurology. Philadelphia, PA, FA Davis, 1985

Michelson D, Faries D, Wernicke J, et al: Atomoxetine in the treatment of children and adolescents with attention deficit/hyperactivity disorder: a randomized, placebo-controlled, dose-response study (abstract). Pediatrics 108:E83, 2001

Milberger S, Biederman J, Faraone SV, et al: Is maternal smoking during pregnancy a risk factor for attention deficit hyperactivity disorder in children? Am J Psychiatry 153:1138–1142, 1996

Ogdie MN, Fisher SE, Yang M, et al: Attention deficit hyperactivity disorder: fine mapping supports linkage to 5p3, 6q12, 16p13, and 17p11. Am J Hum Genet 75:181–188, 2004

Overmeyer S, Simmons A, Santosh J, et al: Corpus callosum may be similar in children with ADHD and siblings of children with ADHD. Dev Med Child Neurol 42:8–13, 2000

Overmeyer S, Bullmore ET, Suckling J, et al: Distributed grey and white matter deficits in hyperkinetic disorder: MRI evidence for anatomical abnormality in an attentional network. Psychol Med 31:1425–1435, 2001

Payton A, Holmes J, Barrett JH, et al: Examining for association between candidate gene polymorphisms in the dopamine pathway and attention deficit hyperactivity disorder: a family based study. Am J Med Genet 105:464–470, 2001

Peterson BS, Leckman JF, Tucker D, et al: Preliminary findings of antistreptococcal antibody titers and basal ganglia volumes in tic, obsessive-compulsive, and attention deficit/hyperactivity disorders. Arch Gen Psychiatry 57:364–372, 2000

Pliszka SR, McCracken JT, Maas JW: Catecholamines in attention-deficit/hyperactivity disorder: current perspectives. J Am Acad Child Adolesc Psychiatry 35:264–272, 1996

Popper CW, Gammon GD, West SA, et al: Disorders usually first diagnosed in infancy, childhood, or adolescence, in The American Psychiatric Publishing Textbook of Clinical Psychiatry, 4th Edition. Edited by Hales RE, Yudofsky SC. Washington, DC, American Psychiatric Publishing, 2003, pp 833–974

Pueyo R, Maneru C, Vendrell P, et al: Attention deficit/hyperactivity disorder: cerebral asymmetry observed on magnetic resonance (in Spanish). Rev Neurol 30:920–925, 2000

Reimherr FW, Wender PH, Ebert MH, et al: Cerebrospinal fluid homovanillic acid and 5-hydroxy-indoleacetic acid in adults with attention deficit disorder, residual type. Psychiatry Res 11:71–78, 1984

Rhee SH, Waldman ID, Hay DA, et al: Sex differences in genetic and environmental influences on DSM-III-R attention-deficit/hyperactivity disorder. J Abnorm Psychol 108:24–41, 1999

Roman T, Szobot C, Martins S, et al: Dopamine transporter gene and response to methylphenidate in attention-deficit/hyperactivity disorder. Pharmacogenetics 12:497–499, 2002

Sacks O: An Anthropologist on Mars. New York, Knopf, 1995

Schachar R, Wachsmuth R: Hyperactivity and parental psychopathology. J Child Psychol Psychiatry 31:381–392, 1990

Schachar R, Mota VL, Logan GD, et al: Confirmation of an inhibitory control deficit in attention deficit/hyperactivity disorder. J Abnorm Child Psychol 28:227–235, 2000

Schmithorst VJ, Wilke M, Dardzinski BJ, et al: Correlation of white matter diffusivity and anisotropy with age during childhood and adolescence: a cross-sectional diffusion-tensor MR imaging study. Radiology 222:212–218, 2002

Schweitzer JB, Faber TL, Grafton ST, et al: Alterations in the functional anatomy of working memory in adult attention deficit hyperactivity disorder. Am J Psychiatry 157:278–280, 2000

Seeger G, Schloss P, Schmidt MH: Functional polymorphism within the promoter of the serotonin transporter gene is associated with severe hyperkinetic disorders. Mol Psychiatry 6:235–238, 2001a

Seeger G, Schloss P, Schmidt MH: Marker gene polymorphisms in hyperkinetic disorder: predictors of response to methylphenidate? Neurosci Lett 313:45–48, 2001b

Seidman LJ, Doyle A, Fried R, et al: Neuropsychological function in adults with attention-deficit/hyperactivity disorder. Psychiatr Clin North Am 27:261–282, 2004a

Seidman LJ, Valera EM, Bush G: Brain function and structure in adults with attention-deficit/hyperactivity disorder. Psychiatr Clin North Am 27:323–347, 2004b

Servan-Schreiber D, Carter CS, Bruno RM, et al: Dopamine and the mechanisms of cognition, part II: D-amphetamine effects in human subjects performing a selective attention task. Biol Psychiatry 43:723–729, 1998

Shaywitz BA, Cohen BJ, Bowers MB Jr: CSF metabolites in children with minimal brain dysfunction: evidence for alteration of brain dopamine. J Pediatr 90:67–71, 1977

Smalley SL, Kustanovich V, Minassian SL, et al: Genetic linkage of attention-deficit/hyperactivity disorder on chromosome 16p13, in a region implicated in autism. Am J Hum Genet 71:959–963, 2002

Sowell E, Peterson B: Cortical abnormalities in children and adolescents with attention-deficit/hyperactivity disorder. Lancet 362:1699–1707, 2003

Spencer T: Norepinephrine: understanding its role in ADHD, in The Current and Emerging Role of Alpha-2 Agonists in the Treatment of ADHD, Vol I: ADHD Etiology and Neurobiology. Hasbrouck Heights, NJ, Veritas Institute for Medical Education, 2006, pp 12–16

Spencer T, Biederman J, Wilens T, et al: Pharmacotherapy of attention deficit hyperactivity disorder across the life cycle. J Am Acad Child Adolesc Psychiatry 35:409–432, 1996

Spencer T, Biederman J, Wilens T, et al: Elevation of dopamine transporter by 30%–40% in attention deficit hyperactivity disorder. Paper presented at the annual meeting of the American Psychiatric Association, New York, May 2004

Sprich S, Biederman J, Crawford MH, et al: Adoptive and biological families of children and adolescents with ADHD. J Am Acad Child Adolesc Psychiatry 39:1432–1437, 2000

Sudderth DB, Kandel J: Adult ADD: The Complete Handbook. Roseville, CA, Prima Publishing, 1997

Sullivan PF, Fifield WJ, Kennedy MA, et al: No association between novelty seeking and the type 4 dopamine receptor gene (DRD4) in two New Zealand samples. Am J Psychiatry 155:98–101, 1998

Teicher MH, Anderson CM, Polcari A, et al: Functional deficits in basal ganglia of children with attention-deficit hyperactivity disorder shown with functional magnetic resonance imaging relaxometry. Nat Med 6:470–473, 2000

Vaidya CJ, Bunge SA, Dudukovic NM, et al: Altered neural substrates of cognitive control in childhood ADHD: evidence from functional magnetic resonance imaging. Am J Psychiatry 162:1605–1613, 2005

Waldman I: Meta-analysis of the DAT-ADHD association. Poster presented at the 3rd international meeting of the Attention-Deficit/Hyperactivity Disorder Molecular Genetics Network, Boston, MA, June 2001

Weiss JL, Seidman LJ: The clinical use of psychological and neuropsychological tests, in The New Harvard Guide to Psychiatry. Edited by Nicholi A. Cambridge, MA, Harvard University Press, 1998, pp 46–69

Wender PH: Attention-Deficit/Hyperactivity Disorder in Adults. New York, Oxford University Press, 1995

Zametkin AJ, Nordahl TE, Gross M, et al: Attention deficit/hyperactivity disorder: the result of abnormalities in fronto-striatal connections. J Am Acad Child Adolesc Psychiatry 26:676–686, 1987

Zametkin AJ, Nordahl TE, Gross M, et al: Cerebral glucose metabolism in adults with hyperactivity of childhood onset. N Engl J Med 323:1361–1366, 1990

CHAPTER 4

ALLIES IN TREATMENT

ENHANCING THE THERAPEUTIC ALLIANCE

A good working partnership between the psychiatrist and any patient is essential for successful treatment. Adult ADHD patients have particular features and special issues that can make the therapeutic alliance more fragile and compromise or destroy treatment. It helps if the psychiatrist has the traditional attributes of a good clinician: consistency, responsive listening, a nonjudgmental attitude, and solid expertise. Working with adults with ADHD requires more than simply being empathic and asking open-ended questions. Such patients may not readily voice their concerns spontaneously and then wait for the professional to respond. Their disorder is a neurological one that has psychological and social consequences. Most of them have multiple diagnoses and intersecting problems. Our challenge as clinicians is to keep the goals of treatment clear and work steadily toward them.

This chapter first explores a way of working to enhance the alliance by using a cognitive rehabilitation model. The next sections deal with four specific aspects of treating these patients that impact the doctor–patient alliance. First is collaborating with the patient, family members, and other members of the treatment team. Second are cultural, ethnic, and racial issues. Next are special legal issues. Concluding the chapter is a fuller discussion of countertransference, especially when the clinician's responses to the patient interfere with treatment.

CONTRIBUTIONS FROM A COGNITIVE REHABILITATION MODEL

One way of enhancing the therapeutic alliance is to rely on a cognitive rehabilitation approach first used with neurologically impaired patients.

This approach has three components: 1) improve cognitive function, 2) develop compensatory strategies, and 3) restructure the patient's environment (Nadeau 2002).

Improve Cognitive Function

Improving cognitive function often requires using medication. It also means helping patients create a structured lifestyle, with regular time for sleep, a sensible diet, and exercise. Issues interfering with this structure, such as substance abuse, poor compliance with medication, or chronically disrupted sleep, need attention and specific remedies.

Develop Internal and External Compensatory Strategies

Helping patients become better organized is vital. Some may profit from a simple daily schedule. Others need technological help like a personal digital assistant. Many patients find their computer is invaluable for helping them schedule themselves and remember commitments. Others will need help from a coach to stay on track.

Restructure the Environment to Maximize Function

Review the patient's environment, from his or her living arrangements to work environment to social network. Adults with ADHD often lag developmentally and need more active intervention than others their chronological age. They may need help with systems to do everything from making and keeping appointments to doing their taxes.

BUILDING ALLIANCES

Collaborating With Family Members

Working with adults with ADHD requires clinicians to work closely with the patient's family members. While keeping a primary commitment to the patient, clinicians can still work with others in the patient's social network. The clinician can explain to ADHD patients that their symptoms impact their entire family system. Many patients already know this. Their being in treatment at all may be due to family pressures. Having family members as allies can improve treatment results, if they understand the goals and interventions involved. This involvement, of course, varies with the needs of the individual patient. College students may not want their parents included. Then the clinician must balance the usefulness of parental involvement against the young adult's need to differentiate and to separate from them. Similarly, the spouse or significant other of an adult patient has much to offer and is often highly motivated to cooperate.

Bringing up the possibility of active collaboration with the family from the beginning of treatment often works well. With ADHD patients, from the start, there is a natural bridge to parents and significant others. It is highly desirable to have historical documentation and corroboration of the patient's past and current clinical status. The clinician can emphasize, with good reason, that the prospects for effective treatment improve if he or she can collaborate with family members. At the same time, the clinician can reassure the patient that he or she will keep confidential any information about the patient that is not fitting or necessary for others to know. Getting signed permission in advance to discuss the patient with any other person is always prudent clinical practice.

Collaborating With Other Mental Health Professionals

Although some psychiatrists provide all the treatment resources to patients, many work as part of a treatment team. The collaborative model is familiar to child psychiatrists and increasingly to adult psychiatrists as well. Some prefer this approach, whereas others use it because of the patient's insurance constraints. It is important for the psychiatrist to have a good working relationship with other professionals, such as social workers and psychologists. One aspect of collaboration includes developing a roster of other clinicians who know about the special nature of adult ADHD patients and work well with them. As in working with other patients, working collaboratively with ADHD adults requires the clinician to maintain regular contact with other professionals involved. Each needs to know what the other is doing.

Collaborating With a Coach

Clinicians working with ADHD adults often cannot track the issues of daily life as closely as many patients need. Doing so requires a degree of responsiveness and an involvement in the practical minutiae of a patient's life that most conventional professionals have not wanted or been able to do. In response to this need, a new kind of caregiver has evolved, a "coach."

The concept of an ADHD coach is still poorly defined. The model comes from athletics, where one person helps another with close contact and practical direction. Some ADHD coaches have professional training, such as in counseling or social work, whereas others do not. There appears to be a niche for their services among adults with ADHD. The field is evolving rapidly, and there are not clear standards for excellence. Many psychiatrists are wary of interacting with other helpers whose role is ill defined and whose expertise is unclear.

An ADHD coach is an active ally, a personal organizer. Typically, coaching starts with a planning phase in which the patient and coach get to know each other and develop specific goals. To succeed, the patient needs to feel that working with the coach is his or her own agenda, not someone else's. Once the pair have a work plan, they decide how often and how to stay in contact: in person, by e-mail, or by phone. The coach helps the patient estimate how long it takes to accomplish specific tasks. He or she builds in reminders of appointments and commitments.

Coaches make goals more specific, concrete, and compelling. Often that means helping the adult with ADHD break tasks down into smaller components. The coach's framework is not "Why did you do that?" but "What other options do you have? How can you do it better?" At the same time, the coach keeps the larger picture and long-term goals in mind.

Feeling demoralized is common for adults with ADHD. The effective coach helps the patient maintain perspective and self-esteem.

Coaching presumes that the ADHD adult has resources and abilities. The coach focuses on actions and measurable outcomes, not on feelings. What is the patient having difficulty with right now? How can he or she work through or around it? The aim is to help the patient to reach his or her own stated goals. "Coaching is not psychotherapy" (Ratey 2002).

When looking for a coach, the patient should interview more than one prospect. It helps if the patient knows what his or her needs are and can be clear about them. The patient should look for someone who matches his or her interests and personality style.

Coaches are less expensive than clinicians, and coaches have more objectivity and less emotional investment than do family members. Coaches can particularly help burned-out spouses. Husbands are grateful if someone helps an ADHD wife run the household effectively and function at work outside the home. Wives appreciate the coach who keeps after the ADHD husband about his domestic and work tasks.

The Attention Deficit Disorder Association is a good source of coaches with special skills (Attention Deficit Disorder Association Subcommittee on AD/HD Coaching 2005). Two national groups train and certify coaches: LifeCoach Inc. (124 Waterman St., Providence, RI 02906;

phone 508-252-4965) and National Coaching Network (P.O. Box 353, Lafayette Hill, PA 19444; phone 610-825-4505) (Doyle et al. 2002). Numerous private organizations offer training and certification, but no central organization or governing body oversees the field or offers licenses. ADHD coaches are more available in major urban areas than in rural regions.

ISSUES OF CULTURE, ETHNICITY, AND RACE

Psychiatrists often use the terms *culture, ethnicity,* and *race* when they discuss aspects of patients' lives. These vital dimensions of human experience influence the way patients see themselves, what they regard as illness, and what kind of treatment they seek or avoid.

The definition of *culture* in this context is "a set of meanings, values, everyday practices, behavioral norms and beliefs used by members of a particular group in society as a way of conceptualizing their unique view of the world…[It] encompasses language, nonverbal expressions, social relationships, manifestations of emotion, religious beliefs and practices, and socioeconomic ideologies. [It] changes and adapts from generation to generation" (Ruiz 2004, p. 527). *Race* is defined as a concept based on common physiognomy, with physical, biological, and genetic connotations. Although the validity of this definition has been questioned, many still accept it. *Ethnicity* is the subjective sense of belonging in a group of people who share a common origin as well as a common matrix of cultural beliefs and practices. Ethnicity is an integral component of one's sense of identity (Ruiz 2004).

Cultural background often influences whether adults seek diagnosis of and treatment for ADHD. Beliefs and behavior about health and illness vary by ethnicity. Persons with common cultural processes and life experiences often share health-related beliefs and behaviors. None of the terms just defined successfully captures the complexity of people's experiences and contexts.

Clinicians who work with diverse patients need cultural competency; that is, they must be able to understand the similarities and differences between themselves and patients. Cultural awareness is the process through which individuals "learn to appreciate and become sensitive to the values, lifestyles, practices and problem-solving strategies of an individual with a different cultural background" (Campinha-Bacote 1994, p. 23). Becoming culturally knowledgeable requires us to learn about the beliefs and values of different cultural and ethnic groups. It means staying open and objective to individuals from different cultural backgrounds (Institute of Medicine 2002).

In the United States, people who have a different skin color than white or who speak a language other than English may be treated differently, in ways that produce poorer health outcomes. This reality may explain the disparate health risks and outcomes of different groups in American society (Institute of Medicine 2002). For example, given the same symptoms, mental health professionals may diagnose black and white patients differently (Garb 1997). The surgeon general's report *Mental Health: Culture, Race and Ethnicity* noted that members of ethnic and racial minorities in the United States live in social and economic inequality. These inequalities impose greater burdens on minorities and detract from their mental health. Members of minority groups have less access to mental health services and are less likely to receive them (U.S. Department of Health and Human Services 2001).

There are no good data on the cultural, racial, and ethnic differences and similarities among boys and girls and men and women who have ADHD (Dulcan 1997).

African Americans and ADHD

Many African Americans suspect that ADHD does not exist. Related to this belief are their concerns that too many children are overmedicated for their symptoms (Strickland et al. 1991). The surgeon general's report mentioned earlier supports the reality of the disorder in African Americans and other ethnic minorities. The report denied overdiagnosis or overprescription of medications for ADHD (U.S. Department of Health and Human Services 2001). Former U.S. Surgeon General David Satcher, M.D., Ph.D., who directed the work that culminated in that report, identified misperceptions about ADHD in the African American community. The disorder is underrecognized and undertreated in African American children and teens, largely because they lack access to comprehensive assessment and appropriate treatment options (New Freedom Commission on Mental Health 2003).

The misperceptions persist. In a recent survey of 262 white and 226 African American parents, the African American parents felt that the disorder was overdiagnosed in their children. Fewer of them (64%) than white parents (79%) would know where to get treatment for the disorder. Twice as many African American parents (59%) as white parents attributed ADHD to sugar in the diet. They were less likely to have their children take medication for ADHD. "In the African American community, the prescription least likely to filled in the first place is an ADHD prescription" (Bailey 2005.

Data from clinical research on African American children and ADHD present an unclear picture. In one school-based study, white children were twice as likely as African American children to be evaluated, diagnosed, and treated for ADHD. The researchers asserted that the "threshold of parental recognition and seeking of services" contributed to this discrepancy (Bussing et al. 2003). In another such study, African American children were identified as having ADHD symptoms at higher rates than white children (Reid et al. 1998). Interestingly, Stevens et al. (2004) found no significant differences in the diagnosis and treatment of African American children compared with whites.

Researchers recently studied children and adolescents treated in 17 mental health care centers in South Carolina. Approximately 40%–45% of the patients in this system are African American. Researchers examined a representative sample of 1,176 patients with a primary diagnosis of ADHD in a 4-month period during 2000. Of the final sample of 164, 82% were boys, average age 9.8 years; 45% were African American; and 46% had a co-occurring diagnosis, most frequently oppositional defiant disorder. Researchers reviewing the charts in this sample found no gender or ethnic differences for meeting the DSM-IV (American Psychiatric Association 1994) criteria for ADHD, for the presence of information regarding the target symptoms of ADHD, or for suitable developmental and medical history. There were also no gender or ethnic differences in whether a rating of serious functional impairment was in the chart, whether the clinician noted symptoms before age 7, or whether a standard diagnostic instrument was used. Even more striking, they noted no gender or ethnic differences among those who were prescribed medication, or in whether medication monitoring was occurring. Finally, they found no gender or ethnic differences in the prescriptions of medications by type, whether stimulants, alpha-blockers, or mood/anxiety medications (Jerrell 2003). Studies of ADHD in African American adults are notable by their absence from the literature.

Several forces keep African American persons from getting treatment for psychiatric disorders such as ADHD. These include the stigma of being a person of color, certain deeply held religious beliefs, distrust of physicians, and language and literacy barriers to suitable care. Suffering among African Americans may, in some ways, be regarded as a given. It is understandable that "the blues," expressed in music, rose from this community. Some African Americans deeply believe that prayer alone can heal psychological distress. Although schizophrenia and affective illness have similar prevalence among African Americans and whites, African Americans are far more likely to be diagnosed as having schizophrenia than whites. African Americans are far less likely to be diagnosed as depressed or to be treated for depression with suitable medication (Adebimpe 2004; Lawson 1996).

Discriminatory practices contribute to the cultural distrust of the mental health profession that many African American persons have. Cultural distrust is "a healthy paranoia" exhibited by people of African descent toward institutions, systems, and individuals that have harmed them in the past and may do so again (Breland-Noble 2004). However, this distrust contributes to their reluctance to consult mental health professionals (Snowden 1999).

African American adults who seek treatment for ADHD also have to surmount family and community pressures.

> "My friends said, 'Man, are you *crazy*?' when I told them I was going to a psychiatrist." Ray, a 28-year-old African American, was to be the first in the family to go to college. "From grammar school, no matter how hard I tried, my grades were uneven. I couldn't pay attention for more than a few minutes. I had trouble sitting still in class. I had to read and reread to make information stick," he said. Likable, ambitious, and a terrific saxophone player, he got enthusiastic letters of recommendation from teachers as he finished high school.
>
> His first year at college he struggled, and he ended up on academic probation. Despite his best intentions, his sophomore year went badly. In his spring semester, he sought evaluation by a psychologist, who diagnosed him with ADHD, predominantly inattentive type. Her recommendations, for extra time on examinations and other interventions, came too late to rescue him academically. He flunked out.
>
> "I could barely get out of bed for 6 months," he said. "I never did anything about the ADHD. Finally I got this entry-level government job. I've done well. My boss keeps saying, 'A smart boy like you needs a college degree.' So I've enrolled at the local community college. But what if I fail again?
>
> "My brother's two sons have been diagnosed with ADHD. I'm sure my dad has it, although he'd never get diagnosed or treated."
>
> Fortunately, Ray responded well and rapidly to treatment. A combination of medication, coaching on organization, and getting appropriate accommodations at college enabled him to do well and to graduate. Now he is considering getting an MBA, and he has a good basis for his educational hopes.

Other African American patients with more financial and other resources still have to struggle with cultural and family issues.

> Personable and well-spoken, Callie comes from a family of successful entrepreneurs. She said, "When I was diagnosed with ADHD in secondary school, my parents' response was, 'Nonsense. Just work harder. We all had to.' I did well enough to get into a fine African American college. The faculty and administration there had the same attitude as my par-

ents. They didn't believe in ADHD, and they didn't offer any help. That was 10 years ago, and now I'm trying to sell life insurance. Clients like me, but they get mad if I'm late because I'm disorganized or get lost. I can't balance my checkbook. How can I help other people run their financial life?"

Hispanics and ADHD

Some of the same extra burdens affect persons of Hispanic descent who have ADHD. Health and the presence of illness are socially defined concepts. What one group considers to be poor health another may not. Some groups are less likely to acknowledge the presence of health problems. In one study, Hispanic parents less frequently than white parents identified their children as having chronic health conditions or special health care needs. However, in that study the Hispanic children identified with special or chronic health issues were much more likely than identified white children to visit the emergency department. They functioned worse day to day because of their health problems (Shenkman et al. 2001). In another study, Hispanics were less likely to report having a "health condition" but more often described themselves as in "fair" or "poor" health. Hispanics may use a different threshold for defining illness or for determining the severity level at which a problem is labeled as a health condition or requires medical attention (Doty and Ives 2002).

Speaking of "Hispanics" as one group minimizes the different cultures among them, for as many as six aggregates exist (Giminez 1989). Each has a different socioeconomic status and degree of integration in the United States. Two are considered minority groups (people of Mexican and Puerto Rican descent) and four are immigrant populations (Cubans, Central American refugees, Central American immigrants, and South American immigrants).

Persons identified as Hispanic have more difficulties receiving health care than do whites, and their problems are compounded if they speak only Spanish (Fiscella et al. 2002). They have lower levels of satisfaction with their health care and more negative physician–patient interactions than whites do (Collins et al. 2002). Overall, Hispanic children are less likely than white children to receive developmental services (Bethell et al. 2001). They are less likely to have one regular health care provider, and their parents are less likely to receive care that is family centered or to be assessed for mental or emotional issues (Bethell et al. 2003).

Compared with whites, Hispanic youths ages 3–16 years are less likely to be diagnosed with ADHD or treated with stimulant medication, according to a recent study (Stevens et al. 2004). Researchers in that study speculated that language barriers, different expectations of child behavior, and less concern about ADHD symptoms may contribute to the less frequent diagnosis and less frequent use of stimulants for affected children.

There is little information about the incidence and treatment of ADHD in Hispanic adults.

> Luis, 27, long suspected that he had ADHD but did not want to admit it. Then he flunked a crucial early set of exams in his Ph.D. program. "I hated the attitude in school that the Hispanic kids were the dumb kids. I was smart. I was also disorganized, and I didn't pay attention. My father used to yell at me, 'Why don't you *listen*?' To please him, I majored in engineering when I started college, but I flunked out. I started again in political science, which I loved. After 7 years in college, I'm in Washington, DC, and in graduate school. I can't fail now."
>
> With full and active treatment of his ADHD, Luis revived his flagging academic career.

Increasingly, material about ADHD is available in Spanish to the Hispanic community in print and on the Internet. This dissemination of information may help.

To be effective, health messages to Hispanics, as to other populations, need to be culturally sensitive. For example, many Hispanics espouse *fatalismo*, the sense that a person can do little to alter his or her destiny (Flores 2000). That concept may impede getting treatment for conditions such as ADHD. Health messages about ADHD and other disorders may work better if they are communicated in the context of another value, *familialismo*. This value expresses the importance of working to ensure the best quality of life for all family members. Such an approach to ADHD in Hispanic communities may ease access to treatment for both children and adults (Bethell et al. 2003).

LEGAL ISSUES AND ADHD

ADHD has many legal ramifications. After all, it affects education, employment, criminal prosecutions, and divorce and custody proceedings, among others. Clinicians working with adults with ADHD need to be clear about their role in the legal issues involved. Most clinicians are familiar with assessing and diagnosing patients for the purpose of treatment. Documenting how a person may qualify for legal accommodation under the law, however, is different. That requires thinking beyond the usual clinical framework and presenting a case that addresses the legal issues satisfactorily.

The principal laws affecting adults with ADHD are the Rehabilitation Act of 1973 and the Americans With Disabilities Act of 1990 (Latham and Latham 2002). The Rehabilitation Act of 1973 banned discrimination against persons with disabilities by the U.S. government, by contractors with that government, and by recipients of federal funds. Notably, the act applied to most American educational institutions. The Americans With Disabilities Act of 1990 attempted to extend these rights to all persons in our society.

To qualify for protection under these laws, an affected person must have a physical or mental impairment. Many legal rulings confirm that ADHD is such an impairment (*Davidson v. Midelfort Clinic, Ltd* [1998]). There must be proof that the disability substantially limits a "major" life activity. Learning and working are examples of major life activities, among others. The Equal Employment Opportunity Commission has added thinking, concentrating, and interacting with others to the list of major life activities. Courts, however, do not always abide by these guidelines (Latham and Latham 2000).

To prove that the patient has a disability, the clinician must document that the patient, because of his or her ADHD, has "substantial" limitations in cited areas. A limitation is substantial when an affected individual is

a. unable to perform a major life activity that the average person in the general population can perform; or
b. significantly restricted as to the condition, manner, or duration under which an individual can perform a particular major life activity as compared to the condition, manner, or duration under which the average person in the general population can perform that same major life activity (Latham and Latham 2002, p. 210).

Making the case for a substantial limitation in the domain of work is difficult. Here the clinician must document that the patient's impairment keeps him or her not just from a particular job but from significant classes of work.

Having to compare a patient with ADHD to an "average person" may be hard to do. It is much easier to determine "average" for physical impairments such as problems with hearing or sight than it is for learning, attentional, and psychiatric impairments.

Once a person has demonstrated that he or she is a qualified individual with a disability, the laws mandate "reasonable" accommodations in the academic and work environments. Reasonable accommodations are of three types: 1) those that ensure equal opportunity in the admissions process to an academic institution or in the application process for a job, 2) those that enable a disabled person to complete a course of study or to do a job, and 3) those that allow individuals with disabilities to enjoy the same benefits and privileges as do those without disabilities.

Typical reasonable academic accommodations modify the non-essential parts of a program so that qualified disabled individuals have the same educational benefits as those without disability. An example would be providing texts in braille for the blind learner. Reasonable workplace accommodations modify the nonessential parts of a job so that disabled qualified persons can do it. Examples include time off for treatment, modified work schedules, and the use of job coaches. The disabled person uses an interactive process with teachers and administrators in the academic setting, or superiors in the workplace, to reach reasonable accommodations. Such a process, however, often requires the disabled person to disclose much, if not all, of his or her medical information.

Clinicians who prepare legal reports for patients with ADHD must first establish that a disability exists. Next is specifying the nature and severity of its impact on the patient's function. Last is proposing what specific strategies and accommodations are necessary because of the patient's disability. These requirements impose a substantial burden on the clinician.

A new source of concern for clinicians is that they may be at risk for legal action if they fail to diagnose and treat ADHD appropriately. There are now anecdotal reports of psychiatrists being successfully tried for not treating the disorder (Adler et al. 2005).

COUNTERTRANSFERENCE ISSUES

Adults who have ADHD present with a wide variety of symptoms. Some are severely ill. Their chaotic life is the outcome of decades of failure and disappointment. Comorbid conditions can be so intractable that it seems impossible ever to address the patient's ADHD. Other ADHD patients have symptoms that need only fine-tuning to help them function at their best.

To best help adults with ADHD, we may have to reach out in unaccustomed ways. We may have to work with family members differently and learn to relate to new mental health workers, such as ADHD coaches. We may have to deal more fully with cultural, racial, and ethnic issues than usual. These may impede acceptance of ADHD as a concept, or they may make it harder for a patient to get treatment or to collaborate fully. Because ADHD has legal aspects and consequences, we may have to work in unaccustomed forensic territory.

The complex challenges of ADHD patients stir strong emotional reactions in clinicians. As with any patient, we need to know how we respond and whether our reactions impair or enhance the patient's progress (Wishnie 2005). Countertransference reactions provide valuable clues to aspects of a patient's situation that may be useful to explore. Whether these reactions are the result of something triggered in the treating doctor or something in the patient, they require understanding and, potentially, action. Allowing for the different personalities, training, and background of clinicians, recurring themes or issues arise in work with adult ADHD patients.

Negative Countertransference Issues

Resentment

ADHD patients bring into their treatment their problems negotiating the tasks of everyday life. They may have a harder time than other patients remembering the correct day and time of their appointments, especially the initial assessment visit. Bills may be lost, accumulate, or be paid late. It may be more difficult for them than for other patients to keep track of their medication. They may not notice that they are about to run out. Many call at the last minute for refills on prescriptions. This lack of notice is even more of a problem in patients taking central nervous system stimulants who need to present a paper prescription to the pharmacy. Clinicians may need to write the prescription in a last-minute flurry, which is annoying. How much of the patient's forgetting is a symptom of his or her underlying difficulty? How much is it part of a pattern of abusing medication (and physicians)? How much does it express the patient's resistance to change? Even if we recognize that the behavior is symptomatic of the patient's problems, and not drug abuse or resistance to treatment, it is hard to remain equable. Staying in the professional role is harder if we are tired or overworked.

Some adults with ADHD come for treatment reluctantly, at the instigation of others. Their motivation is not to change their lives but to stop the nagging of a spouse or intimate partner. Some want a "quick fix": a few milligrams (or more than a few milligrams) of the right central nervous system stimulant, and they will be transformed. Such patients make many clinicians bristle.

Some patients who seek treatment for ADHD have strongly negative feelings about using medication. This resistance, an issue with psychiatric patients with any disorder, needs to be explored and dealt with. Resistance may cause special difficulty in treating ADHD patients, however, because of such clear evidence that medication helps. The clinician treating the adult ADHD patient may feel he or she has even more justification than usual for recommending medication.

Suspicion

ADHD as a diagnosis is still controversial in professional circles as well as lay ones. Some psychiatrists still doubt that ADHD exists, especially in adults. Such professionals tend to omit the disorder in their differential diagnosis, and they may regard patients who come for treatment with suspicion. Reports from the lay press and clinical literature of central nervous system stimulants used as mental "performance enhancers," like steroids for better athletic achievement, fuel this distrust.

Some adults seek treatment for ADHD hoping to find an excuse for their failures in life. On the basis of their disorder, they want specific accommodations to which they feel fully and legally entitled. Working with such patients, however, may require wrestling with questions such as "Am I providing the patient with justifiable supports that enable the patient to do his or her best? Or, because of special accommodations, does the patient have an unfair advantage over others who do not have the disorder? Am I improving the patient's function—or colluding with the patient's entitlements? Is the patient genuinely handicapped, or is he or she malingering, like some persons who present with somatic symptoms?" Answers to these and related questions are not always clear. Distrust of the patient's motives makes it difficult to do our best.

Prejudice

Recent work has focused on the negative reactions that medical professionals and others have to persons of other races, cultures, and ethnicities. These reactions, often unconscious or preconscious, influence us more than we would like to admit. Such attitudes can negatively impact diagnosis as well as treatment. Do we have assumptions about who does or does not have ADHD based on racial, ethnic, or cultural factors? Do those assumptions influence the choices we make in recommending and delivering treatment?

Envy

Some adults achieve worldly success because of their ADHD, not in spite of it. That can stir envy in clinicians, who have reached their place in life through steady application and deferred gratification. By temperament and training, many physicians value order, duty, and responsibility. Meeting the requirements of medical school and residency calls for considerable and consistent attention to detail. Persons who succeed with a much looser approach to life, like some adults with ADHD, can annoy us.

Discouragement

By the time many adults with ADHD present for treatment, they carry considerable burdens. Despite having labored long and hard to contend with their difficulties, they may be overwhelmed. Many have major co-morbidities, especially if no one has recognized or treated their ADHD. Abuse of alcohol and other substances and entrenched anxiety and affective disorders commonly complicate these patients' presentation. Some patients have had considerable psychiatric treatment that was unsuccessful, at least partly because of the unaddressed ADHD. Many patients have children with ADHD who need unusual amounts of attention and care if they are going to thrive. Such adult patients struggle not to be overwhelmed with their problems. So do their clinicians.

Managing Negative Countertransference

We need to avoid the traps of negative countertransference to adult ADHD patients. Responding fully to a patient is difficult if the clinician doubts the validity, or even the existence, of this diagnostic category. We also need to notice if we fail to understand the legal ramifications of the disorder and thus do not provide the documentation patients need. Unjustified or excessive suspicion about the patient's motives in seeking an ADHD diagnosis can be destructive. Treating a patient who has the accoutrements of success may be hard for us, especially when he or she has thrived by an unconventional route or with seemingly little effort. Negative reactions to cultural, racial, and ethnic factors in the patient can cloud our judgment and interfere with providing the best treatment. If the patient's difficulties overwhelm us as they do him or her, it is hard to systematically address what can be helped.

Positive Countertransference Issues

Clinicians can have problems working with ADHD adults because of positive countertransference reactions as well. Many of these patients are engaging, resourceful, and personable. Often they have engrossing life histories and have overcome great obstacles. They charm us, like they do other people. When that happens, however, countertransference problems occur: the doctor feels less objective (Rako and Mazer 1980).

Unwittingly, we can collude with patients in having unrealistic expectations of treatment. Nowhere is this truer than when using central nervous system stimulants to treat the symptoms of ADHD. Sometimes the patient notices improvement after the first doses of the first medication. When the stimulants work well, they produce fast, sustained, and dramatic results. However, even when the stimulants are indicated, some patients do not do well. Fewer adults than children with ADHD respond to these agents. Sometimes we have to try several preparations of methylphenidate and dextroamphetamine, at different dosages. That can be discouraging, especially if the clinician is swept up in the patient's strong wish for rapid improvement.

Positive countertransference is dangerous if the clinician overidentifies with the patient. We may underestimate the severity and complexity of the patient's difficulties and miss other problems. A particular trap is seeing only the ADHD and not checking for or overlooking cyclic mood disorder, especially past hypomanic or manic episodes. The patient may not be aware of such episodes or minimize their importance. A full, systematic history from the individual, supplemented by information from one or more other persons who know the patient well, should be part of every evaluation for ADHD in an adult.

The clinician may encourage unrealistic expectations if he or she shares the patient's hopes of a fast and full response to a treatment without complications. If results are slower or less dramatic than predicted, the patient may feel particularly disappointed. Effective treatment often substantially improves the lives of adults with ADHD. If a patient does not respond to one medication, he or she may respond to another. If necessary, we can try a number of agents, in sequence and in combination. Interventions other than medication also help adults with ADHD. We have a full, rational basis for hope that we can transmit.

Mastering Countertransference Issues

Countertransference requires us to pay attention to our own reactions as well as those of patients. We need to acknowledge, bear, and put our own feelings in perspective, while not acting on them (Rako and Mazer 1980). The seasoned clinician considers how much his or her emotional reactions to the patient are warranted by the patient. Does the patient remind the clinician of an emotionally troublesome person in his or her professional or social life, now or earlier? Whether countertransference feelings are negative or positive, what do they tell the clinician about the patient? If used well, such responses allow us to understand patients viscerally, providing information that is otherwise unavailable. Taking personal time for reflection, having group or individual supervision, and using a trusted colleague as a consultant all help maintain professional equilibrium. If our emotional responses are disrupting treatment, can we explore them in the work with the patient?

By mastering our countertransference, we can formulate fresh, powerful treatment strategies. We may be able to tolerate a patient's symptoms better, without taking them personally. Alternatively, we may need to do the opposite and set firmer limits or expectations. On rare occasions, the clinician may decide that it is not possible to work with the patient. Then the task is maintaining care until the patient successfully engages another professional.

Not all feeling responses to patients are negative or dangerously positive. Part of the pleasure of working with adult ADHD patients is that they are often resourceful and personable. They persevere in life despite major burdens and obstacles. They have much to teach us about courage, resilience, and productive differences between people.

SUMMARY

- Establishing and maintaining a good therapeutic alliance with adult ADHD patients is essential for success, as it is with any psychiatric patient. A good working model comes from one that helps neurological patients undergoing cognitive rehabilitation.
- The treating psychiatrist usefully takes an active stance with adult ADHD patients, who may need more outreach than others. In addition to collaborating with family members and with other mental health professionals, treating adult ADHD patients may involve work with "coaches." These persons provide support and direction to patients on day-to-day matters. Their place in treatment regimens is evolving.
- Cultural factors powerfully influence how people define illness and when and where they seek help for medical conditions. Persons of color in the United States face barriers and impediments to health care that whites do not. Many African Americans are skeptical about the validity of the diagnosis of ADHD in children, and even more so in adults. In the Hispanic community, views of illness and barriers of cost and language may make it harder for these patients to identify and get treatment for ADHD. Recent public health advances and in-

creased health information in Spanish may make it easier for children and adults in these communities in the future. Cultural issues impact the diagnosis and treatment of ADHD in all ethnic and cultural groups, not simply the African American and Hispanic communities. Clearly, these factors complicate diagnosis and treatment of ADHD in adults. Cultural factors need special attention when treatment is not going well.

- Legal factors complicate treatment of the adult ADHD patient. The legal definition of the disorder is different from DSM-IV-TR (American Psychiatric Association 2000) criteria. Clinicians may find that discrepancy confusing, especially when they are documenting patients' needs for special accommodations. To best help their patients, clinicians need to understand the laws that apply to ADHD. Clinicians who support a patient's application to be considered disabled under the law have to think, and document, beyond their usual clinical framework. They have to document a diagnosis that meets legal standards, not just medical definitions. They must specify its impact on the patient's life and function, and propose reasonable accommodations at school or at work that will allow the patient to succeed.
- The special complexities of adult ADHD patients generate strong and varied emotional reactions in clinicians. We need to acknowledge, explore, and work with countertransference issues. Dealing with countertransference, by ourselves or with consultation or supervision, can substantially strengthen the alliance with patients and improve outcomes.

REFERENCES

Adebimpe VR: A second opinion on the use of white norms in psychiatric diagnosis of black patients. Psychiatr Ann 34:542–551, 2004

Adler L, Dodson W, Spencer T, et al: Diagnostic strategies for adult ADHD: working toward a standard of care. Medical Crossfire 6:1–13, 2005

American Psychiatric Association: Diagnostic and Statistical Manual of Mental Disorders, 4th Edition. Washington, DC, American Psychiatric Association, 1994

American Psychiatric Association: Diagnostic and Statistical Manual of Mental Disorders, 4th Edition, Text Revision. Washington, DC, American Psychiatric Association, 2000

Attention Deficit Disorder Association Subcommittee on AD/HD Coaching: The ADDA guiding principles for coaching individuals with attention deficit disorder. Available at: http://www.add.org/articles/coachingguide.html. Accessed December 8, 2005.

Bailey R: Racial differences in the understanding of, and treatment for, attention deficit hyperactivity disorder. Paper presented at the annual meeting of the American Academy of Psychiatry and the Law, Montreal, Quebec, October 2005

Bethell CB, Peck C, Schor E: Assessing and improving health system provision of well-child care: the Promoting Healthy Development Survey. Pediatrics 107:1084–1094, 2001

Bethell CB, Carter K, Lansky D, et al: Measuring and interpreting health care quality across culturally diverse populations: a focus on consumer-reported indicators of health care quality. New York, Foundation for Accountability, March 2003. Available at http://www.markle.org/resources/facct/doclibFiles/documentFile_592.pdf. Accessed March 13, 2006.

Breland-Noble A: Mental healthcare disparities affect treatment of black adolescents. Psychiatr Ann 34:534–538, 2004

Bussing R, Zima BT, Gary FA, et al: Barriers to detection, help-seeking, and service use for children with ADHD symptoms. J Behav Health Serv Res 30:176–189, 2003

Campinha-Bacote J: The Process of Cultural Competence in Health Care. Cincinnati, OH, Transcultural C.A.R.E. Associates, 1994

Collins KS, Hughes DL, Doty MM, et al: Diverse communities, common concerns: assessing health care quality for minority Americans. New York, Commonwealth Fund Report #523, 2002

Davidson v Midelfort Clinic, Ltd., 133 F3d 499 (7th Cir. 1998)

Doty MM, Ives BL: Quality of health care for Hispanic populations: findings from the Commonwealth Fund 2001 Health Care Quality Survey. New York, The Commonwealth Fund, 2002

Doyle BB, Wender PH, Adler L, et al: ADHD in adults: valid diagnosis and treatment strategies. Medical Crossfire 4:30–40, 2002

Dulcan M: Practice parameters for the assessment and treatment of children, adolescents, and adults with attention-deficit/hyperactivity disorder. J Am Acad Child Adolesc Psychiatry 36:85S–121S, 1997

Fiscella K, Franks P, Doescher MP, et al: Disparity in health care by race, ethnicity and language among the insured. Med Care 40:52–59, 2002

Flores G: Culture and the patient–physician relationship: achieving cultural competency in health care. Pediatrics 136:14–23, 2000

Garb HN: Race bias, social class bias, and gender bias in clinical judgment. Clinical Psychology: Science and Practice 4:99–120, 1997

Giminez ME: Latino/"Hispanic"—who needs a name? the case against a standardized terminology. Int J Health Serv 19:557–571, 1989

Institute of Medicine: Speaking of Health. Washington, DC, National Academies Press, 2002

Jerrell JM: Are assessment and treatment influenced by ethnicity and gender? Psychiatric Times 20:1–6, 2003. Available at: http://www.psychiatrictimes.com/p031071.html. Accessed December 6, 2005.

Latham PS, Latham PH: Attention Deficit and the Law, 2nd Edition. Washington, DC, JKL Communications, 2000

Latham PS, Latham PH: What clinicians need to know about legal issues relevant to ADHD, in Clinician's Guide to Adult ADHD. Edited by Goldstein S, Ellison AT. New York, Academic Press, 2002, pp 205–218

Lawson WB: Clinical issues in the pharmacotherapy of African Americans. Psychopharmacol Bull 32:275–281, 1996

Nadeau K: The clinician's role in the treatment of ADHD, in Clinician's Guide to Adult ADHD. Edited by Goldstein S, Ellison AT. New York, Academic Press, 2002, pp 107–127

New Freedom Commission on Mental Health: Achieving the Promise: Transforming Mental Health Care in America. Final Report (DHHS Pub No SMA-03-3832). Rockville, MD, U.S. Department of Health and Human Services, 2003

Rako S, Mazer H: Semrad, the Heart of a Therapist. Northvale, NJ, Jason Aronson, 1980

Ratey N: Life coaching for adult ADHD, in Clinician's Guide to Adult ADHD. Edited by Goldstein S, Ellison AT. New York, Academic Press, 2002, pp 261–277

Reid R, DuPaul GJ, Power TJ, et al: Assessing culturally different students for attention deficit hyperactivity disorder using behavior rating scales. J Abnorm Child Psychol 26:187–198, 1998

Ruiz P: Addressing culture, race and ethnicity in psychiatric practice. Psychiatr Ann 34:526–532, 2004

Shenkman E, Vogel B, Brooks R, et al: Race and ethnicity and the identification of special needs children. Health Care Financ Rev 23:35–51, 2001

Snowden LR: African American service use for mental health problems. J Community Psychol 27:303–313, 1999

Stevens J, Harman JS, Kelleher KJ: Ethnic and regional differences in primary care visits for attention-deficit hyperactivity disorder. J Dev Behav Pediatr 25:318–325, 2004

Strickland TL, Ranganath V, Lin KM, et al: Psychopharmacologic considerations in the treatment of black American populations. Psychopharmacol Bull 27:441–448, 1991

U.S. Department of Health and Human Services: Mental Health: Culture, Race and Ethnicity. A Supplement to Mental Health: A Report of the Surgeon General. Rockville, MD, Substance Abuse and Mental Health Services Administration, 2001

Wishnie HA: Working in the Countertransference: Necessary Entanglements. New York, Jason Aronson, 2005

C H A P T E R 5

TREATING ADULT ADHD WITH MEDICATION

Introduction

MANY STUDIES HAVE SHOWN THAT the most effective treatment for children who have ADHD includes medication. Although there are fewer data for adults, they point to the same conclusion. Many adults dislike taking medication, especially indefinitely. It is helpful to remind them that the long-term effects of untreated ADHD are much worse than the side effects of the medications.

MEDICATIONS THAT HELP ADULTS WITH ADHD

Clearly the central nervous system (CNS) stimulants that help ADHD children—methylphenidate and dextroamphetamine, in varied preparations—also improve symptoms in affected adults. One of the long-acting preparations of dextroamphetamine, Adderall XR, has a U.S. Food and Drug Administration (FDA) indication to treat ADHD in adults as well as children. Another stimulant, pemoline (Cylert), helps in theory but has been withdrawn from the market. Atomoxetine (Strattera) is the only nonstimulant medication that has FDA approval for treating ADHD in adults as well as in children. In addition, some antidepressants help: bupropion (Wellbutrin), tricyclic antidepressants, and monoamine oxidase inhibitors. As is true for other psychiatric disorders, clinicians often use medications to treat ADHD before the FDA gives them a formal indication. In such cases, it is prudent to discuss this situation fully with the patient so that he or she can provide informed consent. The number and variety of medications waiting for and earning FDA approval for the disorder will likely increase.

MEDICATIONS THAT DO *NOT* HELP ADULTS WITH ADHD

Many medications and substances have been tested and found unsatisfactory for ADHD. Often we do not have conclusive data for adults because most of the testing has been in children. *Ineffective* agents include lithium carbonate; amantadine; L-dopa; the amino acid precursors D,L-phenylalanine and L-tyrosine; and caffeine. Other *ineffective* approaches include anti-yeast medications, megavitamin therapy, and dietary manipulation such as amino acid restriction and simple sugar restriction (Spencer et al. 1996).

Many dietary supplements that are popular because they are "natural" have been ineffective when tested for use with ADHD. Among these *ineffective* substances are acetyl-L-carnitine, ginkgo biloba, dimethylaminoethanol, phosphatidylserine (a CNS phospholipid), and essential fatty acids such as gamma-linolenic acid and decosahexanoic acid (Greydanus et al. 2003). Because of their unreliable purity, potential side effects, and lack of efficacy, herbal products such as ephedra have major drawbacks (Greydanus and Patel 2002).

Numerous alternative approaches exist. The following approaches lack controlled trial data to support their use in adult ADHD: essential fatty acid supplementation, glyconutritional supplementation, vitamin supplementation, homeopathic remedies, acupuncture, electroencephalographic biofeedback, vestibular stimulation, and immune therapies (Arnold 1999).

CURRENT STATUS AND FUTURE DIRECTIONS

Although the news about medications for ADHD is good, it is not reason for clinicians to be complacent. As will be seen, the CNS stimulants are often effective, but in their multiple preparations they remain essentially two medications. The new preparations provide a smoother delivery and a longer ride, but they are all methylphenidate or amphetamine. Although atomoxetine has proven useful, it does not rival the efficacy of the stimulants. For patients who do not respond to those medications, or who have comorbidities that preclude using them, we need new medications with new mechanisms of action. Perhaps our developing understanding of the biology of the disorder will make that progress possible (Martin 2005).

PREPARING TO USE MEDICATION

Before prescribing any medication, the clinician needs to know the patient's past treatment history, current and past psychiatric status, and general medical status (see Chapter 2, "Diagnosing ADHD in Adults"). With patients who have significant medical illness or complex existing medication regimens, close collaboration with the primary care physician or another medical specialist may be necessary.

MEDICATION: FIVE PHASES

Just as with other psychiatric patients, there are five phases in working with adult ADHD patients about their medication. These phases are discussed in detail below:

1. *Diagnosis and assessment:* Providing practical information, putting the medication in context as part of full treatment, and desensitizing the patient to taking it
2. *Active treatment:* Helping the patient reach an effective dosage
3. *Maintenance:* Keeping the patient on the medication to achieve the optimal results
4. *Reactivating treatment:* Taking action if the patient regresses or runs into fresh problems
5. *Discontinuation:* Planning how and when the patient will stop taking medication, if that is called for

Phase I: Diagnosis and Assessment

A patient undergoing assessment needs accurate, timely information about the disorder and its treatment. He or she needs a context for medication as part of a larger plan. Help the patient to know how the medicine works, its onset, and its duration. Alert the patient to side effects and what can ease them. Inform the patient how long he or she will be taking the medication and what, if any, are the consequences of long-term use. Provide information about abuse and dependence. Many patients have concerns about these issues, especially when taking the CNS stimulants. In addition to verbal information, patients appreciate written handouts and directions to appropriate Web sites (see Appendix). Many adults with ADHD do little reading, so recommending entire books to them may be unrealistic. Focusing reading recommendations on the patient's specific interests may be more useful.

Delivering factual information is one task of the initial phase of treatment. Another is dealing with patients' feelings about the disorder and the medication for it. In patients with ADHD, such feelings require exploration and discussion. Patients may be struggling with shame about not achieving and with embarrassment about being considered an "airhead" or worse. They may think that they should have outgrown their symptoms. Taking medicine may seem like evidence of failure or defeat.

Patients have particularly strong feelings about some of the ADHD medications, especially the CNS stimulants. People may have such negative opinions about these agents that they may not even be able to try one. Family members may have marked reactions to the diagnosis and its consequences and about every aspect of treatment, including medication. Clinicians have to know about these feelings and deal with them effectively.

The patient looking at the world through the gray-to-black lens of depression is not seeing well or clearly. Regardless of how accurate the facts are about medication, or how cogently they are presented, they may not penetrate the armor of the depressed person. Until the patient is less depressed, he or she may not be able to take a milligram of any medication for ADHD.

Phase II: Active Treatment

When treating ADHD patients with medication, start at a low dosage. Even small amounts of medication may help—and also minimize side effects. Gradually increase the dosage, noting the effect of each increase. When a further increase produces no more improvement, go back to the prior dosage—this is the best one. At each dosage level, weigh the benefits of the medication versus its side effects. Is the patient better off with the medication than without it?

This phase of treatment requires close contact with patients. They should call with an update within a week if all is going well and earlier if they have concerns or side effects. Initial meetings are at 2-week intervals, with longer intervals once the regimen stabilizes.

When the treatment response is best, changes seem natural, not willed. Patients accomplish more with less effort. They wonder how they wasted so much time, with so much angst, before they took medication. One man summarized his new experience of taking a CNS stimulant for ADHD:

> The major aspect is working methodically through tasks without getting frustrated and stressed. I am not working at such a high octane (weird, as they are amphetamines!). I am setting myself reminders for everything naturally. Whereas I had expected to consciously change my habits and utilize the newfound concentration, it seems to have naturally made me change my habits. Early days yet, but a great stride forward. I had one of the most productive working weeks I have ever had.

Patients also need to know what the medicine will *not* do.

One woman said, "I can access my resources when I want to now. Once I start a task I do it better, but I still have to tell my brain what to do."

"This is better," said one man, "but this is not a transformation."

Not everyone responds to medications; perhaps 60% of adult ADHD patients do better with a CNS stimulant, for example. People often have unrealistic expectations.

Phase III: Maintenance

Maintenance is usually the easiest phase of medication usage. In this phase, the patient continues to use the medication as prescribed, with periodic checkups. Maintenance assumes that the patient is doing stably well. Such patients check in every 3 months. Patients need regular follow-up meetings, regardless of which medication they are taking. These follow-ups may be even more important in patients with ADHD, because steady performance and reliability are issues. These meetings are a good time to discuss response to medication, review new options or alternatives to the patient's medicine, check progress on rating scales, and inquire about life satisfaction (Croft 2005).

With any of the agents used for ADHD in adults, there is a chance over time that the medicine will lose its impact. The simplest remedy is to increase dosage and see if clinical efficacy returns. If not, alternate medications may renew effectiveness. This loss of efficacy happens to few adult ADHD patients.

In the past, for patients doing stably well, clinicians could provide prescriptions for 3 months at one time, each marked with a notation, "Do not fill before (X) date." The FDA no longer allows this practice.

Of course, patients taking medications other than the stimulants need only one prescription with refills. Some have insurance coverage that provides them with a 90-day supply, with refills for up to 1 year. A few lucky patients can get a 90-day supply of a CNS stimulant, usually with a mail-in program. Frequent refills and need for replacement of "lost" prescriptions are red flags. Certainly, there is a risk of diversion and misuse, but ADHD patients frequently misplace and lose things, including their medication and their prescriptions.

Phase IV: Reactivating Treatment

How a patient does will determine whether treatment needs to be reconsidered or reactivated. Some patients may be able to stay in maintenance indefinitely. Others, with changed life circumstances and greater pressures, may need their medication regimen changed.

Phase V: Discontinuation

Patients often press for guidelines about stopping their medication. When, if ever, to discontinue medication for ADHD is a matter of debate. Most clinicians expect that patients will need it indefinitely. There is no accepted protocol for discontinuation.

Patients using only a CNS stimulant may find that they use less of the medication or use it irregularly or ad hoc. If they function well without the medicine, fine. Spouses and significant others, however, often notice if patients stop using the medication and ask them to resume it. Most patients who use stimulants within accepted dosage schedules do not have adverse effects when they stop taking them.

The nonstimulant medications provide other challenges. There is little information about discontinuation syndromes in patients stopping either atomoxetine (Strattera) or bupropion (Wellbutrin). As always, prudent clinicians have patients downshift the dosage over a few weeks rather than stop it suddenly.

SUMMARY

- Medication is essential to the most effective treatment for ADHD in adults. CNS stimulants and atomoxetine (Strattera) clearly help, as may antidepressant agents such as bupropion (Wellbutrin), tricyclic antidepressants, and monoamine oxidase inhibitors. No evidence supports the use of other types of medications, "natural" supplements, or dietary restrictions.
- Check the patient's current and past psychiatric and general medical history and treatment. Monitor vital signs.
- During the initial evaluation, and in ongoing treatment, psychoeducation is essential. Provide the patient with factual information about the medication: efficacy, side effects, long-term consequences of use, and issues of dependency and abuse. Explore the patient's feelings about taking medication.
- In the active phase of treatment, titrate medication and monitor for side effects until the optimal dosage is found. Maintain the patient's medication with periodic assessments. Reactivate treatment, including changing the patient's medication needs, if his or her life circumstances change or he or she loses momentum, or both. Discontinue medication with care.

REFERENCES

Arnold LE: Treatment alternatives for attention deficit hyperactivity disorder. J Atten Disord 3:30–48, 1999

Croft HA: Physician handling of prescription stimulants. Psychiatr Ann 35:221–226, 2005

Greydanus DE, Patel DR: Sports doping in the adolescent athlete: the hope, hype, and hyperbole. Pediatr Clin North Am 49:829–855, 2002

Greydanus DE, Pratt HD, Sloane MA, et al: ADD/ADHD: interventions for a complex behavioral disorder. Pediatr Clin North Am 48:622–626, 2003

Martin A: The hard work of growing up with ADHD. Am J Psychiatry 162: 1575–1577, 2005

Spencer T, Biederman J, Wilens T, et al: Pharmacotherapy of attention-deficit hyperactivity disorder across the life cycle. J Am Acad Child Adolesc Psychiatry 35:409–432, 1996

CHAPTER 6

TREATING ADHD WITH CENTRAL NERVOUS SYSTEM STIMULANTS

CENTRAL NERVOUS SYSTEM (CNS) stimulants are medications that structurally resemble the naturally occurring catecholamines dopamine and norepinephrine. Preparations of methylphenidate (Ritalin) and of amphetamine commonly help adults with ADHD. Amphetamine is available clinically in the form of dextroamphetamine (Dexedrine) and in the racemic mixture of the two isomers dextroamphetamine and levoamphetamine (Adderall, Adderall XR).

More than 200 controlled studies document the effectiveness of Ritalin and Dexedrine for ADHD in children. CNS stimulants have been the drugs of choice for the disorder since the earliest reports (Bradley 1937). Much of the support for that practice derives from short studies of latency-age white boys. Now some studies use the stimulants in other age groups, in girls and women, and in minorities. Longer-term studies are under way (Spencer et al. 2004).

The CNS stimulants are now the leading medications used for adults with ADHD. However, there is less of a clinical research base for their use in adults. They may be less effective in adults than they are in children.

THE MULTIMODAL TREATMENT STUDY

Many studies have shown how useful the CNS stimulants are for children with ADHD. The Multimodal Treatment Study of Children With Attention Deficit Hyperactivity Disorder (MTA) was a landmark study (MTA Cooperative Group 1999). This multisite study, funded by the

National Institute of Mental Health, assessed children, ages 7–9.9 years, with the diagnosis of ADHD, mixed type. The project evaluated the impact of different treatment modalities alone and in combination. There were four study arms: medication management, psychosocial and behavior therapy, combined therapy (medication management and psychosocial and behavior therapy), and community care. Researchers randomly assigned 579 children to the treatment groups and followed them clinically for 14 months.

Study children on medication management received full attention. In sequence, the researchers used CNS stimulants: methylphenidate (three times daily), dextroamphetamine, pemoline, and the tricyclic antidepressant imipramine. As well as providing monthly office visits and dosing medicine based on the child's weight, the staff fine-tuned the medication with input from parents and teachers. As a result, each child had the best dosage of the medication for him or her. The families in this group also had readings and advice. The American Academy of Child and Adolescent Psychiatry now recommends this thoughtful approach in its guidelines for ADHD (Greenhill et al. 2002).

In the psychosocial and behavior therapy arm, parents received training in behavioral approaches to ADHD. The child had 8 individual therapy sessions, the family had 27 group therapy sessions, and there were 10–16 teacher consultations. Finally, the child was in a therapeutic summer camp program for 8 weeks.

Each child in the combination arm of the study received all the medication management and the psychosocial and behavioral treatments. Families of children in the community care arm had no active treatment but received a copy of the clinical evaluation that made the ADHD diagnosis and a list of local treatment resources. They could seek active treatment, including medication from local pediatricians or child psychiatrists, but such treatment was outside the boundaries of the study.

At the end of the study, children in all four arms had improved. However, study children taking medication, either alone or with psychotherapy, did significantly better than those who had only psychotherapy. In terms of improved ADHD, children having medication and psychotherapy did no better than those on medication alone. However, the children with combined treatment may have improved more in their non-ADHD symptoms and general function. Of the study medications, stimulants were preferred. By the end of the study, 85.2% of the 289 children in the medication-only and combination therapy groups were taking them (MTA Cooperative Group 1999).

The MTA study results combat claims that physicians overprescribe the CNS stimulants. Of the children in the community care arm, although all were diagnosed with ADHD, only two-thirds later got stimulant medication from a local physician. At the study's end, these children were taking less stimulant (mean daily dosage=22.6 mg) than the children in the medication-only group (mean=37.7 mg) and in the combination therapy group (mean=31.2 mg). Children in community care lacked sustained, close attention, which probably contributed to their poorer outcome. Community pediatricians stopped increasing dosage as soon as the child responded to medication, rather than titrating it to the optimal amount. A separate survey of four American communities documented *underprescription* of stimulants for ADHD in children (Jensen et al. 1999).

In the MTA study, all the children did better, regardless of the treatment provided. Participants in clinical trials usually improve because of the attention from study staff. However, children in the medication-only or the combination therapy group did better, on virtually all measures, than the youngsters who did not take medication, either in the psychological therapy group or the community care group. Intensive psychological treatment alone had no better treatment results than community care that did not include medicine.

The stimulants continue to be the agents of first choice in children with ADHD (Conners et al. 2001). As well as improving schoolwork and behavior, they help improve social deficits. In one study, ADHD adolescents who took CNS stimulants and had psychosocial treatment had better social relationships as well as other improvements (Smith et al. 1998). Follow-up clinical research studies in children show that the short-acting stimulants continue to have beneficial effects for 2–5 years (Charach et al. 2004). In standard clinical practice, they are often helpful for decades.

CENTRAL NERVOUS SYSTEM STIMULANTS HELP ADULTS WITH ADHD

Although there are few standardized clinical trials, the CNS stimulants have been used for 30 years to treat adults (Wood et al. 1976). Only six controlled studies have examined the efficacy of methylphenidate in adults with ADHD (Iaboni et al. 1996; Spencer et al. 2004). There are only three controlled studies of amphetamines in adults (Paterson et al. 1999). In all the studies, the adults tolerated the medications well.

The stimulants help adults, but the results are less impressive than in children. With care, perhaps 90% of children properly diagnosed with ADHD respond to a stimulant without a major adverse event (Goldman et al. 1998). *Response* in studies is a clinically or statistically significant reduction in hyperactivity or improvement in attention. The studies use behavioral ratings of parents, teachers, or researchers. While the standard measure of improvement has been better school grades, the benefits of the stimulants may be even more on behavior and cognition. This latter benefit is critically important for adults with ADHD (Swanson et al. 1993).

In contrast, the response rate to stimulants for adults with ADHD is 60%–70%. About 30% show significant improvement, 40% show some improvement, and 10%–30% do not respond (Greenhill et al. 2002). In early studies, adults seemed to respond poorly to the stimulants, perhaps because of low dosage (up to 0.6 mg/kg of methylphenidate or its equivalent for amphetamine). Assessment methodologies and criteria for improvement differed between early studies.

When clinicians in later studies raised the dosages, results improved. In a 7-week study of 23 adults with ADHD, researchers titrated participants up to dosages of 1.0 mg/kg/day of methylphenidate. In this crossover study, 78% of the patients taking methylphenidate had a robust improvement in symptoms, whereas only 4% of patients on placebo did. At the study's end, the typical daily dosage of methylphenidate was 0.92 mg/kg/day. Patients taking methylphenidate had significantly fewer symptoms across all domains. The beneficial effects were independent of gender, psychiatric comorbidity with anxiety or moderate depression, or a family history of psychiatric disorders (Spencer et al. 1995).

The results of a larger study support these data. This study involved 103 patients in a 6-week randomized, double-blind, placebo-controlled trial of methylphenidate. Participants who took methylphenidate had an average daily dosage of 82 mg. Those on active medication reduced their symptoms by 43% on the ADHD rating scale. Significant improvement occurred in 73% of participants taking methylphenidate versus 23% of those taking placebo (Spencer et al. 2002). A recent follow-up study had the same outcome: 76% of participants taking an average dosage of 82 mg (1.1 mg/kg/day) of methylphenidate had significant overall response versus a 19% response rate in those taking placebo. Patients taking active medication reported much-improved life satisfaction after extended treatment, but not in the first 6 weeks (Spencer et al. 2005).

Studies involving the use of amphetamine for adults with ADHD show similar results. In a study parallel to the 1995 methylphenidate study for adult ADHD, Spencer and colleagues did a controlled trial using a mixed amphetamine salts compound (Adderall: dextro- and levo-amphetamine sulfate, dextro- and levoamphetamine aspartate, and dextroamphetamine saccharate). In the 7-week randomized, double-blind, placebo-controlled crossover study, participants were titrated up to 30 mg of Adderall twice daily. Treatment at an average dosage of 54 mg/day was highly effective. Patients taking active medication lowered their symptoms by 42% on the ADHD symptom rating scale. Significant improvement occurred in 70% of participants taking Adderall, versus only 7% taking placebo (Spencer et al. 2001).

Preliminary results from a controlled, multisite trial of an extended-release form of a mixed amphetamine salts compound (Adderall XR) are also encouraging. This randomized, double-blind, forced-titration study evaluated 255 adults with ADHD. It assessed the efficacy and safety of Adderall XR at 20, 40, or 60 mg once daily compared with placebo. At all dosages, over the 6 weeks of the study, Adderall XR significantly improved symptoms more than placebo (Weisler et al. 2003).

One study of the long-acting stimulant magnesium pemoline (Cylert) in adults with ADHD showed that it was moderately effective. In 2005, however, the U.S. Food and Drug Administration (FDA) recommended that pemoline be withdrawn from the market, because it can cause serious and sometimes deadly liver damage. Clinicians should contact patients taking pemoline promptly to discuss switching to another treatment. The FDA Web site provides more information: http://www.fda.gov/cder/drug/InfoSheets/HCP/pemolineHCP.htm.

The stimulants significantly reduce ADHD symptoms in adults but rarely eliminate them completely. In reviewed studies, less than 10% of patients responded to placebo (Wilens et al. 1995). Patients may respond to the medication within the first 24 hours. Adults with ADHD typically tolerate the medications well and find them effective for months to years. Adults naturally need larger dosages than children do. Although some adults respond to low dosages, higher dosages generally produce better response rates (Elia et al. 1999; Wilens 2003).

Methylphenidate and amphetamine are chemically similar, but perhaps 25% of adults will respond to one and not the other. Generally, patients should try a representative of both the methylphenidate and the amphetamine groups before taking one of the non-CNS stimulants (Greenhill et al. 2002).

HOW DO THE CENTRAL NERVOUS SYSTEM STIMULANTS WORK?

In the brain, information travels along a neuron by an electrical impulse. When the impulse hits the cell membrane, chemical neurotransmitters move into the gap between neurons, the synapse. The released neurotransmitters strike the cell membrane of the postsynaptic neuron, start-

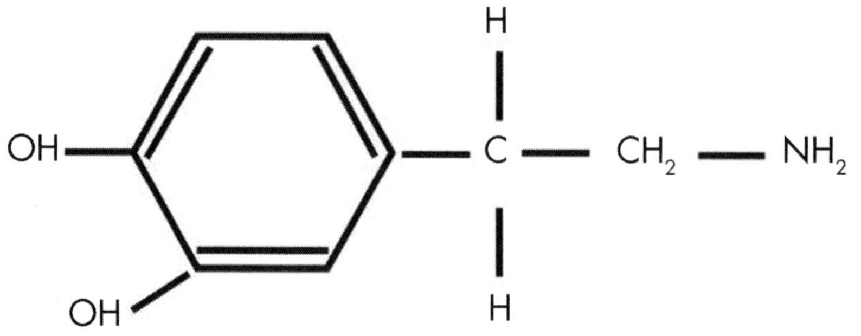

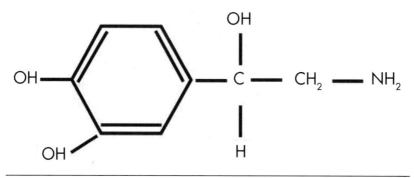

FIGURE 6–1.   Chemical structure of dopamine.

FIGURE 6–2.   Chemical structure of norepinephrine.

ing another electrical impulse. Thus information flows electrically through the neurons, while the neurotransmitters form chemical bridges between them. Of many neurotransmitters, the most important clinically are serotonin, norepinephrine, and dopamine. Methylphenidate and amphetamine structurally resemble dopamine and norepinephrine (Figures 6–1, 6–2, 6–3, and 6–4).

Once in the synapse, the neurotransmitter can strike the membrane of the next neuron, it can degrade biologically, or it can return to the presynaptic neuron by a reuptake process. Transporters called *autoreceptors* run this reuptake process, moving dopamine and other neurotransmitters back into the originating neuron. Anything interfering with reuptake keeps neurotransmitters such as dopamine in the synapse, strengthening the chemical bridge between neurons.

Although the CNS stimulants help patients with ADHD, their exact mechanism of action is still unclear. There are three possible routes. First,

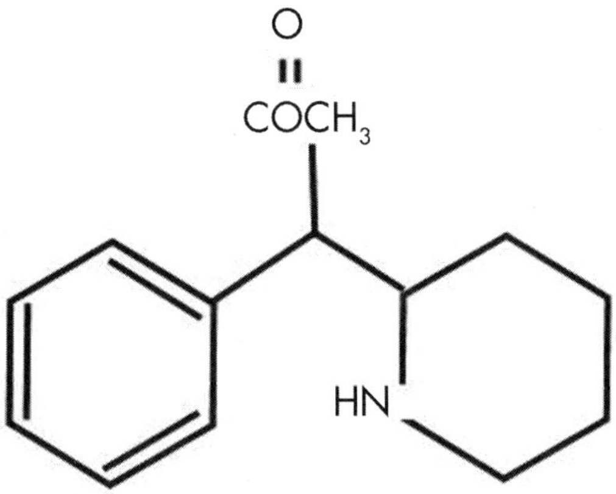

FIGURE 6–3. Chemical structure of methylphenidate.

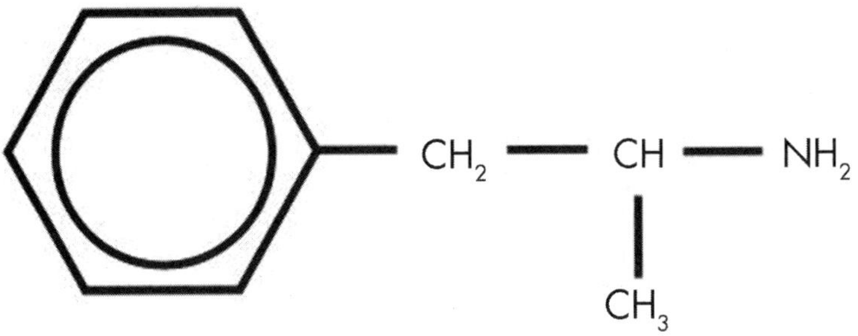

FIGURE 6–4. Chemical structure of amphetamine.

they increase brain levels of dopamine, norepinephrine, and serotonin by blocking their reuptake into the presynaptic neuron. Second, stimulants increase the release of transmitters into the synaptic cleft. Third, they inhibit the breakdown of the neurotransmitters by monoamine oxidase (Solanto 1998).

The stimulants impact both dopaminergic and noradrenergic cortical synapses to improve brain function in ADHD. They are indirect agonists. Rather than stimulating catecholamine receptors directly, they reinhibit the reuptake of the neurotransmitters (Wilens 2006). They alter the activity of dopaminergic systems in the deeper brain structures, the nigrostriatum and mesocortex. They also affect noradrenergic projections from the locus coeruleus to the cortex. Preclinical studies suggest that the dopaminergic activity of the stimulants improves motor activity and reinforcement processes. Their noradrenergic action improves response time and working memory. Persons without ADHD who try a CNS stimulant notice improvement in these areas, but they can perform stably and well without the medicine. The stimulants help the person with ADHD compensate for what he or she does poorly. They do not target a specific neurological lesion (Solanto 1998). Agents that profoundly influence brain serotonin, such as the selective serotonin reuptake inhibitor antidepressants, are not clinically useful in ADHD (Prince and Wilens 2002).

The two sections that follow contain information about the CNS stimulants, methylphenidate and amphetamine. Each section begins with a discussion of how the specific stimulant works and ends with specific information on the commercially available preparations, in alphabetical order. See Table 6–1 for a practical summary of CNS stimulant dosing in the treatment of adult ADHD.

METHYLPHENIDATE STIMULANTS

Methylphenidate impacts two processes that set the level and variation of brain dopamine. Tonic dopamine cell firing maintains the baseline, steady-state extrasynaptic dopamine level. This level sets the overall responsiveness of the dopaminergic system. Phasic dopamine cell firing causes fast dopamine changes that highlight the salience of stimuli. *Salience* means that a stimulus is meaningful, worth attending to.

Methylphenidate induces slow, steady-state increases in dopamine that mimic those produced by tonic firing. By blocking dopamine transporters, methylphenidate amplifies the neurotransmitter's signals overall. For persons who have ADHD, "everyday" stimuli do not generate dopamine responses that signal salience and thus compel interest and attention. At therapeutic dosages, methylphenidate amplifies the salience of mundane stimuli, making even ordinary tasks more interesting.

However, methylphenidate also induces fast dopamine increases, like those from phasic dopamine cell firing. Rapidly increasing methylphenidate, either orally or intravenously, overactivates the dopaminergic system. The drug experience itself becomes more salient, intensely desirable. Stimuli that are not drug related, such as the activities of everyday life, lose intensity and meaningfulness. The stage is set for abuse (Volkow and Swanson 2003).

Methylphenidate binds fairly selectively to the transporter for dopamine, keeping neurotransmitter in the synapse. It increases extracellular dopamine concentrations (Volkow et al. 2001). Dopaminergic neurons cluster thickly in brain sites that control focus and attention.

TABLE 6–1. Central nervous system stimulant dosing for ADHD

Medication name	Form	Starting dose (mg)	Maximum dose (mg/kg/day)	Usual dosing pattern	Duration (hours)
Methylphenidate preparations					
Concerta	tablets	18	2	qd	8–12
Focalin	tablets	2.5–5	1	bid	5–6
Focalin XR	capsules	5	1	qd	8–10
Metadate CD	capsules	20	2	qd	8–10
Ritalin hydrochloride	tablets	5–10	2	bid/tid	4
Ritalin LA	capsules	20	2	qd	8–10
Amphetamine preparations					
Adderall	tablets	5	1.5	bid	5–6
Adderall XR	capsules	5–10	1.5	qd	8–12
Dexedrine	tablets	5	1.5	bid/tid	4
Dexedrine Spansules	capsules	5	1.5	qd	8–12
DextroStat	tablets	5	1.5	bid/tid	4–6

Source. Adapted from information in the *Physician's Desk Reference*, 60th Edition. Montvale, NJ, Thomson Health Care, 2006.

They also stimulate reward circuits when we enjoy ourselves. When, for example, we learn, eat, or make love, dopaminergic neurons release molecules that strike receptors in reward circuit neurons. When the reward signal is just right, we respond, "I like that. Pay attention!" Too much signal, and we feel unpleasantly overstimulated. This response happens when people without ADHD take Ritalin: they feel as though they have had too much caffeinated coffee. Alternatively, too little reward signal, and the experience has little impact or may even be boring.

Cocaine acts intensely in this pleasure system. It blocks about half the dopamine transporters, lessening reuptake. Dopamine rapidly builds up in the pleasure circuit synapses. It registers as "This feels great—got to do this again!"

To the surprise of researchers, methylphenidate blocks 70% of dopamine transporters, even more than cocaine does (Volkow et al. 2001). So why is Ritalin not more addictive? Some researchers think that the ADHD brain has more dopamine transporters. These quickly move dopamine back into the transmitting neuron before it impacts receptors in the reward circuit (Dougherty et al. 1999). Other researchers disagree; the question is unsettled (Van Dyck et al. 2002).

The difference between cocaine and methylphenidate may relate to how fast each is cleared from the brain. When healthy volunteers take methylphenidate or cocaine, both drugs impact the corpus striatum. Both peak at about the same time: 4–8 minutes for methylphenidate, 2–8 minutes for sniffed cocaine. After both drugs, the feelings of pleasure are most intense after 5 minutes and subside in 30–40 minutes. However, methylphenidate maintains its peak brain concentration for 15–20 minutes and cocaine for only 2–4 minutes. Methylphenidate lingers longer, with 50% still present after 90 minutes. In contrast, 50% of the cocaine clears in only 20 minutes (Volkow et al. 1995). Feelings of intense pleasure occur as the concentration of dopamine in the corpus striatum rises. Once it levels, the brain begins to adapt. Cocaine clears so rapidly that the brain cannot adapt; it is ready for another "hit." Methylphenidate, lingering in the striatum, blocks the sensation of pleasure from a new dose.

Oral methylphenidate raises CNS dopamine levels in 1 hour. Inhaled or injected cocaine does that in seconds; the intense, speedy hit is essential to the addictive process. Few people feel high when they take methylphenidate by mouth. Inhaling or injecting it, however, can cause a high. By those routes, it has abuse potential (Vastag 2001).

If persons with ADHD have more brain dopamine transporters, they have less neurotransmitter available to hit key reward circuits. Activities like learning, which delights some people, may produce fewer rewards in ADHD adults. If their attention circuits are understimulated, they have poor motivation and low productivity.

There is another important difference in the ADHD brain: more neurons fire at random than in the normal brain. This higher "background firing rate" produces more brain static and fewer focused signals. Stimuli bombard patients from both inside and outside their head, interfering with concentration.

Methylphenidate reverses both trends. In the synapses, it blocks dopamine transporters, preventing reuptake. More extracellular brain dopamine strengthens signals in the attention and reward circuits. Methylphenidate may lessen background firing rates by cutting "static" and background noise; it makes task-related neurons function better (Kiyatkin and Rebec 1996).

When a person sees a stimulus as meaningful, dopamine cells fire, releasing more transmitter (Hollerman and Schultz 1998). Dopamine affects salience and motivation by amplifying brain signals that information is meaningful. When that happens, we learn better (Berridge and Robinson 1998). People respond better to methylphenidate when they are doing what interests them. Then, the medication amplifies the impact of available dopamine. Thus the response to methylphenidate is not relative. Performance depends on a task's context.

Researchers used positron emission tomography (PET) scans to see how a large oral dose (60 mg) of methylphenidate affected extracellular brain dopamine in healthy volunteers. Methylphenidate significantly blocked dopamine transporters in all participants, but it increased extracellular dopamine in only some (Volkow et al. 2002). How can one explain this? Methylphenidate blocks dopamine transporters, and it also affects dopamine cell firing. This action might explain why not all the persons studied showed increased extracellular brain dopamine. Perhaps only some participants felt that the study task was meaningful (Wightman and Robinson 2002).

These researchers did another experiment to see how methylphenidate impacts salience. They gave some adult volunteers 20 mg of oral methylphenidate and others placebo. They used PET scans with [^{11}C] raclopride, a D_2 dopamine receptor radioligand that competes with endogenous dopamine for binding. Then they looked at what happened to extracellular dopamine in the brain of healthy adults doing a salient task compared with the results when the volunteers did a neutral task.

The salient task required participants to solve mathematical problems, earning money for each correct answer. As expected, participants taking methylphenidate showed increased extracellular brain dopamine while they were doing the salient task. Subjects taking placebo did not. In addition, the researchers assessed participants' subjective interest in the salient task. Those who took methylphenidate reported more interest in the math task, and more motivation to do it, than those who took placebo. Increased dopamine went along with higher subjective interest in the salient task.

Then researchers looked at methylphenidate and extracellular dopamine when participants did a neutral task. This time the subjects just viewed cards, without remuneration. Volunteers taking methylphenidate did not show increased extracellular dopamine when they did the neutral task. It was less meaningful, less salient. The researchers concluded that methylphenidate enhances the salience of a stimulus by increasing dopamine. Methylphenidate may enhance the increase of dopamine already induced by the stimuli themselves, making the stimuli yet more salient and improving performance (Wightman and Robinson 2002).

In the treatment of ADHD, how methylphenidate enhances motivation may be even more important than how it affects performance. Enhanced motivation may explain why stimulants improve performance in normal individuals. It also suggests why unmedicated children with ADHD perform satisfactorily when they regard a task as salient (Grinspoon and Hedblom 1975). The study supports using methylphenidate to treat persons with ADHD. It also validates the truism that people learn better when tasks are meaningful. Any strategies that make schoolwork more interesting improve learning, whether or not a person has ADHD (Volkow et al. 2004).

Methylphenidate exists as four optical isomers, but it is available in commercial preparations as a 50:50 mixture of D-*threo* and L-*threo* enantiomers. The L-*threo* enantiomer is quickly metabolized in the gastrointestinal tract and liver. Food enhances absorption. The D-*threo* enantiomer travels to the brain, where it is concentrated in the corpus striatum and metabolized by esterases into ritalinic acid over 2–4 hours (Cho and Segal 1994). Because only one isomer reaches the brain, methylphenidate is only half as potent as amphetamine (Greenhill et al. 1996). Because of its kinetics, methylphenidate not only has a fast effect, but it can also have rebound symptoms when it wears off: an unpleasant mix of sadness, irritation, and lethargy. Using a small dose of immediate-release methylphenidate late in the day may reduce rebound. There are few drug–drug interactions with methylphenidate, except with the monoamine oxidase inhibitor (MAOI) antidepressants.

Concerta

Each tablet of Concerta (osmotic-release oral system methylphenidate) has an outer coat that contains 22% of the medication and two inner compartments that contain the remaining 78%. Once the patient ingests the tablet, the outer coat dissolves, and the first impact of the medicine is felt within 1 hour. The tablet absorbs fluid from the gut through its semipermeable membrane. As the membrane expands, the medicine is extruded through a tiny hole at the end of the tablet. The increasing concentration of medication in the bloodstream that results gives the best effect (Swanson et al. 2003). The person feels the impact for 10–12 hours, having the effect of three consecutive doses of methylphenidate. Concerta has the longest duration of action of extended-release preparations. The structure of the tablet is virtually tamper proof, minimizing abuse (Jaffe 2002).

Concerta may deliver its first dose less effectively than other long-acting formulations of methylphenidate (Gonzales et al. 2002; Lopez et al. 2003a). To allow for this, some clinicians suggest that patients take a dose of immediate-release methylphenidate with their morning Concerta. On the other hand, Concerta provides the best coverage of ADHD symptoms through the afternoon. This preparation is now approved for use by adolescents at a dosage of up to 72 mg/day (McBurnett 2003).

Concerta has advantages beyond a convenient dosage schedule. For some purposes, such as driving an automobile, it may work better than immediate-release methylphenidate. Concerta's sustained efficacy may improve the driving skills of adolescents and young adults with ADHD, who are notoriously poor behind the wheel. A recent study of ADHD teenagers taking Ritalin or Concerta compared their behavior while they used a driving simulator. Study adolescents who took Ritalin were more likely to brake inappropriately on the open road, run through stop signals, or drive with more erratic speed control. They were more likely to drive off the road or across the midline or to have more collisions. The researchers also asked the teenagers to record their actual driving behavior in daily diaries. Those taking Ritalin took more risks. They complained that their driving skills dropped sharply at 8 P.M., when their last dose of medicine wore off. In contrast, the ADHD teenagers taking Concerta drove from 8 P.M. to midnight as well as did a low-risk group of men ages 55–59 years (Cox et al. 2004).

In a yearlong controlled clinical trial, 6.9% of participants taking Concerta discontinued it because of adverse effects, including tics, appetite suppression, insomnia, and hostility. Other side effects included abdominal pain, headache, and emotional lability (Wilens and Pelham 2003). If the patient takes it too late in the day, he or she may not be able to get to sleep. Generally, however, patients tolerate it well, with no adverse affect on growth or on vital signs.

Focalin and Focalin XR

Conventional commercial preparations of methylphenidate contain two mirror images, naturally occurring forms: a right-handed, or "D," enantiomer, and a left-handed, "L" form. The D-enantiomer is the biologically active form. Now marketed as Focalin (dexmethylphenidate), its dosage is half that of conventional Ritalin. It has demonstrated efficacy in children (Srinivas et al. 1992). Some clinical researchers suggest that Focalin may have a longer duration of action than conventional methylphenidate (Keating and Figgitt 2002). Others suspect it may be more beneficial than conventional Ritalin, with fewer side effects, but that argument is not settled. Focalin is now available in an extended-release preparation as Focalin XR, which allows for less frequent dosing (Wilens 2005). In this formulation, it has approval from the FDA for the treatment of ADHD in adults.

Metadate CD and Metadate ER

Metadate is available as controlled-delivery capsules (Metadate CD) and extended-release tablets (Metadate ER). The CD capsules, in 10-, 20-, and 30-mg strengths, provide active methylphenidate for up to 8 or 9 hours. Each capsule contains immediate- and delayed-release beads. In the Metadate CD capsule, 30% of the methylphenidate is available immediately, and the rest is released over 6–10 hours. Patients having trouble taking medicine as a pill or intact capsule can break the Metadate capsule and sprinkle it over food (Swanson et al. 2004).

In one study of healthy adults, in the first 6 hours after administration of medication, those taking Metadate CD had higher plasma methylphenidate than those taking equivalent Concerta (Gonzalez et al. 2002). The second pulse of methylphenidate may have reduced bioavailability and therefore reduced efficacy.

Metadate ER is available in 10- and 20-mg tablets. The tablets are well absorbed. The patient has to swallow the tablet whole; crushing or chewing the tablet destroys its extended-release property. This preparation is identical to Ritalin SR, which is discussed below.

On a once-a-day schedule, Metadate, Ritalin LA, or Concerta works well for patients with 8-hour workdays. That length of time may be too short for patients with longer workdays, but supplemental Ritalin can be used for extra coverage (Biederman et al. 2002).

MethyPatch

Methylphenidate now comes in a transdermal skin patch. In recent studies of children with ADHD, the patch significantly relieved symptoms when applied for 7–12 hours a day (Hoffman 2003). Removing the patch ends drug delivery, but the behavioral effects may persist for another hour or two. MethyPatch is available in three dosage forms for greater convenience. The dosage is the same as when using methylphenidate as Ritalin. In trials with children, there were few side effects. Data are not yet available about effectiveness in adults.

Ritalin Hydrochloride

Ritalin (methylphenidate), a mainstay in children with ADHD, helps affected adults as well (Spencer et al. 2005). For adults as for children, one dose of Ritalin lasts only 2–4 hours. Many adults consider that a big disadvantage. Fortunately, there are now long-acting versions of methylphenidate. The extended-release preparations are less subject to abuse than the immediate-release products (Wilens and Dodson 2004).

Ritalin LA

Ideally, a long-acting methylphenidate should provide the rapid impact of regular Ritalin. Of the forms available, Ritalin LA produces this result best. Each Ritalin LA capsule contains half immediate-release and half sustained-release beads of methylphenidate. Taking this medication is like having two doses of methylphenidate 4 hours apart. It provides particularly good coverage in the morning. Ritalin LA delivers the methylphenidate smoothly. Depending on the activity of brain esterases, effects lasts up to 10 hours, typically 8 or 9 hours. Capsules of Ritalin LA come in 10-, 20-, 30-, and 40-mg doses. Having several available dosages allows patients and clinicians to fine-tune the amount and timing of the medication (Spencer et al. 2000).

Ritalin LA holds up well in comparisons with Concerta. In one study, children with ADHD took equivalent doses of Ritalin LA (20 mg) or Concerta (18 mg) or placebo. The behavior of youngsters taking placebo worsened steadily over 8 hours of observation. Children taking either form of the active medication improved. However, in the first 4 hours of the study period, the children taking the Ritalin LA paid more attention and behaved better than the children taking Concerta (Lopez et al. 2003a).

One study comparing Ritalin LA and Concerta in children may have implications for adults. After the first 4 hours, the children taking Ritalin

LA improved more on all three rating scale measures. They answered more mathematics problems correctly than did children taking Concerta (Lopez et al. 2003b). A study of Ritalin LA and Concerta in ADHD adults supported the findings in children. During the first 4 hours after administration, significantly more methylphenidate was released from Ritalin LA (20 mg) than from Concerta (18 mg) (Markowitz et al. 2003). Because Ritalin LA typically acts for less than 10 hours, patients taking it often need more than one dose for full-day coverage.

Ritalin SR

The sustained-release form of Ritalin was the first longer-acting preparation of methylphenidate commercially available. However, Ritalin SR has a slower onset of action than Ritalin and loses its clinical effect after about 5 hours (Pelham et al. 1987). The tablets lose their extended-release capacity if crushed, chewed, or divided. Few clinicians use Ritalin SR.

Which Preparation Should You Use?

Few studies compare formulations of methylphenidate, so clinicians try first one and then another. Among current preparations, Concerta and Ritalin LA offer the most. Patients can usually know rapidly what works best for them. Some may need to try the amphetamine stimulants and the other available medications as well.

The cost of medications always concerns patients, especially when taking medications needed for long-term use. Insurance companies want subscribers to take the cheapest generic medication. Some patients strongly prefer name-brand preparations. These have better quality control. Furthermore, the generics contain dyes and additives that some patients tolerate poorly.

AMPHETAMINE STIMULANTS

Amphetamine is the basis for the other group of CNS stimulants used for ADHD. The amphetamine molecule exists in nature in two mirror-image forms. Like methylphenidate, it binds dopamine transporters and prevents reuptake. Amphetamine also blocks dopamine storage in the vesicles of the presynaptic neuron, fostering release into the cytoplasm and into the synapse (Wilens and Spencer 2000). Enhanced dopamine action in the dorsal prefrontal cortex may improve attention, concentration, executive function, and wakefulness. Amphetamine's action in other brain regions, such as the basal ganglia, may improve hyperactivity. It also inhibits the synaptic reuptake of norepinephrine (Stahl 2004).

Unlike methylphenidate, amphetamine undergoes moderate metabolism by several mechanisms in the liver and is excreted in the urine. The total dosage of amphetamine and the urine acidity largely determine the duration of its action (Cho and Segal 1994). Both isomers of amphetamine are biologically active. Because it is twice as potent as methylphenidate, dextroamphetamine doses are half those of Ritalin (Ding et al. 1997). Like methylphenidate, dextroamphetamine is rapidly absorbed and begins affecting behavior within 30 minutes (Greenhill et al. 2002).

Dozens of studies show that dextroamphetamine is safe and effective to treat ADHD in children (Greenhill et al. 1999). Although few formal trials use it in adults with ADHD, the results are similar. One randomized, double-blind study of 68 adults with ADHD found that patients responded significantly better to dextroamphetamine than to placebo (Paterson et al. 1999).

Adderall

Adderall, a long-acting amphetamine product, contains equal milligram portions of neutral sulfate salts of dextroamphetamine and amphetamine with *d*-amphetamine saccharate and *d,l*-amphetamine aspartate. Adderall acts promptly, within half an hour, and its clinical impact lasts 5 or 6 hours.

Although as little as 5 mg of Adderall twice a day may help adults, the effective dosage range is wide. In a 16-week study of 24 adult outpatients with ADHD, participants started at 5 mg twice a day, which was titrated up to an optimal dose. Thirteen participants (54%) responded well, whereas nine (38%) were poor responders or nonresponders (Horrigan and Barnhill 2000).

In another controlled study of 47 adults with ADHD, participants took either placebo or mixed amphetamine salts (Adderall) at up to 30 mg twice a day for 7 weeks. Treatment with Adderall at a mean dose of 54 mg/day was very effective; 70% of patients taking the active medication improved "very significantly," whereas only 7% of participants taking placebo did (Spencer et al. 2001).

If a patient likes the effects of Adderall and tolerates it well, increase it systematically to find the best dosage. Patients do not necessarily take the same amount in the morning and in the afternoon. Adderall has the usual stimulant side effects. Anxious patients may feel more symptomatic. Sometimes "regular" Adderall is called Adderall IR (immediate release) to differentiate it from Adderall XR (extended release).

Warn patients that if the prescription is written for "Adderall," the pharmacy may substitute the generic "mixed amphetamine salts." More than one patient has worried that he or she has received the wrong medicine when that phrase is on the label.

Adderall XR

Adderall XR (extended release) has the FDA indication for treating ADHD in adults as well as children. The medication acts for 10–12 hours. The capsules are available in several dosages, from 5 mg to 30 mg. If needed, patients can open the capsule and sprinkle the medicine on food.

Each capsule has two types of Adderall-containing beads. The immediate-release beads have an active drug core and a protective coating that dissolves promptly after ingestion. The pH-sensitive polymer coat of the delayed-release beads dissolves in the higher pH (approximately 5.5) of the small intestine, about 4 hours after ingestion. The extended-release formulation delivers the medication smoothly over the day. Patients should not crush or chew capsules. Typically they take the medication once a day, in the morning, with or without food (Tulloch et al. 2002). Adderall XR is hard to abuse, but some people crush the capsules and then take the contents all at once or snort them (Rush 2003).

Adderall XR has proved its usefulness in children. One study compared placebo; 10 mg of immediate-release Adderall; and 10, 20, or 30 mg of Adderall XR. The higher the dosage of active medication, the greater the improvement (McGough et al. 2000). A large study of Adderall XR in 6- to 12-year-old children with ADHD supported these findings. In this study, a clear dose–response relationship was found in all measures of efficacy with 10, 20, and 30 mg daily doses of Adderall XR. Boys and girls taking Adderall XR improved significantly within the first week and more with each increase. The single morning dose produced improved behavior throughout the day. Changes in blood pressure and pulse were not clinically significant (Biederman et al. 2002).

A third study, the Long-Acting Adderall Community Assessment Trial, evaluated the effectiveness of Adderall XR for children with ADHD over 7 weeks at 378 sites nationwide (Ambrosini et al. 2000). The 2,968 children were between 6 and 12 years of age and already taking stable doses of Adderall IR or any methylphenidate formulation. Researchers evaluated how the children were doing on their prestudy regimen. They converted each daily dosage of the youngster's medication (e.g., 30 mg of Adderall IR or 54 mg of Concerta) into the equivalent dosage of Adderall XR (30 mg). Then they fine-tuned the dosage of Adderall XR depending on the child's response. By the end of the study, the children were functioning better overall and had a better quality of life. Parents and physicians alike preferred the results with Adderall XR to those of prior regimens, even though they had been satisfactory. Once-daily dosing clearly helped.

Another study of Adderall XR in childhood ADHD showed that it kept its effectiveness over 18 months. Children took up to 30 mg a day (Chandler et al. 2002).

Adderall XR is effective for adults with ADHD. In one study, adults with ADHD took 30 mg of Adderall XR daily. No difference was found in the rate and extent of its absorption, whether the person took it as an intact capsule after fasting overnight, after a high-fat breakfast, or sprinkled on soft food after fasting overnight (Tulloch et al. 2002).

Another study compared Adderall XR with placebo in 255 ADHD adults (mean age=39 years). The 191 participants given active medication took 20, 40, or 60 mg/day of Adderall XR, and 64 subjects were given placebo. Compared with patients taking placebo, patients taking any Adderall XR significantly improved. Measures 12 hours after taking the medication showed sustained improvement. Side effects were mild to moderate and tended to drop off after the first week (Weisler et al. 2003).

Adult ADHD patients in another study took Adderall XR titrated over 4 weeks to 60 mg/day. About two-thirds reported that their symptoms were much or very much improved (Wilens et al. 2003). Yet another study of adult ADHD patients given a forced titration of dosage of Adderall XR to 60 mg/day had the same results. Patients with mild ADHD responded well to dosages of 20 mg/day; those with severe ADHD needed up to 60 mg/day (Faraone et al. 2004). The results of these studies support using substantial dosages of stimulant medication with adults. Adults fare better with larger dosages. If pharmacists object to higher dosages of the CNS stimulants, we can remind them that the original schedules were for children.

One study looked at the impact of Adderall XR on the driving habits of 19- to 25-year-olds who had ADHD. The investigators used a sophisticated driving simulator that assesses skills such as situation awareness, hazard perception, risk assessment, and decision making under time pressure. The driving scenarios included realistic auditory and visual displays of highway and city driving, with changes in terrain and traffic. The 19 participants with ADHD were randomized to double-blind treatment with placebo or once-daily Adderall XR for 3 weeks and 3 weeks of crossover treatment. Driving performance and symptom level both significantly improved with Adderall XR compared with placebo. Researchers rated 67% of Adderall XR–treated patients as "very much improved" or "much improved" on the Clinical Global Impression–Improvement scale. No placebo-treated adult received those ratings (Kay et al. 2004).

In another study, when researchers switched adult ADHD patients doing well on Concerta to equivalent dosages of Adderall XR, the patients' ADHD symptoms improved even more than with Concerta. The patients maintained their gains for a full 2 years (Chandler 2003).

Dexedrine and DextroStat

Although its chemical structure is much like that of methylphenidate, dextroamphetamine sulfate (Dexedrine) has a 5- to 6-hour duration of action, compared with Ritalin's 2–4 hours. Patients taking Dexedrine are less aware of it "kicking in" and stopping than with Ritalin. Its smoother kinetics makes it easier to tolerate. Even so, patients taking Dexedrine can have rebound symptoms. It can cause typical stimulant side effects: gastrointestinal upset, loss of appetite, headache, irritability, rise in pulse and blood pressure, and insomnia. Although these side effects tend to subside with time, they can be severe. For adults, the typical effective dosage is 15–20 mg of dextroamphetamine taken up to three times a day (Cyr and Brown 1998).

An alternate preparation of dextroamphetamine sulfate is DextroStat, which may kick in a little faster. DextroStat is available as 5- and 10-mg tablets. Its peak plasma levels are about 2 hours after ingestion, compared with 3 for Dexedrine. As with Dexedrine, patients require twice- or thrice-daily dosing; the total daily dose is the same as for Dexedrine.

Dexedrine Spansules

Dexedrine Spansules are bead-filled capsules that give an initial dose of amphetamine followed by sustained release. Peak plasma level is 8 hours after ingestion. The time-release mechanism of Dexedrine Spansules is not always effective. However, studies comparing it with Ritalin, Adderall, dextroamphetamine sulfate, and pemoline show sustained efficacy (R.S. James and Sharp 2001).

Other Amphetamine Stimulants

Pemoline

This CNS stimulant, once available as Cylert, has been withdrawn from use. The FDA recommended its withdrawal because pemoline can cause fatal liver toxicity.

Methamphetamine (Desoxyn Gradumet SR)

Although methamphetamine has the FDA indication for the treatment of ADHD, it has the highest potential for abuse and addiction among the available stimulants. Do not use it.

USING CENTRAL NERVOUS SYSTEM STIMULANTS IN ADULT ADHD

Reasons *Not* to Use a Central Nervous System Stimulant

There may be good reasons not to use a stimulant. The patient may have already tried one or more of them and had a bad reaction or found them ineffective. Is the patient currently abusing alcohol or other drugs? Does he or she have a history of doing so? We cannot use these medications in patients who have a history of or current illicit use or abuse of stimulants. Exceptions to the rule are when the patient is abstinent or in a controlled setting or when we can supervise him or her closely. We have to be alert to abuse or diversion of the medication by family, household members, or friends. A special concern is misuse in young adults. One estimate is that 13% of college students have inhaled crushed tablets of methylphenidate (Rush 2003).

Patients with an active psychotic disorder should not take stimulants. Generally, persons taking MAOI antidepressants should not take stimulants either. That combination can make blood pressure skyrocket.

What about the patient who has seizures? Stimulants actually do not worsen seizures. Still, the prudent clinician ensures that the epileptic patient is stable on anticonvulsant medicine before adding CNS stimulants to treat ADHD (Greenhill et al. 2002).

In general, do not use the stimulants in persons who have a prior history of sensitivity to them. Other contraindications are glaucoma, symptomatic cardiovascular disease, hyperthyroidism or hypertension, and uncontrolled seizures. Screen for those conditions before prescribing the stimulants. If the patient does not have recent data, request that he or she have an evaluation by his or her primary care physician.

Even if the patient has one or more medical conditions, the stimulants may still work fine. However, coordinating treatment with the primary care physician or specialist may be necessary. The stimulants quicken pulse and raise blood pressure. In a vulnerable patient, they may cause or worsen hypertension. This effect can happen also when nonstimulants are used to treat ADHD. In one series of 25 adults with ADHD, new-onset cases of systolic or diastolic hypertension (blood pressure ≥140/90 mm Hg) occurred in 8% of participants taking placebo and 10% of those taking active medication, stimulant or nonstimulant (Wilens et al. 2005). If a stimulant or other medicine helps the ADHD but the patient becomes hypertensive or has worsened hypertension, the primary care clinician or specialist can provide antihypertensive medication. A sensible routine is to check the blood pressure and pulse of patients before starting them on any medication for ADHD—CNS stimulant or other—then monitor vital signs periodically, at least once every 3 months.

Preparing the Patient for Treatment

A review of studies using stimulants showed that of 174 participants, 28% responded best to amphetamine, 16% responded best to methylphenidate, and an additional 41% responded equally well to either stimulant. Some do not respond to either (Arnold 2000). The Texas Medication Algorithm Project calls for trying one form of methylphenidate and one form of dextroamphetamine before moving on to treatment with the nonstimulants (Pliszka et al. 2000). The first medication may be the right one, but finding the best dosage of the best medication may take several trials. Some patients have more side effects than others at equivalent dosages of the medications (Elia et al. 1999).

What symptoms does the patient most want to improve? Inattention? Distractibility? Not persisting with a task? If those symptoms improve, he or she is likelier to persist with treatment, including taking medication.

> Said one patient, "I was always moving around, getting up and down. I was so busy getting ready to settle down to work that I never got any work done. All that extra activity has simply stopped."

The quieting effects of psychostimulants on the impulsivity, hyperactivity, inattention, and emotional lability of ADHD are different from the caffeine-induced focusing of attention, the antianxiety effects of the benzodiazepines, or the tranquilizing effects of antipsychotic agents. All these agents act by different neurochemical and neurophysiologic mechanisms to produce different effects (Popper et al. 2003).

Warn patients that adverse events can occur rapidly. However, side effects are usually minor, do not last long, and tend to ease over time. They stop after patients stop taking the medicine.

Patients sometimes ask if it is necessary to monitor blood levels. The answer is no; numerous studies have shown that stimulant blood levels do not predict response (Dulcan 1990).

As well as reducing the core symptoms of ADHD, treatment with CNS stimulants often leads to improved social skills and better self-esteem. Medication alone is rarely enough. Most patients need changes in external structure and support to maximize results (Jensen et al. 2001).

Using Adderall XR

The patient begins by taking 10 mg of Adderall XR each morning for the first week and 20 mg/day for the second week. Responsible, collaborative adult patients often know rapidly what the effect of a dosage is. They can try the next higher dosage earlier than a week.

Especially when the patient is beginning to take medicine, he or she should use it 7 days a week. Once we know the optimal continuous dosage, we can decide about intermittent or occasional usage. Although some patients feel they should take a break from the medication, there is no good physiological reason for this view. The patient who feels much better when not taking the medicine probably does not have the optimal dosage. Such patients usually do better at a lower dosage.

Any patient may be overwhelmed by too much verbal information from the clinician. This response is even more striking with ADHD patients, who often cannot follow someone else's verbal communication. Written or printed instructions allow the patient to know what dosage he or she is taking, at what time, and how often. Check to be sure that the patient understands. Expect more than the usual confusion about your instructions to and communication with patients who have ADHD.

The amount of the initial prescription anticipates the number of capsules the patient will need for 2 weeks, typically about 25. The directions on the prescription (e.g., "Take two capsules, once a day") are for the pharmacy staff. Patients are to follow your written schedule, not what it says on the label of the bottle. Patients appreciate having enough capsules to cover an initial trial, while not having to pay for a large supply of unused medicine if it does not agree with them.

The patient should call with an update within 1 week, or promptly if he or she is having bad or unexpected side effects. Writing down the reactions to a given dosage helps specify whether or what improvement is taking place. Patients need help remembering to take the medication, even once daily. Taping the capsule to the toothbrush the last thing at night may remind the patient to take it the next morning. One patient taped her capsule to the toilet seat each night, a strategy that was "100% successful" (Weiss and Weiss 2004).

On the follow-up visit 2 weeks later, discuss the patient's response. Having a patient's significant other attend this and other follow-up meetings will help you to fill out the progress report. Are there side effects, such as disruptions of eating or sleeping, stomachaches, headaches, or edginess?

If the patient is tolerating the medicine well, he or she continues to increase the dosage of Adderall XR by 10-mg increments weekly. Some patients can titrate up every 3–4 days, whereas others prefer the schedule of weekly increases. Anxious patients may go slower. The patient drops back a dosage level when he or she notices no further improvement at the higher amount or when the side effects are intrusive. More medicine is not necessarily better. The best dosage gives the most improvement with few to no side effects.

Some patients insist the medicine does not last as long as it is supposed to. They notice 8–10 hours of improved function with Adderall XR, for example, rather than the advertised 10–12 hours. Other patients feel that the medicine lasts longer than expected.

Some clinicians use weight as a guide, dosing amphetamine up to 0.5 to 1 mg/kg/day, to 60 mg/day or more. Others feel that dosage by weight is not a useful guide for adults (Greenhill et al. 2002). Although there is no standard effective daily dosage of Adderall, adult patients often take 30–50 mg/day (Horrigan and Barnhill 2000). If anything, the issue in treating adults is underdosing them with their CNS stimulant (Biederman et al. 2002).

Once the patient has a suitable dosage, it can be fine-tuned by 5-mg amounts. In follow-up visits, more information emerges. Does the medicine fail the patient at particular times of day? What is the impact on the patient's relationships, especially with his or her spouse? Are there tasks that need coverage, such as automobile driving, that patients may forget to discuss? Prescribing medicine is rarely as straightforward as marching steadily through dosages of Adderall XR and finding the magical right one.

Starting With Adderall

Instead of starting with a long-acting medication, some adult patients prefer the shorter impact of Adderall IR tablets. Until they know what a stimulant feels like, some patients want to avoid effects that last up to 12 hours. With such a patient, start with a low dosage of Adderall, such as 5 mg once every morning. This makes side effects unlikely or mild. Taking the medicine—and not having unpleasant side effects—eases patients' fears.

If this amount has no effect, the patient increases it to 10 mg/day after 3 or 4 days to a week, and then by further 5-mg increments every 3 or 4 days to a week, until finding the optimal dose. Then the patient takes that amount twice a day, 5–6 hours apart. Even then there may be fine-tuning of dosage. Some patients prefer to take a different amount in the morning than in the afternoon.

Some patients will prefer then switching to Adderall XR, taking the total daily dosage by capsule in the morning. Others prefer the tighter control that the shorter-acting preparation provides.

Many people find the CNS stimulant helpful but not a cure-all. Sometimes one dose a day is not enough, even with Adderall XR. The medicine does not last as long as expected, or the patient has an extended workday. One strategy is to divide the total daily amount of Adderall XR into two doses, taken a few hours apart. Alternatively, supplement the once-daily morning dose of Adderall XR with a low dose of Dexedrine or regular Adderall in the late afternoon. Detailed questions in follow-up are important. Patients may function best if they follow a morning dose of Adderall XR with afternoon Adderall, but they may resent two copayments for two different medications.

Starting With Concerta

Some patients, who consider Ritalin as the gold standard, want to start with an agent in the methylphenidate group. In that case, or if they have had a poor or uncertain result from taking Adderall or Adderall XR, they usually welcome trying one or more of the Ritalin derivatives.

Many adults prefer a long-acting methylphenidate such as Concerta. Start with 18 mg once a day, increasing the dosage to 36 mg in a week or less. If the patient tolerates the medication well, raise the dosage to 54 mg/day of Concerta. Increase the dosage by 18 mg every week or so until the patient reaches the optimal dosage. The highest usual dosage is 144 mg (roughly equivalent to 60 mg of Adderall XR). The usual dosage range of methylphenidate in adults is 1–2 mg/kg/day, or about 72–108 mg of Concerta (Biederman 2002).

Some patients prefer a short-acting methylphenidate. Adults are often sensitive to small doses and to small changes of dosage. Start these patients at a low dosage, 2.5 mg of Ritalin twice a day for a week. The weekly incremental increase is 2.5 mg. When the patient notices no change after a dosage increase, then the lower amount is probably the effective one (Dodson 2003). Few adult patients use Ritalin as their sole medication, but it is a handy supplement at the end of the day.

Some patients establish their effective dosage of methylphenidate using Ritalin and then want to switch to Concerta. For these, match the total dosage of Ritalin in milligrams per day to the corresponding, one-dose amount of Concerta. Because of its structure, the Concerta tablet is heavier. Thus the 18-mg dose of Concerta is roughly equivalent to 10–15 mg of Ritalin, 36 mg of Concerta is roughly equivalent to 20–30 mg of Ritalin, and 54 mg of Concerta is roughly equivalent to 30–45 mg of Ritalin.

Concerta acts slower than Ritalin, commonly in about 1 hour. Some clinicians tell patients who are taking Concerta to set their alarm an hour early. When they waken, they take their medicine and then go back to sleep. When they wake again, the Concerta will be fully active in their system. Another rapid-action stratagem is for the patient to take a small dose of Ritalin with the Concerta.

Typically a patient knows within a few weeks if Concerta helps. Once an effective daily dosage is established, we modify how the patient takes the medication. Some patients will stay with once-daily dosing. Others prefer two doses, one at 8 A.M. and another at noon. That provides coverage for the long workday some patients have. As an alternative strategy, supplement the Concerta with doses of Ritalin. Ritalin is handy for the patient who forgets a dose of Concerta and needs medication but wants to be able to go to sleep as usual.

How much Ritalin or its equivalent should an adult ADHD patient take? In children, the usual target daily dosage is 1 mg/kg, or about 1 mg per 2 pounds. For an adult weighing 155 pounds, that is about 70 mg of methylphenidate a day. Although some adults use as little as 5 mg once or twice a day, others need 100 mg/day or more. For optimal response, it may be necessary to increase the dosage beyond the FDA-approved levels. For methylphenidate, the approved level is up to 2 mg/kg/day; for amphetamine, up to 1.5 mg/kg/day (Wilens et al. 2002). Patients may need, or be able, to use the medication at dosages outside this range. In these cases, discuss the issues with the patient. Document in the chart that the discussion took place and that the patient understood the rationale for and concerns about such use.

Fine-Tuning

In taking CNS stimulants for ADHD, patients need to think in terms of blocks of time. A regular workday may be 12 or more hours, not 8 hours. Some patients work during the day and are in class until 10 or

10:30 P.M. Even if they are not at work or in school, adults with ADHD have difficulties in their social activities. There are abundant good reasons, such as driving an automobile, for example, for them to take medication during nonwork hours.

Until the patient finds the best dosage, we meet at least once a month. When the patient has established a usual dosage schedule, we fine-tune it. Some patients prefer a standard dosage every day. Others want more flexibility. Almost all adult ADHD patients use medication responsibly. Patients doing stably well follow-up once every 3 months. They call sooner if their life is not going well or if their spouse or life partner is concerned.

Most patients taking a CNS stimulant for ADHD find their optimal dosage and maintain it. Some clinicians note that it may take as long as 1 year to establish the right dosage, during which time a natural tolerance occurs (Wilens 2005). In such cases, increase the dosage and monitor the patient closely. Repetitive needs to raise the dosage suggest either that the medicine is losing its impact or that the patient is abusing it, or both. For either reason, it is sensible to switch to another medication. Such problems are rare.

Sometimes patients ask about drug holidays, that is, simply not taking their medication for a few days or more. Although ADHD is an everyday problem, best dealt with by continuous medication, such holidays can be instructive. The patient has fresh evidence of the usefulness of the medication. Even more dramatic can be the response of the spouse.

Once patients have established an effective dosage, they rarely increase the amount they need. Over time they tend to use less medicine rather than more. Discontinuation is usually simple. Theoretically, patients should be able to stop using the medication when they want to. However, it is better to taper the dosage for a few days before stopping.

PRACTICAL CAVEATS FOR TAKING STIMULANTS

Dividing or Breaking Up the Medicine

Patients may be tempted to divide or cut up their medication. However, some preparations of the stimulants lose their special qualities if they are divided: Concerta and Ritalin SR.

Seizures

The CNS stimulants do not usually cause seizures or make them more likely. However, if a patient has a seizure, he or she should stop taking the medication and should notify the clinician.

TABLE 6–2.   Foods that alter absorption of central nervous system stimulants[a]

Fruit juices
Sports drinks
Granola bars
High-vitamin cereals
Lemonade
Oral suspension antibiotics
Toaster pastries
Protein bars
Soft drinks (including colas)
Vitamin preparations, including vitamin C

[a]These foods should be avoided before and after taking a central nervous system stimulant.
Source.   Shire Pharmaceuticals package insert for Adderall XR. Wayne, PA, Shire, 2002.

Gastrointestinal Disease

Be vigilant with patients who have a narrowed gastrointestinal tract due to disease or to stricture. Giving them stimulants can cause gastrointestinal obstruction.

Substances That Alter Absorption

Patients should not take the stimulants with substances that are organic acids. All the stimulants are strong chemical bases, with a pH between 12 and 13. If they are in the small bowel with an organic acid, such as ascorbic acid or citric acid, the stimulant will not be absorbed. Taking the medication with a glass of orange juice delays its getting into the bloodstream. Some clinicians tell patients to avoid foods or beverages that contain citric acid or vitamin C for 1 hour before and after each dose (Dodson 2003). Patients need to check labels because many products contain citric acid as a preservative. Specific foods to avoid just before and after taking a CNS stimulant are listed in Table 6–2. Other clinicians feel that the effect of citric acid on absorption is too small to warrant special measures (Wilens 2005).

Safety With Other Medications

It is usually safe to take the CNS stimulants with other medications. The stimulants do not affect the cytochrome P450 system and therefore are safe for use with other psychotropics (Biederman et al. 2003). For example, they are safe to take with atomoxetine (Strattera) (Brown 2004).

Many ADHD patients take antidepressants for anxiety or depression, or both. The CNS stimulants have long been used at low dosages to bolster the effect of antidepressants. The CNS stimulants are safe to take with antidepressants, *except with MAOIs.* Combining a stimulant with an MAOI can cause catastrophic rises in blood pressure. In rare cases, with careful monitoring even this combined use is possible. Few clinicians are likely to try it, however (Feinberg 2004).

Patients need to be vigilant about combining medications they take for asthma with stimulants. Pseudoephedrine, systemic (but not inhaled or intranasal) steroids, theophylline, and albuterol are also causes for concern. While taking albuterol, asthmatic patients should temporarily stop their ADHD stimulant. As with pseudoephedrine, the concern is about added demand on the cardiovascular system.

The Elderly

As adults take these medications longer, concerns will arise about use in the elderly. Although the CNS stimulants may require fine-tuning at that stage, they are still useful. The stimulants are not metabolized via the cytochrome P450 isoenzyme system, and they do not interact with medications that involve that system. They are safe for use by the elderly (Dodson 2004).

SIDE EFFECTS

Central Nervous System

Stimulation

Stimulant medications stimulate the brain. Paradoxically, these medications help ADHD patients focus, pay attention, and calm down. On occasion, however, a patient will feel unpleasantly edgy or irritable.

> One female graduate student taking Adderall reported, "I can study effectively for hours. I remember what the lecturer says. I'm more productive, I'm handing things in on time. This stuff is great—but I've turned into a complete bitch."

For such effects, some clinicians prescribe a beta-blocker such as propranolol, 20 mg/day, in the morning. If a patient needs repeated doses, the long-acting 60- or 80-mg formulation of propranolol is an option (Wilens 2001).

On the other hand, patients may feel too flat, drugged, or "like a zombie." This effect usually occurs when the patient is taking too much medicine; it subsides at lower dosages.

Insomnia

For many ADHD patients, long-standing insomnia reflects the restlessness and hyperactivity of the disorder. In one retrospective study of 217 adults with ADHD, sleep problems were a more frequent problem than inattention: 72% reported initial insomnia, 82% had disrupted sleep, and 70% reported nighttime somnolence. Any of the stimulants tended to improve sleep in this group (Dodson 1999). It is important to know before patients start taking medication what their usual sleep pattern is. If they already have insomnia, it may worsen when they take CNS stimulants. If they do not have insomnia, they may develop it.

In one study of children with ADHD, the frequency of delayed sleep onset in those taking a stimulant was almost three times that in children on placebo (Stein 1999). Some adults with ADHD who take stimulants have poor sleep. The sleep problems may reflect their ADHD, another psychiatric illness such as depression or bipolar disorder, or a primary sleep disorder, as well as possibly being a reaction to the stimulant. Medication wearing off at night may cause a rebound effect that interferes with sleep (Kooij et al. 2001).

Patients rapidly learn how late in the day they can take their CNS stimulant and still fall asleep and stay asleep. Typically, that means by 4 or 5 P.M. if they are taking Ritalin, earlier for one of the longer-acting CNS stimulants. With further experience, some patients take their morning dose earlier or decrease their afternoon dose, or both. Some can take their medication late in the day and still sleep soundly. For some ADHD patients, taking the CNS stimulants during the day improves sleep at night.

> Said one woman, "I sleep like a dead person now. Maybe that's because I'm getting so much more done every day. At night I can relax, not go to bed and worry."

One study of eight adults taking stimulants found that their sleep quality improved and that they moved around less while they slept (Kooij et al. 2001). Patients taking stimulants for ADHD worry that the medicine will make their sleep worse. Once they are taking their optimal dosage, they may be relieved to find that they can nap. Before treatment, many ADHD patients are too restless, tense, and tuned-in to stimuli both inside and outside themselves. With the medication they are likelier to nap, and this eases their worry that it causes insomnia (Dodson 2004).

Patients with stimulant-related insomnia should try taking their medicine earlier in the day. Patients having initial insomnia of more than 1 hour, or who are sleeping a total of less than 7 hours a night, may need to decrease the dosage. This is particularly true of the last dose of the day, if they are using multiple doses. Some patients who take a long-acting stimulant in the morning may usefully take a low-dose, short-acting stimulant at night. For some, that eases the transition to sleep; others complain that it makes their initial insomnia worse.

Exercise helps many people sleep better as well as improving concentration and energy. Cognitive-behavioral interventions are often useful: progressive muscle relaxation, breathing exercises, and other techniques to foster deep relaxation. Stable routines and good sleep hygiene also help. Many patients go full-out all day, do not downshift before bed, and then are surprised that they cannot sleep. Simple factors make a difference: turning off the television, turning lights down. Other helpers are having a quiet room that is the right temperature and using soothing rituals such as bathing, reading, or listening to music. Taking time for personal relationships, from talking companionably to making love, also makes for better rest.

Medication helps insomnia when other remedies do not. The soporific zolpidem (Ambien), 5–10 mg at bedtime, typically provides 5 or 6 hours of sleep without a drug hangover. Although the FDA has approved Ambien only for short-term use, up to 10 days or so, many psychiatrists find it useful over the long term. Over time, patients may become dependent on it, at least psychologically. A few patients feel that it interferes with their memory. Ambien CR, 6.25–12.5 mg at bedtime, typically provides 6–8 hours of sleep.

The soporific eszopiclone (Lunesta) at dosages of 1, 2, or 3 mg at bedtime helps patients sleep for 7–8 hours. Aside from an unpleasant taste in the mouth on arising, patients have few side effects.

A new hypnotic, ramelteon (Rozerem), differs from others by being the first melatonin receptor agonist. Its postulated mechanism of action is to stabilize the circadian rhythm rather than to sedate the brain. Its 8-mg dosage is standard, regardless of the age of the patient. Information is not yet available on transitioning patients to Rozerem from regular use of Ambien or Lunesta. Approved for long-term use, and not a controlled substance, ramelteon is an interesting compound. How effective and well tolerated it is remains to be seen (Takeda Pharmaceuticals 2005).

Sometimes patients sleep better if they rely on the sedative effects of antidepressant medications, such as mirtazapine (Remeron). In one study, 14 of 16 ADHD patients taking mirtazapine for stimulant-related insomnia reported significant improvement. Their mean age was 27.4 years, the age range 12–47 years. The mean final dosage of mirtazapine was 9.4 mg/day. At the end of the 6-week study, all the patients continued taking it (Adler et al. 2000). Mirtazapine sedates because it works as an antihistamine; this effect may be more pronounced at lower dosages. It does not lessen sexual drive or worsen sexual function. The medicine is not addicting. Many patients complain that it sedates them through the day. The other most common side effect is weight gain, which can be considerable.

Another sedating antidepressant, trazodone (Desyrel), is also a sleep aid at 25–200 mg, taken at bedtime. Although many psychiatrists use it for this purpose, there are few data in the literature about its efficacy. Some patients feel dulled or "zonked out" the day after they take it. The medication can induce arrhythmias, especially in patients with a history of cardiac disease. In men, trazodone can induce priapism (persistent or unwanted erections). In rare cases, the priapism may require surgical drainage of the penis and cause permanent impotence (S.P. James and Mendelson 2004).

Another medication for stimulant-induced insomnia is the antihypertensive agent clonidine (Catapres). Low doses at bedtime, such as 0.1 or 0.15 mg, help adults and children but may lower the adult's blood pressure (Wilens and Spencer 2000).

Yet another standby is diphenhydramine (Benadryl), 25–50 mg at bedtime. Many patients who take it feel persistently drugged into the next day.

Difficulties can arise when the clinician and patient see insomnia just as a chemical problem. More pills will not help if the insomnia is more than a symptom of ADHD or a drug side effect. Sometimes the problem is larger and requires exploration.

Rebound

Rebound produces heightened irritability, temper outbursts, difficulty with making transitions, and lowered capacity to tolerate frustration. With immediate-release preparations, it occurs typically 3–4 hours after a given dose. Assess the overall stimulant response. If it has been minimal or poor, consider discontinuing the medicine and trying another. Alternatively, change the timing of when the patient takes the medicine. Use multiple doses of medicine or change the preparation the patient takes.

Tics

Children with ADHD have a high incidence of tics, as much as 32%–50% (Comings and Comings 1990). Over time, tics decrease, and few adults still have them (The Tourette's Syndrome Study Group 2002). Stimulants may worsen tics in adults (Castellanos 1999).

Personality Change

Some patients complain that although the medicine helps them to function better, they "aren't themselves." Patients want to be "spontaneous" but also have better behavioral self-control. They may find that they do not *want* to "lock on" to what is in front of them, thus being unable to change focus or attention. The same is true for their emotions. The clinical challenge is adjusting the patient's dosage for the desired effect. Reducing the dosage may lessen the patient's feeling of being dulled or blunted (Arnold and Jensen 1995).

> One college student said, "I get better grades when I take medicine, but I lose *me* in the process. I'm just not as funny." Kyle's wisecracking endeared him to his friends. We found a medication regimen that allowed him "time off" to be his unfettered self.

Tolerance

Some clinicians estimate that 15%–20% of patients develop tolerance to a stimulant, whereas others rarely encounter tolerance at all (Horrigan 2001). If tolerance develops, one strategy is to discontinue the medication and switch to an alternate agent in the same class. After a month or so, challenge the patient with the original effective medication at the prior best dosage. Some patients need a rotating stimulant schedule: on one medication for a few weeks or months, switching to an alternate, and then going back.

Hypomania or Mania

Stimulants can activate latent or underlying bipolar disorder. The best preventive measure is taking a careful history and screening with an instrument such as the Mood Disorders Questionnaire. The presence or history of hypomania or mania is another important area of inquiry in the initial evaluation and another reason to include parents or significant others in the process. The patient is likely to forget hypomanic episodes, minimize their importance, or see them as a longed-for "normal" state in contrast to his or her more usual depressed self. Patients who become hypomanic or worse require a mood stabilizer and discontinuation of their ADHD medication. Once the mood disorder is controlled, then attention can return to the ADHD (Stahl 2004).

Emergence of Significant Depression, Lability, or Anxiety

Assess the patient for toxicity or withdrawal symptoms. Given the patient's overall response to the stimulant, is it worth continuing? Evaluate the patient for comorbidity and treat it accordingly—for example, with antidepressants and psychotherapy or cognitive-behavioral treatment. Consider reducing or discontinuing the stimulant.

Psychosis

There are no case reports in adults of stimulant-related cases of psychosis at therapeutic dosages. Prudent dosage schedules and careful clinical monitoring should lessen the risk that psychosis will occur (Popper et al. 2003). If an adult patient does become psychotic, discontinue the stimulant and assess the patient to be sure you are accurately diagnosing the comorbid condition. Then begin alternate appropriate treatment for the psychotic condition (Wilens and Spencer 2000).

Other Side Effects

Some patients taking a stimulant have a faster resting pulse, typically 5–10 beats per minute. Most do not notice the increase, and they maintain their exercise tolerance. Several patients taking CNS stimulants have trained successfully for marathons or other activities with high cardiovascular demand. Occasionally stimulants can cause cardiac arrhythmias.

Hypertension

Because the CNS stimulants constrict blood vessels, they can also raise blood pressure. However, the increase is rarely significant, usually only 3–5 mm Hg (Wilens and Spencer 2000). Check blood pressure and pulse before a patient tries a CNS stimulant and then regularly thereafter. However, for patients with hypertension or borderline blood pressure, stimulants have more impact on blood pressure. Coordinate treatment with the patient's primary care physician or cardiologist. Patients with uncontrolled hypertension or symptomatic cardiovascular disease should not take stimulants (Wilens et al. 2003).

Other medications may combine with the stimulant to raise blood pressure.

One female patient was doing clinically well with Adderall when her blood pressure unexpectedly rose. What changed? "I have the usual stresses: trying to keep my weight down, fighting with my ex over custody, struggling with an impossible boss." She paused. "I forgot about my allergies! This spring has been the worst. I've been taking Sudafed by the handful." Once consulted, her internist stopped her pseudoephedrine-containing preparations. With an alternate treatment for her allergies and with regular exercise, she became normotensive while continuing to take the CNS stimulant.

Headache

Patients taking stimulants may complain of headache, especially when they start the medication. Sometimes skipping breakfast is the cause. If headache persists, over-the-counter remedies can help. Sometimes headaches respond to a low dosage of a calcium channel blocker such as verapamil (Calan), in either standard or extended-release form (Dodson 2003). Operationally, try decreasing the dosage of the stimulant for a few days and then increasing it again. In some cases, it is better to switch preparations than to fight continually with headache.

Cold Hands

Vasoconstriction can cause cold hands as well as high blood pressure. In the winter, vasoconstriction can cause considerable discomfort and interfere with fine motor tasks. One patient at college in New England regularly wore gloves indoors in the winter.

Gastrointestinal Symptoms

Patients may experience abdominal discomfort, nausea, or a hollow feeling in their stomach. People who have a "nervous" or sensitive stomach may be more susceptible. Taking the medication after meals, and sometimes a light snack, eases the discomfort. These symptoms often lessen over time.

Note a patient's eating patterns before he or she begins taking a CNS stimulant, then see what impact the medicine has. In one study, 9.7% of 155 children taking methylphenidate and 21.9% of 374 children given mixed amphetamine salts had significant loss of appetite (Biederman et al. 2002; Greenhill et al. 2002). Less than half of adult patients have loss of appetite. If appetite loss occurs, it is typically transient, and patients lose only a few pounds. Preliminary prospective data in adults taking Concerta showed that they lost weight during the first 3 months but regained it in the next 9 months (Wilens and Pelham 2003). A small number of patients lose a lot of weight and have to remind themselves to eat.

They schedule meals for when their medicine has worn off. Frequent small meals may maintain weight better. Having high-calorie supplemental food, such as nutrition bars, helps. Most patients, however, do not have this problem.

> One ADHD patient, desperate about her obesity, spoke for many others when she said, "Where's this wonderful loss of appetite I'm supposed to have?"

Height

There is concern that stimulants cause diminished stature in youngsters. Controlled follow-up studies have found that height tends to become normal by late adolescence, even in those still taking a CNS stimulant (Spencer et al. 1998b). The impact of stimulants on height is not an issue in adults.

QUEST FOR THE OPTIMAL DOSAGE

The CNS stimulant dosage that best controls the symptoms that most bother the patient may also cause undesirable side effects. Inquire about the time sequence of a side effect. Knowing when it starts, when it peaks, and when it wanes or stops may provide suggestions for remedies. For peripheral autonomic side effects, a beta-blocker may help. At times, however, it is necessary to reduce the dosage or switch to another agent if the side effects are too burdensome (Stahl 2004).

WOMEN'S ISSUES: PREGNANCY, CHILDBEARING, AND NURSING

Women with ADHD become pregnant. Those who have poor impulse control may be at more risk for unplanned pregnancies. The eightfold higher incidence of ADHD among adoptees over the base rate reflects how often women with ADHD have unwanted pregnancies and put the babies up for adoption (Deutsch et al. 1982). Women also become pregnant while they are taking the CNS stimulants. A review of 12,000 stimulant-exposed pregnancies found no evidence of teratogenicity (Briggs et al. 1998).

Although there are no controlled studies in humans, the amphetamines are in risk category C. ADHD patients should discontinue use of any *d,l*-amphetamine medication before becoming pregnant. Some newborn infants whose mothers took amphetamine during pregnancy have had withdrawal symptoms. Some of the drug makes its way into breast milk, so the usual recommendation for nursing mothers is to either discontinue the medication or bottle-feed. Discontinue the medication if the nursing infant becomes irritable (Stahl 2004).

DRUG INTERACTIONS

Because the stimulants affect blood pressure, watch their impact in combination with other agents. Desipramine, for example, can markedly raise brain concentrations of amphetamine and amplify its cardiovascular effects. In contrast, amphetamines may antagonize the antihypertensive effects of medicines such as *Veratrum* alkaloids. Norepinephrine reuptake inhibitors (e.g., venlafaxine, duloxetine, atomoxetine, and reboxetine) can raise amphetamine's impact on the CNS and the cardiovascular system.

Gastrointestinal acidifying agents (e.g., ascorbic acid, fruit juices, guanethidine, reserpine, and glutamic acid) *lower* plasma amphetamine levels. Gastrointestinal alkalinizing agents (e.g., bicarbonate) and urinary alkalinizing agents (acetazolamide, some thiazides) *increase* plasma levels of amphetamine and potentiate its actions.

Antipsychotics (e.g., haloperidol, chlorpromazine, and, theoretically, second-generation or "atypical" agents) inhibit the stimulatory effect of amphetamines.

MAOIs slow the absorption of amphetamines, potentiating their action. Headache and hypertension can result. Rarely hypertensive crisis, hyperthermia, and death can occur. Do not use the amphetamines with an MAOI or within 14 days of MAOI use unless you are expert and monitor the patient carefully (Stahl 2004).

LONG-TERM CONSEQUENCES

Patients often worry about what will happen if they take a CNS stimulant for months or years. Children do not seem to have adverse effects. Their growth may lag a little, but they reach the same height as their nonmedicated peers (National Institutes of Health 1998). However, we have not been treating enough ADHD adults with CNS stimulants long enough to know the outcome of chronic use.

SUDDEN-DEATH CONTROVERSY

Do Mixed Amphetamine Salts Cause Sudden Cardiac Death?

In 2005 the Canadian government caused a major controversy by withdrawing Adderall from the marketplace. As their rationale, officials cited sudden cardiac death among persons taking Adderall. The FDA, which reviewed the same data, maintained that there was not a causal association between such deaths and patients taking mixed amphetamine salts.

In all the reported cases of sudden cardiac death, the patient was taking mixed amphetamine salts in either the immediate- or extended-release form. However, the rate of spontaneous sudden cardiac death in children and adolescents taking *no* medication is approximately 3/100,000 per year. The risk of sudden cardiac death in children and adolescents taking mixed amphetamine salts is 20/4.4 million patient exposures, a rate of 0.3–0.5/100,000 per year. In sudden cardiac death in children and adolescents, the profile of cardiac defects is the same, whether or not they are taking amphetamine. There is no evidence of a causal association between sudden cardiac death and using mixed amphetamine salts. Therefore, there is no reason to withdraw the medications from the marketplace (Wilens 2005). Later in 2005, the Canadian government reversed its ruling, making Adderall again available.

A Black Box Warning for All Central Nervous System Stimulants?

In February 2006, the controversy flared anew. In the United States, an expert advisory panel recommended that the FDA require all CNS stimulant medications to carry a black box warning. Such a warning conveys that the medication can cause serious complications, including sudden cardiac death. In response, officials from the American Psychiatric Association recommended that there be rapid, further study of the data. However, American Psychiatric Association officials asserted that a black box warning would be "premature, and may be linked to needless alarm" (American Psychiatric Association 2006). At this writing, the outcome of the recommendation to the FDA is still unclear. Regardless, the controversy reminds clinicians considering CNS stimulants to screen the medical histories of their patients and to monitor patients' physical status, especially for cardiovascular disease. This precaution will naturally be more important in adults than it is in children.

Assessing Cardiac Health in the Patient With ADHD

Assess cardiac health before prescribing any stimulant to any patient. Guidelines exist for children and adolescents (Gutgesell et al. 1999). When evaluating a child, the clinician should establish whether there is any cardiac disease, congenital or acquired. Check for a family history and for current cardiac symptoms or disease in family members. Monitor use of other medications, including nonprescription or over-the-counter agents. Inquire about routine medical history. If there is a suspicion of heart disease, order an electrocardiogram, but one is not warranted routinely. Watch for worrisome symptoms: palpitations, chest pain, syncope, seizures, and symptoms intensifying after exercise.

Notify parents and children about the side effects of medication. Include the fact that there have been occasional deaths of children who were taking the medicine, but that no causal association exists. Document the discussion and note whether the patient (or parents, or both) seemed to understand and agreed to follow your recommendations. In following up, ask about the same physical symptoms. When in doubt, refer the child or adolescent for cardiovascular assessment (Wilens 2005).

Adults with ADHD warrant even closer inquiry about cardiovascular issues or concerns. Any current or past symptoms of cardiac disease should trigger referral for cardiovascular workup. The patient should complete the workup and have specific cardiologic notice that it is safe or warranted before taking the CNS stimulant. Also routinely take the patient's blood pressure and pulse before starting any stimulant medication for ADHD, and monitor them regularly (Wilens 2005).

ABUSE AND ADDICTION

One factor that complicates work with the CNS stimulants is that "they're addictive." Given this street reputation, it is easy to understand why patients with ADHD are wary of them.

Nonmedical Use and Abuse of Prescribed Central Nervous System Stimulants

Abuse of prescription medications, especially controlled substances, is common. Nonmedical use of prescription medications is the second most common category of illicit drug use according to federal government statistics (Substance Abuse and Mental Health Services Administration 2004). A recent survey cited 22 million Americans as having substance abuse. In this survey, 1.4 million Americans used the stimulants for nonmedical purposes, second only to antianxiety medications, which care abused by 1.8 million people. Given the greater number of prescriptions for the antianxiety medications, stimulants may be the most commonly abused psychiatric medications in the United States (Higgins and Powell 2005).

While there is little evidence that ADHD patients who take prescribed CNS stimulants abuse them, there are individual exceptions.

> Hank, 30, started taking mixed amphetamine salts (Adderall) when he was treated for ADHD in early adolescence. In high school, he experimented with and abused street drugs, including Ecstasy, but he continued Adderall as well. As an adult, he sought out physicians, saying he was new to the area and wanted to continue his ADHD treatment. He claimed that all that worked for him was a combination of Adderall and bupropion (Wellbutrin). He mentioned bupropion as a cover for the stimulant. He used 60 mg of Adderall as a loading dose and then took an additional 10 mg every 1–2 hours throughout the day. He usually stopped it after a total dosage of 180–200 mg in one binge. Typically, he felt sick after he reached this total dosage, but he has not had any serious medical problems.

One survey of college students (average age=20.1 years) found that in the previous 12 months, almost one-third had used one or more CNS stimulants without a prescription. Their most common reasons were "to improve intellectual performance" (23.3%), "to be more efficient on assignments" (22.0%), and "to use in combination with alcohol" (19.3%) (Low and Gendaszek 2002). In another college student study, 21% of the participants under the age of 24 reported using methylphenidate, 13% intranasally (Babcock and Byrne 2000). Estimates of nonmedical use of amphetamine are even higher. College students repeatedly assert that they use the medications to enhance intellectual performance, much like athletes use anabolic steroids to improve physical performance (DuPont and Bensinger 2005).

Among the stimulants, immediate-release products are more likely to be abused than extended-release preparations. Drug abusers can get high on oral doses of the immediate-release products if they take them at higher than therapeutic amounts. It is comparatively easy to crush and snort immediate-release methylphenidate or dextroamphetamine or to dissolve them in water and inject them. When dissolved and injected, methylphenidate as Ritalin can cause euphoria. However, the result can be severe difficulties in the eyes, lungs, and heart, because the talc particles in the tablets become microemboli and cause ministrokes (Greenhill 2005).

People can readily crush some extended-release products, such as those that use coated beads, converting them to immediate-release preparations. People can then snort the drug or dissolve it and take it intravenously. Osmotic-release oral system methylphenidate (Concerta) is not easily crushed. If it is crushed and then dissolved in water, the solution still contains substantial amounts of polymer. Animals subjected to this intravenous administration have died of pulmonary hypertension. There is substantially less nonmedical use of Concerta than of other forms of methylphenidate (DuPont and Bensinger 2005).

Studies document the ready availability of many drugs through Internet pharmacies, which have few controls. Skyrocketing drug purchases on the Internet concern public health and law enforcement officials. There is little specific information about sales of the CNS stimulants over the Internet, however (Wilford et al. 2005).

Substance Abuse Tendencies in Persons With ADHD

Proportionally, more people in the ADHD population abuse alcohol and other substances than do their non-ADHD peers. Caffeine is an everyday widespread substance of use and abuse. It helps with concentration and focus, and many untreated ADHD patients use it. Caffeine has disadvantages. After an initial jolt, the effect rapidly tapers. Some people develop tolerance. In large amounts, it irritates the gastrointestinal tract. Many patients need less caffeine once treated for ADHD. Their gut settles down. The more stable blood levels of the CNS stimulants, especially the long-acting ones, give relief from the roller-coaster effect of caffeine.

More people with ADHD use nicotine than in the general population. Nicotine is a powerful drug with complex effects on the CNS. Some people relax; others find that they concentrate better and are more productive. Persons with ADHD start smoking earlier, smoke more cigarettes, and have more difficulty discontinuing nicotine use than do others (Pomerleau et al. 1995).

Many people use alcohol in moderation to relieve stress and enhance eating and socializing. However, the malignant shift to abuse or dependency is more common in persons who are frustrated and unhappy. This describes many adults with untreated ADHD. Alcohol can appeal to the ADHD adult when its depression of the CNS slows him or her down and makes it easier to function.

Combating Patient Fears About Addiction

Stably taking CNS stimulants to treat ADHD is not addiction. Drug abusers use drugs to get high and to escape. In the process, they rapidly become tolerant, needing higher dosages to reach the same effect (Croft 2005). Using the drug outside of medical supervision, they come to crave the fast hit. Increasingly, they organize their life around the drug experience. Avoiding discontinuation becomes their first or only priority (Salzman 1997).

In contrast, the great majority of ADHD patients take medication to feel normal, not to feel high. They want relief from feeling overstimulated, not more stimulation. Once they find a dosage that works, ADHD patients maintain it. Rarely do they need to increase the dosage of a stimulant to preserve its effect. Most patients do not like taking medication. They want the smallest effective dosage for the shortest time. The biggest problem is remembering to take the medication, not craving it. They do not feel good if they take more than the recommended dosage. Over time most adults with ADHD take less of the CNS stimulants rather than more. Rather than feeling driven to repeat doses, as happens with addicts, most ADHD patients forget to take their medicine and need reminding. The common practice of taking drug holidays among these patients is the opposite of driven overusage. No study of the use of stimulants by adults with ADHD has found worrisome rates of euphoria (Faraone and Wilens 2003).

> Only one of my patients has said, "At the dose that works best for my ADHD, I have a little buzz. On days I don't take it, I miss it more than I like to admit." Whether or not he is taking the medicine, he behaves prudently. His original work has brought him widespread acclaim. Other medicines, at other dosages, do not help his ADHD. He has not increased his dosage. His usage remains steady, and his life is a model of responsible behavior.

Does Treating ADHD With Stimulants Lead to Drug Abuse?

Many persons with ADHD abuse drugs. The frequency in reported studies in the literature ranges from 27% to 46%; many clinicians feel these percentages are conservative (Spencer et al. 1998a). It would be disastrous to foster abuse by giving addicting drugs to vulnerable people, especially adolescents.

Experts insist that early treatment with stimulants *protects* adolescents with ADHD from developing a drug abuse problem. A recent landmark study pointed out that 18% of a control group of community adolescents qualified for a diagnosis of substance abuse disorder. Of the ADHD adolescents being medicated for ADHD, 25% had substance abuse, but 75% of the unmedicated ADHD adolescents were drug abusers.

One meta-analysis of six studies of the substance abuse risk in adolescents and young adults with ADHD showed that *stimulant treatment reduced patients' risk of substance abuse nearly twofold over that of patients with untreated ADHD.* Not treating ADHD adolescents makes it more likely that they will develop substance abuse disorders later (Wilens et al. 2003).

Abuse of the CNS stimulants is real, especially among teenagers. The culprits are not usually the ADHD patients but their friends who want to get high. In one study of schoolchildren prescribed stimulants for ADHD, fully one in five was approached by other children to give or sell them their medication (Croft 2005). The newer, longer-lasting stimulants are hard to abuse. The paste-like consistency of Concerta, for example, keeps it from providing the quick hit that abusers want. However, resourceful people have figured out how to abuse even the longer-lasting preparations.

Working With the Adult Who Has Substance Abuse and ADHD

A substance-abusing patient with ADHD presents special challenges. Treating the substance abuse comes first. Most clinicians insist that the patient be stably abstinent before treating the ADHD, especially with a CNS stimulant. Although there is no standard period of required abstinence, 3 months or more free of drugs of abuse seems sensible (Wilens 2003). The presence of drug abuse is *not* an absolute contraindication to using psychostimulants for ADHD (Dulcan 1997).

> At 26, Dirk was sick of his chaotic life. He had dropped out of college, baffled by how hard it was to study even when he wanted to. Enterprising and resourceful, he started his own business, but his disorganization and impulsivity hampered him. Increasingly he needed alcohol or marijuana for sleep. Soon he was smoking marijuana throughout the day. Evenings and weekends he drank a lot with friends.
>
> The clinician who evaluated Dirk for ADHD shocked him by labeling his alcohol and marijuana use as addictions. The doctor agreed to try atomoxetine but not any stimulant until Dirk demonstrated that he abstained from substance abuse. He responded to the challenge and stayed clean. With comprehensive treatment that included medication for his ADHD and continued abstinence from other substances of abuse, he stabilized. His business flourished.

Many ADHD patients with a history of substance abuse work long and hard to overcome their addictions. Their abstinence is precious. The idea of taking a CNS stimulant worries them, naturally, so the clinician needs to proceed with particular caution. These patients may do best to start treatment with a non-CNS stimulant. If they never want to risk using a CNS stimulant, that is fine. Their sobriety makes everything else possible.

Patients with a history of drug abuse who are now abstinent can cautiously use the CNS stimulants. Clinicians usually know rapidly, within days to weeks, if the medicine is going to help. If not, discontinue it promptly. If the medicine works, the patient continues it while being monitored for possible substance abuse.

> Jack, age 42, had a long history of alcohol abuse, depression, and social anxiety. Finally, after considerable effort and regular attendance at Alcoholics Anonymous meetings, he had 9 months of abstinence. Able for the first time to look beyond his alcohol abuse, Jack reviewed patterns of erratic performance that started in grammar school and continued through a failed attempt at college. His impulsivity was a severe problem. As a young man, he had impregnated three different girls in less than a year. His driving record, even when he was sober, was so bad that he had to pay high rates to get any insurance. As an adult, even when not drinking, he was losing things, paying bills late, and botching the myriad details of everyday life. Sensitive and labile, he was prone to temper outbursts that he later regretted. His symptoms and history fit the diagnosis of ADHD, combined type.
>
> Having reviewed the treatment options, we took the calculated risk of trying CNS stimulants. On Adderall, 20 mg twice daily, Jack rapidly made gains. He held a tough new job for 9 months and then jumped to another one that more than doubled his pay. Tearful, his mother called to verify his good news. "Whatever this medicine is that you have given him, you have changed his life."

The key element in succeeding with the patient who has abused substances is the therapeutic alliance. Are the two of you an effective team? The patient who continues to abuse substances requires reevaluation and a change of treatment focus. The CNS stimulants are clearly contraindicated. Is even Strattera safe to use? The clinician's alliance with key others in the patient's life may be a decisive factor. If the alliance is strong, the combination of the clinician and family members or significant others may help the patient successfully address the substance abuse and then, again, take up treatment for ADHD. With other patients, entrenched substance abuse is an insuperable obstacle.

ARE WE OVERPRESCRIBING CENTRAL NERVOUS SYSTEM STIMULANTS?

Is ADHD an excuse for lazy and irresponsible Americans? Are we over-diagnosing and overtreating? Although we do not have good statistics on adults, we do for children. The prescription of Ritalin to children and adolescents increased by 2.5 times between 1990 and 1995. Most experts feel that this change is not a result of overprescription, but rather a result of clinicians being more aware of ADHD and more willing to treat it once they diagnose it (Goldman et al. 1998).

Prescribing patterns vary greatly. There may well be overprescribing in locales, such as in highly competitive urban areas. One study of public schools in two southeastern Virginia cities found that 8%–10% of children in grades 2–5 were receiving ADHD medication during the school day, which is two times the expected rate (LeFever et al. 1999). On the other hand, a survey of four different American communities found that 5.1% of the 1,285 children who were studied qualified for a diagnosis of ADHD. Of those who qualified, only 12.5% had been treated with medication in the prior year. Less than 70% of those with the diagnosis were getting any treatment at all (Jensen et al. 1999). We have a way to go before we treat all the children with ADHD who could benefit from medication, much less the adults.

COSTS AND MARKETING ISSUES

In the U.S. market, costs vary widely for the stimulants. (See Table 6–3 for prices in the Washington, DC, area at the time of writing.) Prices for medication needed for one month range from just over $40 (for generic mixed amphetamine salts) to almost $240 (for Concerta).

Since their introduction in 2000, long-acting stimulant preparations have been replacing the short-acting ones. Recently, long-acting agents had 68.3% of the market share: Adderall XR, 22.9%; Concerta, 22% (IMS Health 2004). Reflecting their equal efficacy and tolerance, methylphenidate and dextroamphetamine preparations do about equally well. Within the classes of long-acting agents, marketing may help Concerta have a bigger market share than Ritalin LA or Metadate CD and may help Adderall XR lead over Dexedrine Spansules. Cost seems to be central for short-acting agents; generic preparations of both methylphenidate and dextroamphetamine do best in the marketplace.

TABLE 6–3. Cost of a month's supply of central nervous system stimulant[a]

Medication brand (generic)	Strength (mg)	Form	Number	Cost	
				Brand	Generic
Concerta	36	tablets	60	$235.29	NA
Focalin	10	tablets	90	$114.99	NA
Focalin XR	20	capsules	30	$111.79	NA
	10	capsules	30	$111.79	NA
Metadate CD	30	capsules	60	$150.69	NA
Ritalin (methylphenidate hydrochloride)	20	tablets	90	$151.79	$65.79
Adderall (mixed amphetamine salts)	30	tablets	30	$71.49	$40.19
Adderall XR	30	capsules	30	$133.99	
Dexedrine (dextroamphetamine)	5	tablets	180	$98.29	$80.39
Dexedrine Spansules (dextroamphetamine)	15	capsules	60	$260.29	$90.09

[a]Assumption: daily dosage=60 mg of methylphenidate or its equivalent, or 30 mg of dextroamphetamine or its equivalent.

Source.   Survey of pharmacy prices in Washington, DC, by B.B.D. and Colin Doyle, January 2006.

SUMMARY

- Among the medications available to treat ADHD in adults, the CNS stimulants are likely the most effective. In the synapse, they interfere with the reuptake of neurotransmitters, especially norepinephrine and dopamine. They facilitate neurotransmitter release and inhibit their breakdown. Generally well tolerated, they are the medications of first choice. Do *not* use CNS stimulants with the patient who is psychotic; who has uncontrolled bipolar disorder; who has glaucoma, hypertension, or active cardiac disease; or who is actively abusing alcohol or other drugs.
- When an ADHD adult tries a CNS stimulant, good clinical practice mandates an adequate trial with an appropriate dosage of at least one of the methylphenidate medications and one of the dextroamphetamine preparations. Adults typically start with a long-acting preparation, such as Adderall XR or Concerta, at low dosage daily, and titrate up. Underdosage is the most common problem in adults. When patients respond well, their work and social function improve.
- Most adults with ADHD, like most children with the disorder, can take a CNS stimulant safely and effectively for years. Few adult ADHD patients abuse or become dependent on CNS stimulants. These drugs are generally safe for long-term, continuous use.
- Although effective, the stimulants have their drawbacks, such as side effects. The stimulants have a relatively narrow spectrum. Effective for the core symptoms of ADHD, they do not treat the comorbid conditions that ADHD adults commonly have. Even when helpful, medication is just one part of comprehensive treatment.

REFERENCES

Adler LA, Braverman L, Ginsberg D: Efficacy of mirtazapine in stimulant associated insomnia. Poster presentation at the Society of Biological Psychiatry 55th Annual Convention, Chicago, IL, May 2000

Ambrosini PJ, Lopez FA, Chandler MC, et al: An open-label community assessment trial of Adderall XR in pediatric ADHD. Poster presentation at the annual meeting of the American Academy of Child and Adolescent Psychiatry, New York, October 2000

American Psychiatric Association: APA statement on the FDA's hearing on ADHD and rare adverse events (press release). Washington, DC, American Psychiatric Association, February 10, 2006

Arnold LE: Methylphenidate vs. amphetamine: a comparative review. J Atten Disord 3:200–211, 2000

Arnold LE, Jensen PS: Attention deficit disorders, in Comprehensive Textbook of Psychiatry, Vol VI. Edited by Kaplan HI, Sadock BJ. Baltimore, MD, Williams & Wilkins, 1995, pp 2295–2310

Atomoxetine (Strattera) for ADHD. Med Lett Drugs Ther 45:11–12, 2003

Babcock Q, Byrne T: Student perceptions of methylphenidate abuse at a public liberal arts college. J Am Coll Health 49:143–145, 2000

Berridge KC, Robinson TE: What is the role of dopamine in reward: hedonic impact, reward learning, or incentive salience? Brain Res Brain Res Rev 28:309–369, 1998

Biederman J: Practical considerations in the stimulant drug selection for the ADHD patient: efficacy, potency and titration. Today's Therapeutic Trends 20:311–328, 2002

Biederman J, Lopez FA, Boellner SW, et al: A randomized, double-blind, placebo-controlled, parallel-group study of SLI381 (Adderall XR) in children with attention-deficit/hyperactivity disorder. Pediatrics 110:258–266, 2002

Biederman J, Chrisman AK, Dodson W, et al: Adult ADHD: spelling out the clinical strategies. Medical Crossfire 5:29–45, 2003

Bradley C: Behavior of children receiving Benzedrine. Am J Psychiatry 94:577–585, 1937

Briggs GG, Freeman RK, Yaffe SJ: Drugs in Pregnancy and Lactation, 5th Edition. Philadelphia, PA, Williams & Wilkins, 1998, pp 53–58

Brown TE: Atomoxetine and stimulants in combination for treatment of attention deficit hyperactivity disorder: four case studies. J Child Adolesc Psychopharmacol 14:131–138, 2004

Castellanos FX: Stimulants and tic disorders: from dogma to data. Arch Gen Psychiatry 56:337–338, 1999

Chandler MC: A two year trial of the effectiveness of Adderall XR. Paper presented at the annual meeting of the American Psychiatric Association, San Francisco, CA, May 2003

Chandler MC, Lopez FA, Biederman J: Long term safety and efficacy of Adderall XR in children with ADHD. Platform presentation at the annual meeting of the American Psychiatric Association, Philadelphia, PA, May 2002

Charach A, Ickowicz A, Schachar S: Stimulant treatment over five years: adherence, effectiveness and adverse effects. J Am Acad Child Adolesc Psychopharmacol 43:559–567, 2004

Cho AK, Segal DS: Amphetamine and Its Analogs. San Diego, CA, Academic Press, 1994

Comings DE, Comings BG: A controlled family history of Tourette's syndrome, I: attention deficit hyperactivity disorder and learning disorders. J Clin Psychiatry 51:275–280, 1990

Conners CK, March JS, Frances A, et al: Treatment of attention-deficit hyperactivity disorder: expert consensus guidelines. J Atten Disord 4(suppl):S1–S128, 2001

Cox DJ, Merkel RL, Penberthy JK, et al: Impact of methylphenidate delivery profiles on driving performance in adolescents with attention-deficit/hyperactivity disorder: a pilot study. J Am Acad Child Adolesc Psychiatry 43:269–275, 2004

Croft HA: Physician handling of prescription stimulants. Psychiatr Ann 35:221–226, 2005

Cyr M, Brown CS: Current drug therapy recommendations for the treatment of attention deficit hyperactivity disorder. Drugs 38:1442–1454, 1998

Deutsch CK, Swanson JM, Buell KH, et al: Overrepresentation of adoptees in children with ADD. Behav Genet 12:231–238, 1982

Ding YS, Fowler JS, Volkow ND, et al: Chiral drugs: comparison of the pharmacokinetics of [11C] D-*threo* and L-*threo*-methylphenidate in the human and baboon brain. Psychopharmacol (Berl) 131:71–78, 1997

Dodson WW: Psychostimulants and sleep in adult ADHD. Paper presented at the annual meeting of the American Psychiatric Association, Washington, DC, May 1999

Dodson WW: Treatment of ADHD. Point Counterpoint 2:4, 2003

Dodson WW: Practical daily techniques for the treatment of adult ADHD. Current ADHD Insights 3:11–140, 2004

Dougherty DD, Bonab AA, Spencer TJ, et al: Dopamine transporter density in patients with ADHD. Lancet 354:2132–2133, 1999

Dulcan MK: Using psychostimulants to treat behavioral disorders of children and adolescents. J Child Adolesc Psychopharmacol 1:7–20, 1990

Dulcan MK: Practice parameters for the assessment and treatment of children, adolescents and adults with attention deficit disorder. J Am Acad Child Adolesc Psychiatry 36(suppl):85S–121S, 1997

DuPont RL, Bensinger M: Use and abuse of prescribed CNS stimulants. Psychiatr Ann 35:214–220, 2005

Faraone SV, Wilens T: Does stimulant treatment lead to substance abuse disorders? J Clin Psychiatry 64(suppl):5–13, 2003

Faraone SV, Biederman J, Spencer TJ, et al: Dose-response efficacy of Adderall XR in adults with ADHD. Poster presentation 66 at the 17th annual U.S. Psychiatric and Mental Health Congress, San Diego, CA, November 2004

Feinberg SS: Combining stimulants with monoamine oxidase inhibitors: a review of uses and one possible indication. J Clin Psychiatry 65:1520–1524, 2004

Goldman LS, Genel M, Bezman RJ, et al: Diagnosis and treatment of attention deficit hyperactivity disorder in children and adolescents. JAMA 279:1100–1107, 1998

Gonzalez MA, Pentikis HS, Anderl N, et al: Methylphenidate bioavailability from two extended-release formulations. Int J Clin Pharmacol Ther 40:175–184, 2002

Greenhill LL: The science of stimulant abuse. Psychiatr Ann 35:210–214, 2005

Greenhill LL, Abikoff HB, Arnold LE, et al: Medication treatment strategies in the MTA study: relevance to clinicians and researchers. J Am Acad Child Adolesc Psychiatry 35:1304–1313, 1996

Greenhill LL, Halperin J, Abikoff H: Stimulant medications. J Am Acad Child Adolesc Psychiatry 38:503–512, 1999

Greenhill LL, Pliszka S, Dulcan MK, et al: Practice parameters for the use of stimulant medications in the treatment of children, adolescents and adults. J Am Acad Child Adolesc Psychiatry 41(suppl):26S–49S, 2002

Grinspoon L, Hedblom P: The Speed Culture: Amphetamine Use and Abuse in America. Cambridge, MA, Harvard University Press, 1975

Gutgesell H, Atkins D, Barst R, et al: Cardiovascular monitoring of children and adolescents receiving psychotropic drugs: a statement for healthcare professionals from the Committee on Congenital Cardiac Defects, Council on Cardiovascular Disease in the Young, American Heart Association. Circulation 99:979–982, 1999

Higgins ES, Powell RA: Stimulant abuse and HIPAA: case example. Primary Psychiatry 12:53–56, 2005

Hoffman M: A transdermal form of methylphenidate for the treatment of attention deficit hyperactivity disorder. Paper presented at the annual meeting of the Society for Developmental and Behavioral Pediatrics, Buffalo, NY, February 2003

Hollerman JR, Schultz W: Dopamine neurons report an error in the temporal prediction of reward during learning. Nat Neurosci 1:304–309, 1998

Horrigan J: Effective dosing of stimulants. ADHD Point Counterpoint 3:1–4, 2001

Horrigan J, Barnhill J: Low dose amphetamine salts and adult attention-deficit hyperactivity disorder. J Clin Psychiatry 61:414–417, 2000

Iaboni F, Bouffard R, Minde K, et al: The efficacy of methylphenidate in treating adults with ADHD, in Scientific Proceedings of the American Academy of Child and Adolescent Psychiatry. Philadelphia, PA, American Academy of Child and Adolescent Psychiatry, 1996, pp 27–33

IMS Health: U.S. ADHD market share as a percentage of individual prescriptions (press release). Fairfield, CT, IMS Health, 2004

Jaffe SL: Failed attempts at intranasal abuse of Concerta (letter). J Am Acad Child Adolesc Psychiatry 41:5, 2002

James RS, Sharp WS: Double-blind, placebo controlled study of single-dose amphetamine preparations in ADHD. J Am Acad Child Adolesc Psychiatry 40:1268–1276, 2001

James SP, Mendelson WB: The use of trazodone as a hypnotic: a critical review. J Clin Psychiatry 65:752–755, 2004

Jensen PS, Kettle L, Roper MT, et al: Are stimulants overprescribed? treatment of ADHD in four U.S. communities. J Am Acad Child Adolesc Psychiatry 38:797–804, 1999

Jensen PS, Hinshaw SP, Swanson JM, et al: Findings from the NIMH Multimodal Treatment Study of ADHD (MTA): implications and applications for primary care providers. J Dev Behav Pediatr 22:60–73, 2001

Kay G, Pakull B, Clark TM, et al: The effect of Adderall XR treatment on driving performance of young adults with ADHD. Poster presentation 54 at the 17th annual U.S. Psychiatric and Mental Health Congress, San Diego, CA, November 2004

Keating GM, Figgitt DP: Dexmethylphenidate. Drugs 62:1899–1904, 2002

Kiyatkin EA, Rebec GV: Dopaminergic modulation of glutamate-induced excitations of neurons in the neostriatum and nucleus accumbens of awake, unrestrained rats. J Neurophysiol 75:142–153, 1996

Kooij JJ, Middelkoop HA, van Gils K, et al: The effect of stimulants on nocturnal motor activity and sleep quality in adults with ADHD: an open-label case study. J Clin Psychiatry 62:952–956, 2001

LeFever GB, Dawson KV, Morrow AL: The extent of drug therapy for attention deficit hyperactivity disorder among children in public schools. Am J Public Health 89:1359–1364, 1999

Lopez F, Silva RR, Pestreich L, et al: Comparative efficacy of Ritalin LA, Concerta and placebo in children with ADHD across the school day. Paper presented at the annual meeting of the American Academy of Child and Adolescent Psychiatry, Miami, FL, October 2003a

Lopez F, Silva R, Pestreich L, et al: Comparative efficacy of two once-daily methylphenidate formulations (Ritalin LA and Concerta) and placebo in children with attention deficit hyperactivity disorder across the school day. Paediatr Drugs 5:545–555, 2003b

Low KG, Gendaszek AE: Illicit use of psychostimulants among college students. Psychology, Health, and Medicine 7:283–287, 2002

Markowitz JS, Straughn AB, Patrick KS, et al: Pharmacokinetics of methylphenidate after oral administration of two modified release formulations in healthy adults. Clin Pharmacokinet 42:393–401, 2003

McBurnett K: Safety and efficacy of Concerta, a once-daily OROS formulation of methylphenidate in adolescents with ADHD. Paper presented at the 15th annual CHADD International Conference, Denver, CO, October 2003

McGough JJ, Biederman J, Greenhill LL, et al: Analog classroom assessment of SL1381 for the treatment of ADHD. Poster presentation at the annual meeting of the American Academy of Child and Adolescent Psychiatry, New York, October 2000

MTA Cooperative Group: A 14-month randomized clinical trial of treatment strategies for attention-deficit-hyperactivity disorder. Arch Gen Psychiatry 56:1073–1086, 1999

National Institutes of Health: Diagnosis and Treatment of Attention Deficit Hyperactivity Disorder. NIH Consensus Statement Vol 16 No 2. Bethesda, MD, National Institutes of Health, 1998

Paterson R, Douglas C, Hallmayer J, et al: A randomised, double-blind, placebo-controlled trial of dexamphetamine in adults with attention deficit hyperactivity disorder. Aust N Z J Psychiatry 33:494–502, 1999

Pelham WE Jr, Sturges J, Hoza J, et al: Sustained release and standard methylphenidate effects on cognitive and social behavior in children with ADHD. Pediatrics 131:71–78, 1987

Pliszka SR, Greenhill LL, Crismon ML, et al: The Texas Children's Medication Algorithm Project: report of the Texas Consensus Conference Panel on medication treatment of childhood attention-deficit/hyperactivity disorder: part I: attention-deficit/hyperactivity disorder. J Am Acad Child Adolesc Psychiatry 39:908–919, 2000

Pomerleau OF, Downey KK, Stelson FW, et al: Cigarette smoking in adults diagnosed with attention deficit hyperactivity disorder. J Subst Abuse 7:373–378, 1995

Popper CW, Gammon GD, West SA, et al: Disorders usually first diagnosed in infancy, childhood, or adolescence, in The American Psychiatric Publishing Textbook of Clinical Psychiatry, 4th Edition. Edited by Hales RE, Yudofsky SC. Washington, DC, American Psychiatric Publishing, 2003, pp 833–974

Prince JB, Wilens TE: Pharmacotherapy of adult ADHD, in Clinician's Guide to Adult ADHD: Assessment and Intervention. New York, Elsevier Science, 2002, pp 165–186

Rush C: Subjective effects of modafinil and conventional psychostimulants. Currents in Affective Illness 23:5–9, 2003

Salzman C: The benzodiazepine controversy: therapeutic effects versus dependence, withdrawal and toxicity. Harv Rev Psychiatry 4:279–282, 1997

Shire: Adderall XR (package insert). Wayne, PA, Shire, 2002

Smith BH, Pelham WE, Evans S, et al: Dosage effects of methylphenidate on the social behavior of adolescents diagnosed with attention-deficit/hyperactivity disorder. Exp Clin Psychopharmacol 6:187–204, 1998

Solanto MV: Neuropsychopharmacological mechanisms of stimulant drug action in ADHD. Behav Brain Res 94:127–152, 1998

Spencer T, Wilens T, Biederman J, et al: A double-blind, crossover comparison of methylphenidate and placebo in adults with childhood onset attention-deficit hyperactivity disorder. Arch Gen Psychiatry 52:434–443, 1995

Spencer T, Biederman J, Wilens TE, et al: Adults with attention-deficit/hyperactivity disorder: a controversial diagnosis. J Clin Psychiatry 59(suppl):59–68, 1998a

Spencer T, Biederman J, Wilens TE: Growth deficits in children with attention-deficit/hyperactivity disorder. Pediatrics 102:501–506, 1998b

Spencer T, Biederman J, Wilens TE: Effectiveness and tolerability of Ritalin LA in adults, in Scientific Proceedings of the American Academy of Child and Adolescent Psychiatry. Philadelphia, PA, American Academy of Child and Adolescent Psychiatry, 2000

Spencer T, Biederman J, Wilens TE, et al: Efficacy of a mixed amphetamine salts compound in adults with attention-deficit/hyperactivity disorder. Arch Gen Psychiatry 58:775–782, 2001

Spencer T, Biederman J, Wilens T, et al: Efficacy of methylphenidate in adults with attention-deficit/hyperactivity disorder. Paper presented at the annual meeting of the American Academy of Child and Adolescent Psychiatry, San Francisco, CA, October 2002

Spencer T, Biederman J, Wilens T: Stimulant treatment of adult attention-deficit/hyperactivity disorder. Psychiatr Clin North Am 27:361–372, 2004

Spencer T, Biederman J, Wilens T: A large double blind randomized clinical trial of methylphenidate in the treatment of adults with ADHD. Biol Psychiatry 57:456–463, 2005

Srinivas NR, Hubbard JW, Quinn D, et al: Enantioselective pharmacokinetics and pharmacodynamics of *dl-threo*-methylphenidate in children with attention deficit hyperactivity disorder. Clin Pharmacol Ther 52:561–568, 1992

Stahl SM: Essential Psychopharmacology: The Prescriber's Guide. London, England, Oxford University Press, 2004

Stein MA: Unraveling sleep problems in treated and untreated children with attention-deficit/hyperactivity disorder. J Child Adolesc Psychopharmacol 9:157–168, 1999

Substance Abuse and Mental Health Services Administration: 22 million in U.S. suffer from substance dependence or abuse. Bethesda, MD, Substance Abuse and Mental Health Services Administration, 2003. Available at: http://www.samhsa.gov/news/newsreleases/030905nr_NSDUH.htm. Accessed December 12, 2004.

Swanson JM, McBurnett K, Wigal T, et al: The effect of stimulant medication on children with attention-deficit/hyperactivity disorder: a "review of reviews." Except Child 60:154–162, 1993

Swanson JM, Gupta S, Lam A, et al: Development of a new once-a-day formulation of methylphenidate for the treatment of attention-deficit/hyperactivity disorder: proof-of-concept and proof-of-product studies. Arch Gen Psychiatry 60:204–211, 2003

Swanson JM, Wigal SB, Wigal T, et al: A comparison of once-daily extended-release methylphenidate formulations in children with attention-deficit hyperactivity disorder in the laboratory school (the Comacs Study). Pediatrics 113:206–216, 2004

Takeda Pharmaceuticals: Ramelteon (Rozerem) (package insert). Lincolnshire, IL, Takeda Pharmaceuticals, 2005

The Tourette's Syndrome Study Group: Treatment of ADHD in children with tics: a randomized controlled trial. Neurology 58:527–536, 2002

Tulloch SJ, Zhang Y, McLean A, et al: SLI381 (Adderall XR), a two-component, extended-release formulation of mixed amphetamine salts: bioavailability of three test formulations and comparison of fasted, fed, and sprinkled administration. Pharmacotherapy 22:1405–1415, 2002

Van Dyck CH, Quinlan DM, Cretella LM, et al: Unaltered dopamine transporter availability in adult attention-deficit/hyperactivity disorder. Am J Psychiatry 159:309–312, 2002

Vastag B: Pay attention: Ritalin acts much like cocaine. JAMA 286:905–906, 2001

Volkow ND, Swanson JM: Variables that affect the clinical use and abuse of methylphenidate in the treatment of ADHD. Am J Psychiatry 160:1909–1918, 2003

Volkow ND, Ding Y-S, Fowler JS, et al: Is methylphenidate like cocaine? studies on the pharmacokinetics and distribution in the human brain. Arch Gen Psychiatry 52:456–463, 1995

Volkow ND, Wang G, Fowler JS, et al: Therapeutic doses of oral methylphenidate significantly increase extracellular dopamine in the human brain. J Neurosci 21:RC121, 2001

Volkow ND, Wang G, Fowler JS, et al: Relationship between blockade of dopamine transporters by oral methylphenidate and the increases in extracellular dopamine: therapeutic implications. Synapse 43:181–187, 2002

Volkow ND, Wang G-J, Fowler JS, et al: Evidence that methylphenidate enhances the saliency of a mathematical task by increasing dopamine in the brain. Am J Psychiatry 161:1173–1180, 2004

Weisler RH, Biederman J, Chrisman AK, et al: Long term safety and efficacy of once-daily Adderall XR in adults with ADHD. Paper presented at the annual meeting of the American Psychiatric Association, San Francisco, CA, May 2003

Weiss MD, Weiss JR: A guide to the treatment of adults with ADHD. J Clin Psychiatry 65(suppl):27–37, 2004

Wightman RM, Robinson DL: Transient changes in mesolimbic dopamine and their association with "reward." J Neurochem 82:721–735, 2002

Wilens TE: Update on diagnosis and treatment of attention deficit hyperactivity disorder. Currents in Affective Illness 20:5–12, 2001

Wilens TE: Drug therapy for adults with ADHD. Drugs 63:2395–2411, 2003

Wilens TE: Treatment of pediatric ADHD with stimulants. Paper presented at ADHD Across the Life Span, Boston, MA, March 2005

Wilens TE: ADHD medication mechanism of action: neurotransmitter cause and effect, in The Current and Emerging Role of Alpha-2 Agonists in the Treatment of ADHD, Vol I: ADHD Etiology and Neurobiology. Halbrouck Heights, NJ, Veritas Institute for Medical Education, Inc, pp 16–22, 2006

Wilens TE, Dodson W: A clinical perspective of attention-deficit/hyperactivity disorder into adulthood. J Clin Psychiatry 65:1301–1313, 2004

Wilens TE, Pelham W: ADHD treatment with once-daily OROS methylphenidate: interim 12-month results from a long-term open study. J Am Acad Child Adolesc Psychiatry 42:424–433, 2003

Wilens TE, Spencer T: The stimulants revisited. Child Adolesc Psychiatr Clin N Am 9:573–603, 2000

Wilens TE, Biederman J, Spencer TJ, et al: Stimulants and ADHD. Psychopharmacology (Berl) 15:270–279, 1995

Wilens TE, Biederman J, Spencer T: Attention deficit/hyperactivity disorder across the life span. Annu Rev Med 53:113–131, 2002

Wilens TE, Faraone SV, Biederman J, et al: Does stimulant therapy of ADHD beget later substance abuse? a meta-analytic review of the literature. Pediatrics 111:179–185, 2003

Wilens TE, Hammerness PG, Biederman J, et al: Blood pressure changes associated with medication treatment of adults with attention-deficit/hyperactivity disorder. J Clin Psychiatry 66:253–259, 2005

Wilford BB, Smith DE, Bucher R: Prescription stimulant sales on the Internet. Psychiatr Ann 35:241–252, 2005

Wood DR, Reimherr FW, Wender PH, et al: Diagnosis and treatment of minimal brain dysfunction in adults: a preliminary report. Arch Gen Psychiatry 33: 1453–1460, 1976

CHAPTER 7

TREATING ADHD WITH NONSTIMULANT MEDICATIONS

ALTHOUGH THE CENTRAL NERVOUS SYSTEM (CNS) stimulants are the medications of first choice for adults with ADHD, there are other options.

REASONS TO AVOID THE CENTRAL NERVOUS SYSTEM STIMULANTS

Many patients simply do not want to take CNS stimulants. Having to get the medication, remembering to take it every day, and putting up with side effects is already a chore. Having mixed or negative feelings about the medicine itself makes the situation worse.

> One patient said, "Speed is still speed, whether or not you are prescribing it as medication."

It is a problem if patients or family members disapprove of the stimulants. It is also a problem when they like them too much. If the patient or others in his or her social network are abusing drugs or other substances, proceed carefully. You do not want to worsen a substance abuse situation in a family or social network. Drug-abusing patients who have ADHD must abstain from their substances of choice before receiving any stimulant. If others in the patient's social system abuse drugs, be sure that the patient or his or her friends and relatives do not divert or sell the medication you prescribe. At colleges and universities, for example, there is a brisk market for stimulants, and not just at examination time.

Sometimes patients insist that they have tried the stimulants already and that the medications do not work for them. Before moving away from these agents, however, look fully into the history. Has the patient tried medicines in both the methylphenidate and dextroamphetamine groups? The patient may have tried only a single preparation of one medication, taken less than the optimal dosage, or taken the medication for only a short time. Many adults who were diagnosed with and treated for ADHD have had such experiences, but these occurrences are not a good reason for ruling out the stimulants.

However, at times the stimulants are not the agents of first choice. Sometimes the patient or family members intensely resist using them. Sometimes there is a problem with substance abuse. Some patients have tried the available CNS stimulants at sufficient dosage for sufficient time and simply not found them helpful.

> Abram, a college senior, said, "I was diagnosed with severe ADHD when I was 3. I was completely out of control. I got kicked out of school after school. I even got thrown out of a therapeutic boarding school. Medicine? I was taking Ritalin when I was 4. Since then I've tried every one of the damn CNS stimulants. Long-acting as well as regular. I don't know why people like them. I hate them. They make me feel speedy, and so compulsive."

The ADHD medications that are not CNS stimulants have advantages. They are not drugs of abuse. They do not need a fresh paper prescription every month. The patient does not feel like a felon in front of a hostile pharmacy clerk. The nonstimulants are useful for patients who have current or past substance abuse.

On the other hand, the nonstimulant medications used for ADHD have disadvantages. Patients have to take them regularly every day. The nonstimulant medications do not have the dosage flexibility of the CNS stimulants. Although patients do not abuse nonstimulant medications, the challenge is to have patients keep using them at all. Side effects can pop up the first day or two that the patient takes the medicine, often weeks before he or she knows whether the medication helps.

> "Now let me get this straight," said one male graduate student. "When I take this medicine I may feel sick to my stomach, I may not be able to pee, and...what *exactly* is going to happen to my sex life?"

Even allowing for these problems, some nonstimulant medications clearly help adults and children with ADHD. Others are worth trying. Some medications have not lived up to early hopes. This chapter ends with observations about non–CNS stimulant medications or other substances that patients should avoid.

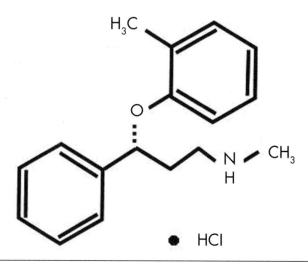

FIGURE 7–1. Chemical structure of atomoxetine (Strattera).

NONSTIMULANT MEDICATIONS EFFECTIVE FOR ADHD

The only nonstimulant medication with the U.S. Food and Drug Administration's (FDA's) official indication for treating attention deficit disorder in adults is atomoxetine (Strattera). The chemical structure of atomoxetine is shown in Figure 7–1. This selective norepinephrine reuptake inhibitor increases the availability of dopamine and norepinephrine in the prefrontal cortex, the brain site for sustained focus and intellectual work (Bymaster et al. 2002). The intended use of atomoxetine was as an antidepressant, but it failed in clinical trials. However, it is helpful with ADHD.

Atomoxetine (Strattera)

Atomoxetine has demonstrated its efficacy in children and adolescents in four acute, randomized, double-blind, placebo-controlled studies. It had a moderate impact on ADHD symptoms and a low incidence of side effects (Spencer et al. 2004). It also helps adults with ADHD. In a double-blind, 6-week, placebo-controlled crossover study of adults with ADHD, 11 of 21 patients treated with Strattera were rated as "much" or "very much" improved. The study design paralleled the earlier studies of methylphenidate and dextroamphetamine in adults (Spencer et al. 1998).

In trials involving a total of 536 ADHD adults who took a mean daily dosage of 95 mg of atomoxetine, symptoms of inattention, hyperactivity, and impulsivity all lessened. Patients taking active medication showed significantly more improvement on all measures than did those on placebo. These patients noted improvements as early as the first week; most responded within 3 weeks. Overall, they rated improvement of their symptoms as moderate. The most frequently used dosage was 90 mg/day (40% of patients); 38% of the participants required more (120 mg/day); and 22% required less (60 mg/day). Patients generally tolerated the medicine well, with just over 20% of patients complaining of dry mouth or insomnia (Michelson et al. 2003).

In an open-label study of adults with ADHD, two-thirds of the participants who took Strattera for 48 weeks showed at least a 30% reduction in symptoms on the Conners' Adult ADHD Rating Scale, a standard rating instrument. They had few side effects. Patients who took Strattera at 40 mg twice a day improved more than did those taking it as a once-daily, 80-mg dose (Biederman et al. 2004). A later report showed that participants maintained their benefits over 97 weeks of administration (Adler et al. 2005).

How Atomoxetine Works

In the synapse, atomoxetine blocks presynaptic transporters. It has a strong affinity with norepinephrine transporters, modest affinity with serotonin transporters, and no affinity with dopamine transporters. Although theoretically a selective norepinephrine reuptake inhibitor, atomoxetine also affects dopamine levels. In the prefrontal cortex, it increases both extracellular norepinephrine and dopamine. It lingers there, providing sustained levels of neurotransmitters for longer than its half-life leads us to expect. Atomoxetine is rapidly absorbed, with peak plasma concentrations within 1–2 hours. Food does not appreciably affect its absorption (Bymaster et al. 2002).

Dosage of Atomoxetine

Strattera is available as 25-, 40-, and 60-mg tablets. Most adult patients tolerate a starting dosage of 40 mg, once a day for a week. If that goes well, increase the dosage to 40 mg twice a day. Some patients prefer the convenience of a single daily dose of 80 mg once a day, as the manufacturer suggests. The twice-daily dosage may cause fewer side effects, but it requires remembering to take the medicine more often. Reassess after the patient has been taking the 80-mg dosage for a month. If the patient is doing well, continue as before. If gains are unimpressive but the patient is tolerating the medicine well, increase the dosage to 100 mg daily (in a single dose or divided doses) and follow up closely.

If side effects are problematic, restart with a lower dosage: 25 mg once a day for a week, 40 mg daily for the next week, and then 80 mg daily. Although some patients profit by taking only 25 mg/day of atomoxetine, a few need the maximum dosage of 120 mg/day. Most adults with ADHD who do well on Strattera take 100 mg/day or less.

Some clinicians use the patient's weight in dosing atomoxetine, starting with the dosage closest to 0.5 mg/kg/day. If the patient tolerates the medication well, after 3–4 days the dosage is increased to 1.4 mg/kg/day. The typical full dosage is 100 mg for a 70-kg adult (155 lbs).

To patients, taking Strattera feels different than taking a CNS stimulant. It is more like taking an antidepressant. Response takes time, side effects may occur before benefits do, and improvement may be gradual and more diffuse. Patients need encouragement to keep taking the medication. A lucky few notice some effect in the first week or so. Most need to take atomoxetine for 1 month or longer before deciding how helpful it is. If it is not helpful within 6–8 weeks, it may not help at all.

Advantages of Atomoxetine

The effects of atomoxetine (Strattera) feel continuous, steady, and stabilizing—unlike the "on" and "off" feelings that patients report with the CNS stimulants, even the long-acting preparations. Patients are not aware of blood level fluctuations. They do not report a "crash" at the day's end, as can occur with stimulants.

Patients do not abuse atomoxetine. In the nucleus accumbens, which largely lacks norepinephrine transporters, dopamine reuptake inactivates dopamine. Unlike the stimulants, atomoxetine does not increase dopamine in this part of the brain, which may be why it lacks abuse potential (Stahl 2004). Patients rarely divert Strattera to others; there is not much street demand for it. Atomoxetine does not interact with alcohol to increase the intoxicating effect.

Atomoxetine has minimal impact on blood pressure and pulse in adults. Children may show a small, transient increase in both blood pressure and pulse. It does not cause cardiac conduction problems. Patients taking it do not need routine electrocardiograms and laboratory tests unless they already have heart disease that requires monitoring (Wernicke and Kratochvil 2002). Abrupt discontinuation, at least in children and adolescents, does not lead to any significant adverse effects (Brown and Wernicke 2002). It is safe in overdose; people do not kill themselves if they take a large amount accidentally or on purpose.

Although no deaths have occurred in patients taking Strattera that were linked to the medicine, there is new concern that it causes liver damage, although rarely.

Patients with bipolar disorder can do well while taking atomoxetine. There is little worry that the drug will precipitate manic episodes. It does not worsen anxiety, so it may be a good choice for the anxious patient. Unlike the CNS stimulants, atomoxetine does not seem to cause or worsen tics (Heil et al. 2002).

A small group of patients may respond better to atomoxetine than to the CNS stimulants. In one study of ADHD children who did not respond to methylphenidate, 51% improved with atomoxetine (Newcorn 2004).

Less sexual drive may occur. Although for most patients that side effect is unwelcome, for others it has advantages.

> Abram reported: "Strattera is great. I can think about my options now instead of just being run by my impulses. I can stay with one girlfriend and enjoy her, instead of feeling like I have to lay every girl on campus. It's a relief."

Disadvantages of Atomoxetine

Less efficacy.   When atomoxetine helps ADHD patients, the impact is usually mild to moderate, less pronounced than when a CNS stimulant is effective. Studies in children comparing atomoxetine with Adderall XR show that more children improve on the CNS stimulant. Parents liked the impact of both medications but preferred that of Adderall XR (Wigal and Steinhoff 2004). Clinical observations of adults with ADHD show a similar pattern.

Delayed onset.   The clinical impact of Strattera is slower than that of the CNS stimulants. In patients who have had symptoms for decades, a few more weeks may make little difference. Having to wait is hard, however, especially when the stimulants are faster.

Concern about suicidal ideation in children.   Six of 1,357 children and adolescents taking Strattera in placebo-controlled trials developed or worsened suicidal ideation. The FDA has required the manufacturers to provide a black box warning to this effect. Experts are skeptical of a causative relationship, however (Pizzi 2005).

Side effects.   Side effects show up promptly, often in the first few days. As is typical for the side effects of most antidepressants, those of atomoxetine tend to lessen with time. Splitting the total dosage into two doses daily can help.

Increased norepinephrine can cause irritability, dry mouth, nausea, decreased appetite, and constipation. In a recent study of children with ADHD, those who took atomoxetine (mean dosage=1.56 mg/kg) had a slight delay of sleep onset at night. However, the delay was significantly longer in participants taking methylphenidate (mean dosage=1.12 mg/kg) (Sangal 2005). Sometimes patients taking atomoxetine feel sedated, and they prefer taking the medication at night. Occasionally they have difficulty starting their urinary stream or even have urinary retention. This affects men more often than women.

> "So that's what that was! I thought I was losing my manhood or something," sputtered one strapping young athlete. His previous doctor had not warned him about the urinary side effects of atomoxetine.

Patients taking Strattera can have sexual side effects: decreased libido, problems with potency, and delay in reaching orgasm or inability to ejaculate.

Children taking atomoxetine show a modest initial slowing of growth velocity, followed by near-normal growth rates during a 2-year exposure (Spencer et al. 2002). Among adults, impact on growth is not an issue.

Some patients taking Strattera alone or with a CNS stimulant have had modest increases in heart rate and blood pressure that were not clinically significant. Patients had no QTc changes on cardiograms when taking atomoxetine. Many prudent clinicians record pulse and blood pressure before starting a patient on Strattera and monitor them as long as the patient takes the medication (Wernicke et al. 2002).

Atomoxetine can damage the liver: in rare cases, a chemical hepatitis and severe liver injury occur. None of about 6,000 patients in clinical trials had this difficulty. However, of the more than 2 million patients who have taken atomoxetine, two treated for several months developed markedly elevated bilirubin and hepatic enzymes. These side effects occurred without other explanatory factors. In one patient, who developed markedly elevated hepatic enzymes and bilirubin levels, these abnormalities recurred when he tried taking atomoxetine again, and stopped when he discontinued it (Lilly Research Laboratories 2004). Such reactions may occur several months after starting therapy with atomoxetine. Laboratory values may worsen for several weeks after the drug is stopped.

Currently we cannot accurately estimate the true incidence of such events. Neither of the reported patients died; both recovered fully and did not require a liver transplant. However, severe drug-related liver injury may progress to acute failure, resulting in the need for a liver transplant or in death. In evaluating patients, note preexisting hepatic risk factors such as chronic persistent hepatitis B and high baseline liver function test values. It is unclear whether routine monitoring of hepatic function is warranted (Spencer 2005). We do need to teach patients signs of liver dysfunction: pruritus, dark urine, jaundice of the skin, yellowed whites of the eyes, right upper quadrant tenderness, and unexplained flu-like symptoms. If they have any of these symptoms, they should immediately notify their clinician, discontinue Strattera, and get laboratory testing of their liver function. Patients taking Strattera who develop any evidence of liver injury should not take the medicine again.

Combining ADHD Medications or Switching to Atomoxetine

Some adults with ADHD doing well on a CNS stimulant may try Strattera also, to see if the combination give a better clinical result. They can simply add it to their stimulant, increasing the Strattera dosage on the usual schedule. It may be a month or more before the impact of the combination is clear. Some patients who like the results of the added Strattera then want to try it as monotherapy. These patients can try doing without their stimulant on two separate weekends. If that goes well, on the third weekend the patient discontinues the stimulant for good and sees if he or she maintains progress on Strattera alone.

Some patients who switch to Strattera continue their stimulant medicine but take less of it, by as much as half. They keep the stimulant handy for a big project or a long workday. Does the patient want to take both medicines indefinitely? Some do, although that complicates their regimen.

> A lawyer patient taking Adderall for his ADHD asked about Strattera, which was helping his son's ADHD. After a month of taking both medications, he reported he liked the combination. He said, "I just feel more…solid." He has continued taking Strattera daily, adding Adderall when he has a brief to finish or another significant deadline to meet.

For patients doing well on atomoxetine alone who want to add a CNS stimulant, prescribe the stimulant according to the usual schedule. Within a few weeks, patients can usually tell if they like the combination. Although Ritalin and Strattera both increase blood pressure and heart rate, in one clinical study the combination had no more impact than either alone (Kratochvil et al. 2002). The prudent clinician, of course, will monitor the patient's vital signs.

There are special precautions about combining a selective serotonin reuptake inhibitor (SSRI) antidepressant and atomoxetine. Fluoxetine (Prozac) and paroxetine (Paxil) inhibit the metabolic pathway with the 2D6 form of the cytochrome P450 system. Adding either of them can raise blood levels of atomoxetine, causing more side effects. If the patient is taking fluoxetine or paroxetine, start with a low dosage of atomoxetine, increase it to the therapeutic dosage, and watch for increased Strattera side effects. Expect to end up using a lower dosage of atomoxetine, perhaps half. This interaction is not a problem for patients taking escitalopram (Lexapro) or sertraline (Zoloft) with atomoxetine.

There is no standard length of treatment with atomoxetine. As with other medications for ADHD, patients may usefully take it for months, years, or indefinitely. ADHD symptoms return gradually after a patient stops taking Strattera. The symptoms do not rebound, as they can after the patient stops a CNS stimulant. When patients stop taking Strattera, they do not have a discontinuation syndrome (Michelson et al. 2002).

A summary of atomoxetine's drug–drug interactions is in Table 7–1.

Cost

At the time of writing, the cost of a month's supply of atomoxetine (40-mg dose, 60 capsules) was $266.99 (pharmacy data, Washington, DC, January 2006). Because atomoxetine is not a controlled substance, the convenience of the medication may somewhat offset its high cost.

Summary

To date, Strattera seems helpful but less effective than the CNS stimulants for adult ADHD patients.

Bupropion (Wellbutrin)

Special qualities of the antidepressant bupropion (Wellbutrin) make it an appealing treatment option for ADHD. The chemical structure of bupropion is shown in Figure 7–2. Bupropion inhibits the reuptake of norepinephrine. Because dopamine is inactivated by norepinephrine reuptake in the frontal cortex, bupropion can increase dopamine there (Stahl 2004). Studies demonstrate that different formulations of bupropion, marketed as Wellbutrin, Wellbutrin SR, and Wellbutrin XL, have similar availability, efficacy, and tolerability (GlaxoSmithKline 2005).

TABLE 7-1.   Atomoxetine (Strattera): drug–drug interactions

Drug name	Recommendations
Acetylsalicylic acid	No dosage adjustment necessary
Albuterol (Proventil)	Additional cardiovascular effects. Administer Strattera with caution to patients taking albuterol po or iv.
Desipramine (Norpramin)	Coadministration safe and well tolerated. No dosage adjustment recommended.
Diazepam (Valium)	No dosage adjustment necessary
Ethanol	No increased adverse events. No dosage adjustment recommended.
Fluoxetine (Prozac) Paroxetine (Paxil)	Plasma concentrations of atomoxetine rise after fluoxetine and paroxetine dosing. You may need to adjust the dosage of Strattera; as little as half may suffice.
Methylphenidate (Ritalin)	Coadministration safe and well tolerated, with no additive effects on heart rate or blood pressure.
Omeprazole (Prilosec) or magnesium and aluminum hydroxide (Maalox) agents affecting gastric pH	These did not affect the bioavailability of Strattera. No serious or clinically adverse events reported during coadministration. No dosage adjustment necessary.
Monoamine oxidase inhibitor (MAOI) medications	DO NOT COADMINISTER WITH STRATTERA. Treatment with Strattera can begin 2 weeks after discontinuing an MAOI.
Phenytoin (Dilantin)	No dosage adjustment necessary
Warfarin (Coumadin)	No dosage adjustment necessary

Source.   Prescribing information. Indianapolis, IN, Eli Lilly Company, 2002.

Bupropion Helps Patients With ADHD

At standard dosages, bupropion is moderately helpful for ADHD in children, adolescents, and adults (Spencer et al. 2004). It does not have an FDA indication for such use, however. Typical effective dosages are up to 200 mg twice a day of Wellbutrin SR and up to 450 mg once a day of the newer Wellbutrin XL preparation. Many patients prefer the convenience of once-daily dosing and the smoother delivery of the medication over time, which Wellbutrin XL provides.

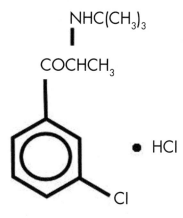

FIGURE 7–2.   Chemical structure of bupropion (Wellbutrin).

In one study, 19 adults with ADHD took an average dosage of 360 mg of bupropion (as Wellbutrin) daily for 6 weeks. Seventy-four percent had moderate to marked improvement. At follow-up 1 year later, most of the responders were still doing well (Wender and Reimherr 1990). An open-label study of bupropion in adults with ADHD showed that the medication, at an average dosage of 360 mg/day, maintained its usefulness for at least 1 year (Wender and Reimherr 1990). A controlled drug-comparison study with methylphenidate showed that bupropion produced "comparable but consistently weaker" therapeutic results (Barrickman et al. 1995).

In another 6-week study, adult ADHD patients took up to 200 mg twice a day of sustained-release bupropion. They had a 42% reduction in symptoms, compared with the 24% reduction in a matched group who took placebo (Wilens et al. 2001). In a third study using sustained-release bupropion to treat ADHD in adults, the antidepressant demonstrated efficacy comparable to that of methylphenidate (Kuperman et al. 2001).

A recent study evaluated the efficacy of bupropion (as Wellbutrin XL) in 162 adults ages 18–60 years who had moderate to severe ADHD (Wilens et al. 2004). Matched patients received either placebo or Wellbutrin XL at dosages ranging from 150 mg/day to 450 mg/day over the 8-week study. The mean final dosage of bupropion was 309 mg/day; most patients were titrated to the maximum dosage of 450 mg/day. By the end of week 2, more patients had responded to bupropion than to placebo across the three main symptom areas of ADHD. These results continued throughout the study. Both observers and participants agreed that bupropion had greater efficacy than placebo. Participants taking bupropion noted improvement across 12 hours, daily. Mean reductions in Clinical Global Impression–Severity scale scores were significantly greater with extended-release bupropion starting at week 4 and continuing thereafter. Although four patients discontinued treatment with bupropion because of side effects, none of the patients taking placebo did. Participants generally rated side effects as mild.

Bupropion causes no cardiac conduction delays. There are few drug–drug interactions, and the side effect burden is generally low. It has less impact on sexual drive and function than most other antidepressants. The medication can feel unpleasantly activating; some patients feel jittery, restless, or edgy. Anxious patients, in particular, tolerate it poorly. Some develop headaches and dizziness. A few patients taking the medication develop panic attacks. If patients take Wellbutrin too late in the day, they may have difficulty getting to sleep or maintaining sleep. For ADHD patients, many of whom already have trouble sleeping, this worsening is a major drawback.

Other side effects result from the peripheral actions of norepinephrine: dry mouth, constipation, anorexia, and sweating. Bupropion also can raise blood pressure. Although the increase is usually small, any change is of concern in a patient with marginal or high blood pressure. Routinely take the blood pressure of patients before starting them on any form of bupropion, and monitor it thereafter. Rarely, bupropion is associated with hypomania or mania. Typically, side effects subside with time.

The most serious problem with bupropion is the increased risk of seizure. Although patients taking any amount of Wellbutrin can have a seizure, the incidence rises significantly at dosages higher than 450 mg/day, the highest recommended dosage.

Using Bupropion (Wellbutrin) for ADHD

Before prescribing bupropion for ADHD, be sure the patient knows that this is an off-label use of the medication. The patient must understand the consequences of the medication not having the official FDA indication for ADHD. Patients should indicate that they understand and agree to use bupropion in this manner. Having them sign a standard form to this effect is prudent clinical practice.

Patients trying Wellbutrin XL for adult ADHD start by taking 150 mg each morning. If they tolerate the medicine well, after a week they increase it to 300 mg/day. After 3 or 4 weeks, if the patient's response is weak but he or she is tolerating the medicine well, the dosage may be increased to the maximum recommended, 450 mg/day. Remind patients not to break or chew the Wellbutrin XL tablets, because doing either changes the controlled-release properties. Patients who find Wellbutrin helpful for their ADHD take it indefinitely.

> Although she had been stably abstinent from alcohol for many years, Faith, age 55, was scared to use any CNS stimulants to treat her newly diagnosed ADHD. "I'm worried about my sobriety," she said. Wellbutrin XL, at 300 mg/day, noticeably improved her ADHD symptoms as well as her mood.

Combining Wellbutrin with stimulants may provide good results. Patients using both medications may be able to lower the dosage of their stimulant. The two may complement each other, especially in impulsive/aggressive patients. However, monitor blood pressure carefully in patients taking the combined regimen.

Bupropion is another option for ADHD adults who have a past history of substance abuse, especially of CNS stimulants. One study examined its use for adults with ADHD and cocaine dependence (Levin et al. 2002). In a 12-week study, subjects who took 400 mg daily of bupropion in three divided doses showed significant reductions in ADHD rating scale scores ($P<0.01$). Interestingly, the 11 men studied showed an average reduction in cocaine craving of 46% ($P<0.001$) over the study period.

Another study showed similar good results with adults with ADHD who had abused alcohol and other substances. Participants, who took sustained-release bupropion at an average daily dosage of 379 mg, had significant reductions in ADHD symptoms and no evidence of increased substance use or craving. There was, however, a high attrition rate: 13 of 32 subjects dropped out during the 6-week study (Prince et al. 2002).

Wellbutrin may help ADHD patients with other complications, such as those patients who have coexisting bipolar disorder. In one 6-week study of adults with ADHD and bipolar II disorder, taking bupropion correlated with improved clinical status. The participants, who took a mean dosage of 363 mg of Wellbutrin SR a day, showed a 53% decline in ADHD symptoms. No study patients developed a manic episode. In fact, they showed a 74% reduction in manic symptoms as assessed on the Young Mania Rating Scale (Wilens et al. 2003). Bupropion may be a good choice in ADHD patients with comorbid mood instability or in adults with cardiac abnormalities (Gelenberg et al. 1991).

Several clinical studies have used bupropion and sustained-release bupropion to treat depressed patients with bipolar disorder. Reports of mania or hypomania have generally been infrequent; when mania or hypomania occurs, it is usually in a patient with a history of mania. The risk of mania with bupropion seems no greater than that reported for other antidepressants (GlaxoSmithKline 2005). It is always prudent, however, to regulate bipolar patients on a mood stabilizer carefully when prescribing antidepressants for them.

As of January 2006, a month's supply of Wellbutrin XL (300 mg dose, 30 tablets) cost $160.99. The generic equivalent, sustained-release bupropion (150 mg dose, 60 tablets) cost $129.99 (pharmacy data, Washington, DC, January 2006).

Although bupropion in its various formulations seems less effective than the stimulants for the treatment of ADHD, it is a welcome option. Further controlled investigations, especially comparing extended-length bupropion (Wellbutrin XL) with other agents, will make clear where this medicine ranks in managing ADHD in adults.

Other Nonstimulant Medications

Tricyclic Antidepressants

Tricyclic antidepressants are helpful for ADHD in adults as well as in children. Although they are all in the same chemical family, individual tricyclics have different affinities for different neurotransmitters. Desipramine (Norpramin) and nortriptyline (Pamelor) tend to block the norepinephrine transporter, whereas imipramine (Tofranil) is more selective for serotonin. In a 6-week, placebo-controlled trial in 41 adults with ADHD, 19 took desipramine at an average daily dosage of 150 mg. Thirteen of the desipramine-treated patients were "much" or "very much" improved by the end of the study. None of the 22 patients given placebo improved (Wilens et al. 1996).

Although tricyclics do moderate ADHD symptoms in adults, they produce less improvement than the CNS stimulants, and many patients complain about side effects (Wender 1997). Consider using a tricyclic for ADHD if patients are having disruptive rebound effects from psychostimulants, if there is a potential or real problem with drug abuse, if sleep disturbance is prominent, or if there is a strong family history of mood disorder (Popper et al. 2003).

If prescribing a tricyclic antidepressant for an adult with ADHD, start with 25–50 mg/day of desipramine (Norpramin) or its equivalent. Depending on the side effects, increase the dosage by 20%–30% every 4–5 days. Patients may complain of dry mouth, that they are constipated, or that they have difficulty starting their urinary stream. They can have postural hypotension. They may gain unwanted weight. The tricyclics can also depress sex drive, inhibit potency, and delay orgasm. A rare but dangerous side effect of these agents, especially desipramine, is cardiac arrhythmia or heart stoppage. Children seem especially vulnerable (Biederman 1998).

Monoamine Oxidase Inhibitors

Although effective for treating ADHD, the monoamine oxidase inhibitor (MAOI) antidepressants are even harder to use than the tricyclics. Medicines such as phenelzine (Nardil) and tranylcypromine (Parnate) are so difficult to work with that few patients, or psychiatrists, want to deal with them. Patients taking them have to watch what they eat and drink. Tyramine-containing substances in many foods and drinks can combine with an irreversible MAOI to cause a dangerous acute rise in blood pressure. The MAOIs are associated with weight gain and insomnia. Other medications effective for ADHD are far simpler to use and less dangerous.

A new formulation of an MAOI may prove useful for ADHD. In a phase II trial of a selegiline transdermal system, 18 male ADHD patients, ages 6–17, showed significant improvement on standard rating scales. The usual dietary restrictions on foods and liquids containing tyramine were unnecessary, because selegiline (Eldepryl) inhibits brain monoamine oxidase A and B activity without significantly inhibiting gut monoamine oxidase A. This lack of reaction in the gastrointestinal tract reduces the probability of acute hypertensive reactions from dietary tyramine (Blob and Sharoky 2002).

Venlafaxine (Effexor, Effexor XR)

Venlafaxine is an antidepressant with complex action. At low dosages it acts as a serotonin reuptake inhibitor. At 150–300 mg/day, it affects both serotonin and norepinephrine. At even higher dosages, it affects dopamine transporters as well (Stahl 2004). There is little solid evidence that this drug helps patients with ADHD.

However, in one study of adults with ADHD, one-third of the patients took venlafaxine alone, one-third took stimulants alone, and one-third took both medications. All the groups responded, but the venlafaxine patients and the antidepressant-plus-stimulant group did better than those taking stimulants alone (Hornig and Rohan 2002). The long-acting preparation of venlafaxine, Effexor XR, provides smoother delivery of the medication, with few side effects. As can bupropion, venlafaxine can raise blood pressure. Checking blood pressure before treatment and then periodically during treatment is good practice. Combination therapy of Effexor XR with stimulants may help patients with ADHD who are anxious or depressed. These patients bear particularly closer watching for elevations in blood pressure.

Modafinil (Provigil, Sparlon)

Modafinil provides relief for patients who have narcolepsy, sudden daytime episodes of intense sleepiness or sleep. Modafinil affects more discreet areas of the CNS than do the stimulants. It works through the hypothalamus, activating neurons containing orexin A and orexin B, neuropeptides that mediate normal wakefulness and vigilance. Modafinil increases the rate of metabolism in the amygdala and the hippocampus (Engber et al. 1998). Whether modafinil affects the dopamine transporter at all is still unclear (Swanson 2003).

Clinical trials of modafinil (Provigil) in adult ADHD patients have had mixed results. In one study, some patients took a mean daily dosage of 207 mg, whereas others took dextroamphetamine (Dexedrine) at a mean daily dosage of 22 mg. Patients on both active medications improved. Patients taking modafinil generally tolerated it well, occasionally complaining of insomnia, irritability, muscle tension, or lessened appetite (Taylor and Russo 2000). At least in preliminary studies, modafinil lacks the high abuse potential of the stimulants (Jasinski 2000). Studies continue to assess modafinil's effectiveness. The FDA has officially approved its use in children with ADHD (Wilens 2006).

If prescribing modafinil for ADHD, have the patient start taking 50 mg twice daily. Over a week, increase the dosage to a maximum daily dosage of 400 mg. At 100–400 mg/day, Provigil alone may relieve the core ADHD symptoms of distractibility, hyperactivity, and inattention.

Some patients can distinguish the activating effect of modafinil from the focusing effect of the stimulants. In theory, combining the two may have an advantage; some clinicians report good results (Taylor and Russo 2000).

Alpha-Agonists

Clonidine (Catapres) and guanfacine (Tenex) lower blood pressure by affecting norepinephrine. Since the mid-1980s, clinicians have prescribed these medications for ADHD in children. Their role is still controversial, especially if they are the only medication in the regimen.

Clonidine helps relieve ADHD-related insomnia; it is also useful for children who have motor tics. Side effects include headaches and dizziness. A meta-analysis of clonidine in children with ADHD showed some impact, but less than with the psychostimulants (Connor et al. 1999). Although the drug may well help behavioral hyperactivity and impulsivity, as well as moderate aggressive behavior and insomnia, it does not treat the attentional problems of childhood ADHD (van der Meere et al. 1999). At least four patients using Catapres and a CNS stimulant at the same time have died (Swanson et al. 1995). Abrupt discontinuation can cause significant tachycardia, hypertension, and severe ventricular tachyarrhythmias in adults. Even when adults taking clonidine taper the drug slowly, they may have a pronounced rebound of plasma norepinephrine and blood pressure that may last up to 2 weeks after discontinuation (Pliszka 2001).

Guanfacine (Tenex) is longer acting and less sedating than Catapres. Guanfacine particularly impacts norepinephrine receptors in the prefrontal cortex and the locus coeruleus. By modulating the activity of the locus coeruleus, guanfacine may indirectly fine-tune central dopaminergic systems. Preliminary reports show more focused attention. In one clinical study, adults with ADHD received up to 2 mg of guanfacine or 20 mg of dextroamphetamine once daily. Participants reported similar improvement in ADHD symptoms on either medication (Taylor and Russo 2000).

Alpha-agonists may be useful only for the adult with ADHD for whom the clinician can diagnose hyperactivity immediately on first meeting (Doyle et al. 2002). With these agents, monitor blood pressure and heart rate before and during treatment. New evidence suggests that alpha-agonists may improve cognitive function in patients with ADHD. A new formulation of guanfacine is being tested with this benefit in mind (Wilens 2006).

Nicotine and Cholinergic Agents

Persons with ADHD more often smoke cigarettes, and they start smoking them earlier, than their non-ADHD peers. Are they using nicotine to treat their ADHD? Nicotine and related compounds increase the brain availability of acetylcholine, a neurotransmitter important for executive function. Nicotine improves attention and arousal and acts as an indirect dopamine agonist.

In one study, patients with ADHD improved when they wore a nicotine patch. Using nicotine itself is difficult because of side effects at the dosages needed (Shytle et al. 2002). Preliminary evidence was encouraging from a study of adults with ADHD that tested ABT-418, a novel cholinergic activating agent that has structural similarities to a nicotine analogue. Modest improvements in ADHD resulted with a dosage of 35 mg once a day; less severely ill patients improved more. There were mild side effects. Overall, the results encouraged researchers to do more trials with ABT-418 and similar compounds (Wilens et al. 1999).

Some clinical trials use other cholinergic agents, including some that treat Alzheimer's disease, such as Aricept (donepezil) and Reminyl (galantamine). In one clinical study, children with ADHD who took Reminyl, 14 mg twice daily for 1–15 weeks, showed significant improvement (Wilens 2003). A similar study in children with ADHD using donepezil (Aricept) produced some improvement that was not statistically significant. Data are not yet available on the use of these agents in adults with ADHD.

Selective Serotonin Reuptake Inhibitors

Generally the SSRIs do not help patients who have ADHD, although there are isolated case reports of good results (Doyle et al. 2002). SSRIs may even make ADHD symptoms worse by activating behavior or by producing a hypomanic switch. The sexual dysfunction and weight gain associated with these medications also make them unattractive to ADHD patients.

Beta-Blockers

Beta-blockers, which lower blood pressure and slow pulse, have long been used to treat hypertension. At the right dosage, patients feel calmer; professional musicians and actors often use them for performance anxiety or stage fright. One study used the beta-blocker propranolol (Inderal) to treat temper outbursts and "residual" attention deficit disorder in adults (Mattes 1986). In that study, 85% of patients improved, but at astronomically high dosages of the medication (average=528 mg/day). Most clinicians would be reluctant to prescribe propranolol at that dosage for any reason.

Antipsychotic Medications

Antipsychotics may be suitable for adults with ADHD in the context of significant comorbidity, including tic disorders, bipolar disorder, or psychotic conditions (Popper et al. 2003).

MEDICATIONS AND SUBSTANCES THAT ARE INEFFECTIVE FOR ADHD

Many other medications have proved unsatisfactory for treatment of ADHD. Among *ineffective* medications are lithium carbonate; amantadine; L-dopa; the amino acid precursors D,L-phenylalanine and L-tyrosine; and caffeine. Other approaches and substances tested and found *ineffective* include antiyeast medications, dietary manipulation, herbal treatments, and megavitamin therapy (Spencer et al. 1996).

Many dietary supplements are popular because they are "natural." However, when tested for use with ADHD, they have not relieved symptoms. Among these *ineffective* substances are acetylcarnitine; ginkgo biloba; DMAE (dimethylaminoethanol); phosphatidylserine, a CNS phospholipid; and essential fatty acids such as gamma-linolenic acid and docosahexaenoic acid (DHA) (Greydanus et al. 2003). Adult ADHD patients should not take herbal products because of these substances' unreliable purity, potential side effects, and lack of efficacy (Greydanus and Patel 2002).

SUMMARY

- Use medications other than the CNS stimulants when the patient has tried them and found them wanting or when there is a problem with substance abuse.
- Atomoxetine (Strattera), which has the FDA indication, keeps norepinephrine and dopamine available in the frontal cortex. Response to atomoxetine in adults with ADHD is moderate. It occurs after the patient has been taking it for some weeks at the therapeutic dosage, which is usually 80 mg/day. Side effects, including nausea and urinary hesitancy, are usually mild to moderate and ease with time. Atomoxetine is not a drug of abuse.
- Bupropion (Wellbutrin) is also moderately helpful. Other agents to consider include nonserotonergic antidepressants such as tricyclic antidepressants, MAOI antidepressants, and modafinil (Provigil). Some patients benefit from a combination of medications. Alone or with a CNS stimulant, these drugs provide the clinician and patient with a wide range of options. Surely other medications for ADHD will follow (Biederman et al. 2003).

REFERENCES

Adler LA, Spencer TJ, Milton DR: Long-term, open-label study of the safety and effectiveness of atomoxetine in adults with attention-deficit/hyperactivity disorder: an interim analysis. J Clin Psychiatry 66:294–299, 2005

Atomoxetine (Strattera) for ADHD. Med Lett Drugs Ther 45:11–12, 2003

Barrickman LL, Perry PJ, Allen AJ, et al: Bupropion versus methylphenidate in the treatment of attention-deficit hyperactivity disorder. J Am Acad Child Adolesc Psychiatry 34:649–657, 1995

Biederman J: A 55-year-old man with attention-deficit/hyperactivity disorder. JAMA 280:1086–1092, 1998

Biederman J, Chrisman AK, Dodson W, et al: Adult ADHD. Medical Crossfire 5:29–45, 2003

Biederman J, Spencer TJ: Pharmacotherapy of adults with attention-deficit/hyperactivity disorder, in Treating ADHD in Adult Patients. Hasbrouck Heights, NJ, MedLearning, 2004, pp 5–9

Blob L, Sharoky M: Safety and efficacy of the selegiline transdermal system for ADHD. Paper presented at the annual meeting of the American Academy of Child and Adolescent Psychiatry, San Francisco, CA, October 2002

Brown WJ, Wernicke J: Tolerability of atomoxetine discontinuation. Paper presented at the annual meeting of the American Academy of Child and Adolescent Psychiatry, San Francisco, CA, October 2002

Bymaster FP, Katner JS, Nelson DL, et al: Atomoxetine increases extracellular levels of norepinephrine and dopamine in prefrontal cortex of rat: a potential mechanism for efficacy in attention deficit/hyperactivity disorder. Neuropsychopharmacology 27:699–711, 2002

Clinical psychopharmacology online. Currents in Affective Illness 22:6, 2003

Connor DF, Fletcher KE, Swanson JM: A meta-analysis of clonidine for symptoms of attention-deficit hyperactivity disorder. J Am Acad Child Adolesc Psychiatry 38:1551–1559, 1999

Doyle BB, Wender PH, Montauk SL, et al: ADHD in adults. Medical Crossfire 4:30–40, 2002

Engber TM, Dennis SA, Jones BE, et al: Brain regional substrates for the actions of the novel wake-promoting agent modafinil in the rat: comparisons with amphetamine. Neuroscience 87:905–911, 1998

Gelenberg AJ, Bassuk EL, Schoonover SC: The Practitioner's Guide to Psychoactive Drugs, 3rd Edition. New York, Plenum Medical, 1991

GlaxoSmithKline: Data on file. Research Triangle Park, NC, GlaxoSmithKline, 2005

Greydanus DE, Patel DR: Sports doping in the adolescent athlete: the hope, hype, and hyperbole. Pediatr Clin North Am 49:829–855, 2002

Greydanus DE, Pratt HD, Sloane MA, et al: ADD/ADHD: interventions for a complex behavioral disorder. Pediatr Clin North Am 48:622–626, 2003

Heil SH, Holmes HW, Bickel WK, et al: Comparison of the subjective, physiological, and psychomotor effects of atomoxetine and methylphenidate in light drug users. Drug Alcohol Depend 67:149–156, 2002

Hornig R, Rohan W: Comparative effects of venlafaxine and stimulants in adult attention-deficit hyperactivity disorder. Am J Psychiatry 159:1202–1205, 2002

Jasinski DR: An evaluation of the abuse potential of modafinil using methylphenidate as a reference. J Psychopharmacol 14:53–60, 2000

Kratochvil CJ, Neilingenstein JH, Dittmann RR, et al: Atomoxetine and methylphenidate treatment in children with ADHD: a prospective, randomized, open-label trial. J Am Acad Child Adolesc Psychiatry 41:776–784, 2002

Kuperman S, Perry PJ, Gaffney GR, et al: Bupropion SR vs. methylphenidate vs. placebo for attention deficit hyperactivity disorder in adults. Ann Clin Psychiatry 13:129–134, 2001

Levin FR, Evans SM, McDowell M, et al: Bupropion treatment for cocaine abuse and adult attention-deficit/hyperactivity disorder. J Addict Dis 21:1–16, 2002

Lilly Research Laboratories: product information: atomoxetine (Strattera). Indianapolis, IN, Lilly Research Laboratories, December 2004

Mattes JA: Propranolol for adults with temper outbursts and residual attention deficit disorder. J Clin Psychopharmacol 6:299–302, 1986

Michelson D: Atomoxetine for attention-deficit/hyperactivity disorder. Paper presented at the 49th annual meeting of the American Academy of Child and Adolescent Psychiatry, San Francisco, CA, October, 2002

Michelson D, Allen AJ, Busner J, et al: Once-daily atomoxetine treatment for children and adolescents with ADHD. Am J Psychiatry 159:1896–1901, 2002

Michelson D, Adler I, Spencer T, et al: Atomoxetine in adults with attention deficit hyperactivity disorder: two randomized, placebo-controlled studies. Biol Psychiatry 53:1120–1132, 2003

Newcorn J: Differential response to stimulants and to atomoxetine. Paper presented at the annual meeting of the American Academy of Child and Adolescent Psychiatry, Washington, DC, October 2004

Pizzi DM: Black box for suicide possible for Strattera, but experts question actual risk. CNS News, November 2005, p 15

Pliszka SR: Comparing the effects of stimulant and nonstimulant agents on catecholamine function: implications for theories of ADHD, in Stimulant Drugs and ADHD: Basic and Clinical Neuroscience. Edited by Solanto MV, Arnsten AFT, Castellanos FX. New York, Oxford University Press, 2001, pp 332–352

Popper CW, Gammon GD, West SA, et al: Disorders usually first diagnosed in infancy, childhood, or adolescence, in The American Psychiatric Publishing Textbook of Clinical Psychiatry, 4th Edition. Edited by Hales RE, Yudofsky SC. Washington, DC, American Psychiatric Publishing, 2003, pp 833–974

Prince JB, Wilens TE, Waxmonsky JG, et al: An open study of bupropion SR in adults with ADHD and substance abuse disorders. Poster presentation at the annual meeting of the American Psychiatric Association, Philadelphia, PA, May 2002

Sangal B: Effects of methylphenidate and atomoxetine on sleep in ADHD children. Paper presented at the annual meeting of the Associated Professional Sleep Societies, Philadelphia, PA, January 2005

Shytle RD, Silver AA, Wilkinson BJ, et al: A pilot-controlled trial of transdermal nicotine in the treatment of ADHD. World J Biol Psychiatry 3:150–155, 2002

Spencer T: Nonstimulant pharmacotherapy of ADHD. Paper presented at ADHD Across the Life Span, Boston, MA, March 2005

Spencer T, Biederman J, Wilens T, et al: Pharmacotherapy of attention-deficit hyperactivity disorder across the lifecycle: a literature review. J Am Acad Child Adolesc Psychiatry 35:409–432, 1996

Spencer T, Biederman J, Wilens T, et al: Effectiveness and tolerability of atomoxetine in adults with ADHD. Am J Psychiatry 155: 693–695, 1998

Spencer T, Heiligenstein JH, Biederman J, et al: Results from two proof-of-concept, placebo-controlled studies of atomoxetine in children with attention-deficit/hyperactivity disorder. J Clin Psychiatry 63:1140–1147, 2002

Spencer T, Biederman J, Wilens T: Nonstimulant treatment of adult attention-deficit hyperactivity disorder. Psychiatr Clin North Am 27:373–383, 2004

Stahl SM: Essential Psychopharmacology: The Prescriber's Guide. London, England, Oxford University Press, 2004

Swanson JM: Modafinil treats core symptoms of ADHD. Paper presented at the annual meeting of the American Psychiatric Association, San Francisco, CA, May 2003

Swanson JM, Flockhart D, Udrea D, et al: Clonidine in the treatment of ADHD: questions about safety and efficacy. J Child Adolesc Psychopharmacol 5:301–304, 1995

Taylor FB, Russo J: Comparing modafinil to dextroamphetamine in the treatment of adult ADHD. New Research 657. Paper presented at the annual meeting of the American Psychiatric Association, Chicago, IL, May 2000

van der Meere J, Gunning B, Stemerdink N: The effect of methylphenidate and clonidine on response inhibition and state regulation in children with ADHD. J Child Psychol Psychiatry 40:291–298, 1999

Wender PH: Attention-deficit hyperactivity disorder in adults: a wide view of a widespread condition. Psychiatr Ann 27:556–562, 1997

Wender PH, Reimherr FW: Bupropion treatment of ADHD in adults. Am J Psychiatry 147:1012–1020, 1990

Wernicke JF, Kratochvil CJ: Safety profile of atomoxetine in the treatment of children and adolescents with ADHD. J Clin Psychiatry 63(suppl):50–55, 2002

Wernicke JF, Kratochvil CJ, Dittman RR, et al: Overview of the safety data of atomoxetine. Paper presented at the 49th annual meeting of the American Academy of Child and Adolescent Psychiatry, San Francisco, CA, October 2002

Wigal S, Steinhoff K: Analog classroom study of amphetamine extended release and atomoxetine for ADHD. Paper presented at the annual meeting of the American Academy of Child and Adolescent Psychiatry, Washington, DC, October 2004

Wilens TE: Galantamine in childhood ADHD. Paper presented at the annual meeting of the American Academy of Child and Adolescent Psychiatry, Miami, FL, October 2003

Wilens TE: ADHD medication mechanism of action: neurotransmitter cause and effect, in The Current and Emerging Role of Alpha-2 Agonists in the Treatment of ADHD, Vol I: ADHD Etiology and Neurobiology. Hasbrouck Heights, NJ, Veritas Institute for Medical Education, pp 16–22, 2006

Wilens TE, Biederman J, Prince J, et al: Six-week, double-blind, placebo-controlled study of desipramine for adult attention deficit hyperactivity disorder. Am J Psychiatry 153:1147–1153, 1996

Wilens TE, Biederman J, Spencer TJ, et al: A pilot-controlled trial of ABT-418, a cholinergic agent, in the treatment of adults with ADHD. Am J Psychiatry 156:1931–1937, 1999

Wilens TE, Spencer TJ, Biederman J, et al: A controlled clinical trial of bupropion for attention deficit hyperactivity disorder in adults. Am J Psychiatry 158:282–288, 2001

Wilens TE, Prince JB, Spencer TJ, et al: An open trial of bupropion for the treatment of adults with attention-deficit hyperactivity disorder and bipolar disorder. Biol Psychiatry 54:9–16, 2003

Wilens TE, Hudziak JJ, Connor DF, et al: A controlled trial of extended-release bupropion in adult ADHD. Poster presented at the annual meeting of the American Psychiatric Association, New York, May 2004

C H A P T E R 8

COMPREHENSIVE TREATMENT OF THE ADULT WITH ADHD

CLINICIANS NEED TO FULLY evaluate the patient. We need to not only make a diagnosis and go through the differential diagnosis but also to identify which factors in the patient's life enhance treatment and which interfere with it. Which impairments result from which symptoms? Clinical decisions include deciding which impairments to treat, in which order, and how to monitor the patient's response. Many patients think their ADHD only affects them in specific tasks, such as doing their job or studying, but the disorder is there 24 hours a day, 7 days a week. Do they need medication continuously or intermittently? With these and other questions in mind, clinicians can construct a treatment plan that addresses specific targets and note how well the patient responds.

GOAL: ENHANCE RESILIENCE

In recent years, many clinicians have changed and sharpened their therapeutic focus. Formerly it was identifying and dealing with psychopathology. Now the therapeutic goal is both more positive and ambitious: enhancing the patient's resilience. Evidence from a variety of sources, including the study of prisoners of war, shows that persons with specific characteristics have a more adaptive, or even masterful, approach to life (Charney 2006). *Resilience* is the term that best conveys these adaptive characteristics as an entity.

Charney (2006) recently outlined 10 critical psychological elements and characteristics of resilience (Table 8–1). The list starts with optimism, the characteristic of having a positive attitude. Next is altruism,

TABLE 8–1. Components of resilience

Optimism
Altruism
A moral compass
Faith and spirituality
Humor
A role model
Social supports
Facing fear
A life mission
Training

Source. Charney D: "The Psychobiology of Resilience to Extreme Stress." Grand Rounds, Department of Psychiatry, Boston, MA, Massachusetts General Hospital, January 2006.

the quality that suffuses interpersonal generosity. In helping or reaching out to others, we help and strengthen ourselves. Having a moral compass, a set of beliefs that cannot be shattered, is another important characteristic of resilient persons. Related to that factor is faith and spirituality. Some persons express their faith in an established religion or set of religious practices, with prayer and worship services as important elements. For others, spirituality is less defined, less formal, but no less real and no less sustaining. Not surprisingly, humor is a prominent characteristic of resilient people. It enables them to bear, even triumph over, what otherwise would overwhelm or destroy them. The next characteristic of the resilient person is having a role model. Lucky persons have many role models among their parents, siblings and other relatives, teachers, clergy, bosses, coworkers, and friends. Instinctively or deliberately, the resilient among us look for and find role models. Social supports are important, too. Having contact with others you can trust, with whom you can share your most troubled, difficult thoughts and feelings, is another source of strength. Resilient persons find ways to face their fears. They keep forcing themselves to leave their comfort zone, to try new ways of being. They have a mission in life, a sense of their talents and gifts, and a determination to make the most of them. Finally, resilient persons find training, either formally or in varied experiences, to develop and enhance their personal characteristics and their sense of life mastery.

As clinicians, we can work with all our patients to help them become more resilient. That goal has special relevance when working with adults who have ADHD.

TABLE 8–2. Five clinical task areas

Psychoeducation	Teach the patient about ADHD as a neurodevelopmental problem with psychological and social consequences
Comorbid conditions	Address complicating psychiatric conditions[a]
Medication	Establish a stable, effective regimen and ensure adherence[b]
Psychotherapy	Improve the patient's executive functions and feeling state
Environmental interventions	Suggest effective changes in work and social settings

[a]See Chapter 9 ("Comorbid and Treatment-Refractory ADHD").
[b]See Chapters 5–7 ("Treating Adult ADHD With Medication: Introduction," "Treating ADHD With Central Nervous System Stimulants," and "Treating ADHD With Non-stimulant Medications," respectively).

FIVE CLINICAL TASKS

Comprehensive treatment of patients with ADHD involves five clinical task areas: psychoeducation, comorbid conditions, medication, psychotherapy, and environmental interventions (Table 8–2).

TREATMENT STAGES

As with any patient, treating the adult with ADHD begins with assessment and diagnosis and then moves to active treatment. If the patient stabilizes, the next phase is maintenance. Treatment may need reactivation if the patient regresses or if life stresses mount. Ending treatment is the task of termination, which may be indefinite for ADHD patients. Effective treatment often means including significant others and collaborating with other caregivers. It may require referral for specialized treatment, such as cognitive-behavioral therapy (CBT) or psychodynamically oriented psychotherapy in individual or group settings. It may require couples or family treatment. Patients may need complementary mental health professionals such as coaches, social workers, and career or vocational counselors.

The following clinical case, which incorporates material from several patients, illustrates the issues in comprehensive treatment.

> Roger, age 22, sought treatment as he started law school, saying, "I can't study. Instead, I'm watching sports on cable TV or hitting porn sites on the Internet. I'm anxious, and I can't get to sleep. If I flunk out, I won't

be able to face my dad, who's a hotshot corporate lawyer. None of my friends from college are here. I played varsity soccer in college, but now all I do is jog occasionally. Weekends, I've gotten drunk with some classmates. A couple of times I've smoked weed, but I know that's stupid."

"I was the class cutup in school. My parents were always on me for my messy room and my lousy grades. My pediatrician had me evaluated for ADHD when I was 8, but my father wouldn't let me take Ritalin. At college, the professors were flexible about deadlines. Adderall from a friend helped me cram before exams."

"I banged up my mother's car three or four times when I was in high school. The cops never caught my friends and me racing. In college I was careful not to drive when I was drinking or doing weed. I have talked myself out of a bunch of speeding tickets, though."

"In college I volunteered for a poverty law program, which was great, and it got me thinking about law school. With an intensive LSAT prep course and some more Adderall, I scored well enough to get in."

"My social life? I've always been horny. I first had sex when I was 12. In college my girlfriend wouldn't take birth control pills, and I hate condoms. She got pregnant and had an abortion, but then she got pregnant again. She had a second abortion, which I felt bad about, and we broke up. After her, I dated around. None of those girls got pregnant, but I got herpes."

Roger agreed to have me talk with his mother by telephone. She said, "When he was little he was so wild that he spent 3 years in preschool instead of 2. He's less hyperactive now, but he's still disorganized. He's like me, that way. I'm sure my brother has severe ADHD, but he has never been treated." She sent a copy of the psychologist's evaluation from grade school, which diagnosed Roger with ADHD, combined type, and report cards in which Roger was called "erratic" and "an underachiever."

Roger had had symptoms since childhood. His inattention and impulsivity caused difficulty in his academic and social life. On the Adult ADHD Self-Report Scale, he scored a total of 49 out of 72 total points, with 28 points in the "inattentive" range and 21 points in the "hyperactive/impulsive" range. On the Brown Adult Attention Deficit Hyperactivity Disorder Scale, he scored 86, well into the "highly probable" range.

Roger had ADHD, combined type (314.01), and adjustment disorder with anxious and depressed mood (309.28); rule out alcohol abuse (305.00) and cannabis abuse (305.20). Although impulsive and immature, he did not have a personality disorder. His general health was good, other than genital herpes. Moderately stressed, he was facing academic demands without a supportive social network. His global assessment of function was 65. His Clinical Global Impression–Severity score was 4, moderately ill.

STAGE ONE: ASSESSMENT AND DIAGNOSIS

Psychoeducation

The adult with ADHD must come to terms with the diagnosis before medication or other remedies can be tried. ADHD is a neurodevelopmental problem with psychological and social consequences. It is not a character flaw or a moral failing. Until the patient can understand that fact, and collaborate effectively in treatment, he or she will suffer unnecessarily—so will those people near and dear to him or her.

Patients usually have many problem areas and weaknesses. It is important to recognize and capitalize on their strengths as well.

> Seeing his problems in the context of ADHD made Roger's individual and family history more coherent. Although he recognized his weaknesses, he also knew that he was personable and energetic. His competitiveness worked well for him in college, on the soccer field, and in helping clients. A career in law might benefit him and others as well. He liked that combination.

Comorbid Conditions

The following are examples of common problems that may need to be treated before addressing the ADHD. (See Chapter 9, "Comorbid and Treatment-Refractory ADHD."

Anxiety and Affective Disorders

> Roger's symptoms were situational. Other than sleeping badly and studying ineffectively, he was functioning. His energy, appetite, and libido were normal. The assessment process helped him stabilize, and he decided against medication to help him sleep.

Substance Abuse

> Roger insisted that he only used marijuana occasionally. I would not treat him with central nervous system (CNS) stimulants unless he stopped smoking it, and he quit entirely. He agreed not to drink alcohol at all until he had stabilized and was doing well in his studies.

Medication

"With regard to core symptoms of ADHD, we do not yet have a treatment modality that is not pharmacological" (Biederman et al. 2003, p. 7). Some patients, however, strongly prefer dealing with ADHD without medication.

> Roger was reluctant to take medication daily. However, the CNS stimulants had helped him study in college. Given his urgency about law school, he agreed to try medicine systematically.

Psychotherapy

Persons with ADHD have psychological issues. For many patients, the assessment and diagnosis process means accepting the symptoms they have had forever. Others, who seemed to do fine as children, stumble when they grapple with the changes and challenges of adulthood.

Adults who have one or more children diagnosed with and successfully treated for ADHD often consider the diagnosis for themselves. They take hope from their child's improved function. Others have struggled for years, sensing that they were different but resisting the labels of "stupid," "lazy," or "immature." For these patients, finding that they have ADHD is a relief. Their problems have a pattern and a name and treatments that may help.

ADHD patients have a wide range of symptoms. Some gifted patients perform their work brilliantly but at a high emotional price. Others who are less talented work less effectively, at the last minute. The most severely ill may not be able to work well at all. At all points on the spectrum of severity, it is hard for ADHD adults to feel good about themselves. A fortunate few ride their creative thinking and resourceful ways to success. Often unconventional or entrepreneurial, they do not want or need treatment. Many others struggle every day not to feel depressed and demoralized. ADHD is more than just its core features. Poor self-esteem, dysfunctional relationships, and dissatisfaction at work—these are common. Adults with ADHD all have psychological issues—but only some patients will need, and profit by, psychotherapy. Do they need such treatment? If so, which psychotherapy or combination of therapies will work best?

Patients beginning treatment take stock: what has happened to them because they did not have treatment earlier? They have psychological grief work. Some get stuck in depression that requires treatment before they can progress. Others acknowledge the impact of ADHD on their earlier life but then move on promptly.

> Roger said, "Maybe I could have done better, but maybe not. I'm so stubborn. I don't like having ADHD, but it's better than thinking of myself as just a jerk."

After clinicians specify the diagnosis (or diagnoses) on the DSM-IV-TR (American Psychiatric Association 2000) axes, questions may linger. What are the patient's underlying assumptions about himself or herself? What life goals does he or she have? What strengths and weaknesses? How mature is the patient?

Some clinicians use psychodynamic formulations to fill out their understanding. This approach requires assessing the patient's developmental level, assessing his or her ego defense mechanisms, and making clear any preconscious or unconscious motives.

> Engaging but immature, Roger had no history of sustained intellectual effort. Although law school was a considered choice, it meant competing with his father on many levels. Roger had always avoided such competition. His relationships with women were intense and short. Acting out was his principal ego mechanism; he also used avoidance and denial. Although he minimized his substance use, he acknowledged it. When confronted, he did stop. He was a shrewd observer of others, and he had a lively sense of humor. At his best, he sublimated and showed altruism.

Clinicians using a cognitive-behavioral approach look for the patient's schema (i.e., the patient's characteristic thoughts, feelings, and actions) (Beck et al. 1990). Happy, effective individuals do not need to consider their schemas, but ADHD patients struggling to succeed need to know about their internal operations. They may have specific negative beliefs, such as "I jump from one thing to another" or "I can't concentrate." Over time, these beliefs can become an overwhelming load of negativity: "I'm an idiot." In situations in which they fumbled before, persons with ADHD see themselves as inept. Sadness, guilt, and anxiety flood them. As they assess a situation, they exaggerate the likelihood of a bad outcome or underestimate their capacity to cope.

In challenging situations, unable to think rationally and positively, many adults with ADHD spiral downward. They may distract themselves with exercise, computer games, or social interactions. The distractions may themselves turn into problems, such as binge eating or imprudent sex. When they are in a downward slide, adults with ADHD may choose behavior that looks like fun but is often self-destructive. If a patient feels ashamed and depressed after attempting a task and failing, he or she might do something nonessential instead. When circumstances or deadlines push the patient, he or she is unprepared. Worse, the patient may decide the task is hopeless and not even try (McDermott 2000).

> Roger dealt with his feelings of failure by distraction and diversion: by watching sports, drinking more, and masturbating. When he had trouble studying, he castigated himself. Instead of learning to push through his discomfort, he turned away from his books, making failure more likely. He went to bed late and then rushed to class, sleepy and disorganized.

Adults with ADHD may not realize how destructive their cognitive avoidance is. If they can acknowledge their thoughts and fears, they and their clinician can discuss how to break tasks into smaller steps. When patient and clinician meet again, they review. This approach compels the patient to start any part of the dreaded task. Even thinking about beginning is better than paralysis.

> At a complete standstill, Roger decided to try studying in the law school library for 15 minutes. The first time he tried, he did not even manage to get to the library. Instead he was flooded with self-recriminations: he would end up a failure, like his uncle. When he reviewed his thinking, he said, "This is ridiculous!" On his next attempt he went to the library and studied for half an hour before he started criticizing himself. Even so, he recognized that he could do some work.

Patients need realistically hopeful ways of thinking about ADHD. Some authors have proposed that ADHD is an advantage in life (Hartmann 1996). Although that may be true for some, most adults with ADHD who seek treatment view themselves as flawed rather than as gifted. It helps to emphasize that there is much that patients can do to improve their life. The "positive psychology" of Seligman and colleagues has much to offer adults with ADHD (Seligman 2002). Patients need strategies to counter their long-held assumptions and beliefs. They need to practice using their new, strength-oriented view of themselves.

> Looking back, Roger saw that he had some accomplishments and loyal, enthusiastic friends. His energy, upbeat personality, and ability to think on his feet were all assets. He thought that he would be a good lawyer, if he could ever get through law school.

Environmental Interventions

Early in treatment, the clinician can make recommendations about the patient's external environment that can help him or her find the right balance of structure and freedom. This may include referral for vocational testing or other career guidance.

> Roger started using a personal digital assistant (PDA) to schedule himself. Playing on a coeducational soccer team gave him energy, and he slept better. As an added benefit, at soccer he found a new girlfriend, Lauren.

Progress is not simply putting more structure into the patient's life. Too much structure can be burdensome and annoying. The patient wants a good balance between structure and spontaneity.

We discussed Roger's getting an ADHD coach. He liked the concept but disliked the idea of seeing (and paying) another professional. Instead, he said, "How about Lauren? She's 'Miss Organization.' She will get me on schedule." He was right; Lauren was glad to help out.

STAGE TWO: ACTIVE TREATMENT

Psychoeducation

Patients need to retain an accurate picture of their disorder. Under stress, reverting to old thinking may destabilize them.

Comorbid Conditions

Watch for comorbid conditions that may develop or intensify under stress and require active intervention.

> With active treatment of his ADHD, Roger's anxiety and depressive feelings subsided. He stopped smoking marijuana entirely; his only alcohol was beer after his weekly soccer game.

Medication

Sometimes patients are fortunate and rapidly find a good medication regimen.

> When he tried medication, Adderall XR, Roger swiftly improved. Within a few weeks, we found that a once-daily dose of 30 mg worked well for him. He could read for sustained periods ("even civil procedures!" he exulted). His apartment was no longer so chaotic, and he did a better job of abstracting and reviewing cases. His Clinical Global Impression–Improvement scale score was 2, much improved.

Other patients struggle. See Chapter 5 ("Treating Adult ADHD With Medication"), Chapter 6 ("Treating ADHD With Central Nervous System Stimulants"), and Chapter 7 ("Treating ADHD With Nonstimulant Medications") for medication approaches.

Psychotherapy

Patients need help keeping their attention where it belongs. They can hyperfocus on what interests them, often having problems pulling themselves away. Events that impact our assumptions about ourselves usually engage us more than other situations. This is certainly true for adults who have ADHD. Every time a person attends to something emotionally charged, he or she reinforces its importance. This focus can be intensely pleasurable, as in falling in love. The process can also be painful, if the patient fails to do something he or she regards as important.

Patients often struggle to develop an authentic self. Many adults with ADHD hide feelings of turmoil and inadequacy behind a facade of competence. Others cannot even manage to look competent. The therapeutic task is not so much helping ADHD adults to become someone else as it is helping them to "become fully who they are" (Solden 2002).

> Roger's negative self-talk was a mantra: "I'll flunk out. Everyone will know I'm an idiot. I'm tired of being the 'likable but not very bright jock.' How about 'capable young lawyer on his way up,' instead?" he asked.

ADHD patients have significant cognitive problems. Often they cannot keep their sense of perspective. An emotionally compelling aspect of a situation may get their attention, when what they need is to assess the whole. They have problems setting priorities. They may stay hyperfocused on one option, or jump from one to another, losing the big picture. Their impulsivity leads them to jump to conclusions quickly. This happens when dysfunctional beliefs rise more rapidly and forcefully than other ones. It is hard to reach alternative, more adaptive, conclusions (McDermott 2000).

The opposite of cognitive impulsivity, obsessiveness, can also occur. ADHD adults can get stuck in maladaptive ways of thinking or behaving. They ruminate. Their habitual responses, called "overdeveloped" strategies, do not serve them well (Beck and Freeman 1990). For example, a parent angry at a repeatedly late teenager may keep him or her from going out for a while. However, reacting to any conflict by grounding the teenager backfires; it is an "overdeveloped" strategy. Restraint and emotional tolerance, the better parental response, is an "underdeveloped" strategy. When provoked, ADHD adults may not respond thoughtfully and moderately. Impulsive and easily frustrated, they can get hostile and aggressive. Even when ADHD adults control their temper (backing off from an overdeveloped strategy), they may not be able to be reasonable and yet assertive (using an underdeveloped strategy).

Usefulness of Cognitive-Behavioral Approaches

Clinicians may not have the time, energy, and expertise for all the patient's psychological needs. For example, should the clinician consider referral for formal cognitive and behavioral treatment, if that is not in his or her own repertoire? Cognitive treatment helps patients redirect their attention, activate their beliefs in productive ways, and change how they feel. CBT targets behavioral habits and social skills. Patients learn strategies such as stepwise problem-solving, self-monitoring, time management, self-organizational techniques, and anger management (Dulcan 1997). The strong scientific base and problem-solving approach of CBT make it appealing to persons with ADHD. CBT clearly helps children with ADHD, and it has much to offer adults (Hinshaw and Erhart 1991).

Process of Cognitive-Behavioral Treatment

CBT begins with a needs assessment. What are the problems, and what are the goals? Once those are clear, then the therapist and patient develop a plan. When patients can focus their attention, direct their behavior, and control their feelings internally, they can do a better job of changing their external environment.

One cognitive technique is known by the acronym "SPEAR," for "Stop, Pull back, Evaluate, Act, and Reevaluate." In trying situations, patients may need to repeat this sequence to control themselves and their reactions. Another cognitive technique addresses the common complaint that adults with ADHD "forget and lose everything." By the time they put an object down, they are thinking of something else. They need to register the object in their short-term memory by telling themselves where they are putting the object as they place it (e.g., "The car keys are in the wicker basket in the downstairs bathroom"). Behavioral interventions give patients alternative strategies, for example, to prioritize among tasks. Patients can write one task on an individual file card until they have a pile of tasks. Then they go through them all, selecting the highest-priority item. They put that card aside and repeat the process until they have one pile with the items in proper priority (McDermott 2000).

Typically, the clinician gives patients specific tasks between sessions. During follow-up meetings, the two review difficulties and setbacks as well as progress. Out of that review come new approaches. The more specific the patient's goals, the likelier that CBT will be helpful. The typical course is 8–12 weekly sessions, but many patients need more. Initially some patients carry a card that lists skills they practice daily. When patients find that they have become accustomed and familiar with the skills, they review the card weekly. If they slip, then they can go back to the daily schedule (McDermott 2000).

As patients finish CBT, they review how to make their new skills habits. Issues and problem areas persist; what changes is the patients' ability to deal with them. If patients lapse, they regroup, renew their coping skills, and get back on track. Beating themselves up is futile. What works better is looking into what triggered the lapse. Was it the return of an old belief, such as "I'm an idiot; what's the use?"? They can address that with the skills they learned in treatment. If they repetitively lapse, or if they do not understand how or why they trip up, some additional sessions of CBT may help.

In one study of 26 adults with ADHD who had CBT, most did well. Of these patients, 85% were taking medication in combination with their CBT; they felt the combination helped. At the end of their treatment, 69% were rated as "much improved" to "very much improved." The average number of treatment sessions was 36 (Wilens et al. 2002). Other studies validate the usefulness of CBT for adults with ADHD as well.

CBT has been helpful in group as well as in individual settings. One group approach to ADHD adults came from dialectical behavior therapy, a CBT for patients with borderline personality disorder. The structured set of 13 units included education about ADHD, depression and its treatment, better ways of controlling impulses and dysfunctional behavior, improved stress management, and approaches to improving relationships. At the end of treatment there were no dropouts; participants improved mood and had fewer ADHD symptoms (Hesslinger et al. 2002).

One group of researchers is evaluating the results of ongoing CBT. Participants are adults with ADHD who all have a partial response to medication. In the study, half the patients simply continue their medication; half do CBT as well. The 10-week CBT treatment has three core modules and several optional ones. The first module teaches organizational and planning skills. In the second module, patients deal with distractibility. From life experience, each patient knows how long he or she can pay attention; each task segment must fall within that concentration time limit. In the third module, patients work on restructuring their negative, dysfunctional thought patterns. Other, optional modules include dealing with procrastination, anger management, and other issues. Preliminary results show that patients with added CBT have significantly fewer ADHD symptoms and less global severity than those who just continue taking medication.

In recent years, CBT has become increasingly popular. However, succeeding at it requires active, sustained work, which some patients do not want to do or cannot manage to do. Cognitive reframing or trying to change behavior patterns may not help intensely symptomatic patients. They may need some relief or stabilization from medication before they can successfully use CBT.

Outside of major urban centers it may be difficult to find qualified CBT practitioners. An additional difficulty for some patients is that some insurance programs do not consider CBT a reimbursable or medical expense.

Other Useful Psychotherapies

There are patients who will need, and profit by, other forms of psychotherapy such as psychodynamic or insight-oriented treatment. In the pressure for quick fixes, there is often too little of the "meaningful interpersonal work that leads to change and growth in a person's character" (Wishnie 2005, p. 38). Sometimes, sustained, intensive psychotherapy best addresses the difficulties. The need for such treatment often becomes clear in the process of interacting with the patient.

Adults with ADHD, like others, have transference to their clinicians. Positive transferential reactions can make treatment proceed better, unless they are too intense. Negative transference, on the other hand, may require exploration in treatment if it interferes with progress. The clinician's attending to countertransference, especially when patients are failing to progress, can be particularly instructive (see Chapter 4, "Allies in Treatment").

Enlisting Family and Significant Others in Treatment

It is often worthwhile to include key family members in the treatment process. Their being allied with the clinician enhances the chances of success.

> Once he was doing better in law school, Roger brought in his parents. His father, still hostile to the diagnosis of ADHD and to medication for it, admitted that Roger was "finally starting to grow up." After the meeting, heartened by her son's progress, his mother finally got treatment for her own ADHD.

The family is a natural group setting for effective CBT. Using behavioral principles, a family can learn to negotiate and solve problems together (Dulcan 1997).

Environmental Interventions

The clinician continues making suggestions about the patient's environment. These suggestions may help in simple ways, or the changes may be complex—helping a patient find a new way of living or a new kind of work.

> At my urging, Roger established regular hours for studying and for exercise and socializing. He used his PDA to organize his life and sent himself e-mail messages about deadlines. He looked forward to earning a good salary as a lawyer, while having an outlet for his competitiveness and his idealism.

STAGE THREE: MAINTENANCE

In the maintenance phase, the clinician helps the patient sustain good function and remains alert to signals of trouble. There are now longer intervals between visits.

Psychoeducation

The clinician continues to reinforce the basic messages about ADHD. ADHD is an ongoing vulnerability, but it does not mean that the patient is stupid, lazy, or bad.

Comorbid Conditions

During major life transitions, patients often intensify their comorbid symptoms. Work and social issues are important. If comorbid symptoms increase, treatment may have to be more active.

> As he approached final examinations during his first year of law school, Roger said that he was not smoking pot but that he was drinking more. His girlfriend, Lauren, nagged him about it. He became defensive and insisted that his drinking was not dangerous. Although he would not commit to abstinence, he agreed that two drinks would be his maximum on any occasion. He would not drink more often than twice a week. That plan worked, and his relieved girlfriend verified his story.

Medication

During the maintenance phase the patient should have a stable, effective medication regimen. However, changed circumstances change medication needs.

> Most days, Roger felt that one dose of Adderall XR gave him the help he needed to concentrate and to study. As exams approached, his day

lengthened. His concentration lagged in the early evening. After discussing the options, he agreed to try a small supplemental dose of Adderall in the afternoon. This enabled him to keep studying but did not interfere with his sleep. Once exams were over, he kept a small supply of supplementary Adderall but rarely used it.

Psychotherapy

In the maintenance phase of treatment the patient should be doing stably well. Treatment should focus on the patient's doing his or her best.

> As Roger made progress, he lashed himself less often for his failings. "I'm not on law review, but I'm smart enough," he said. He felt that his interpersonal skills would serve him well. School was stressful, and when he was under pressure, he tended to fall behind. Now, however, he restored his emotional and functional balance rapidly, rather than going into a tailspin.

Environmental Interventions

The maintenance phase of treatment can be particularly productive for changes in the patient's environment. His or her greater stability is a good launching pad for changes.

> After his first year in law school, Roger interned with a big firm. Although the firm paid top dollar, it made huge demands. He was criticized for his sloppiness about detail and his lateness with paperwork. He said, "I want to be a litigator, but I still want to have a life."
>
> The summer after his second year, he worked in a small firm where he felt more at home. The firm's tradition of pro bono work appealed to him. His supervisor complimented him on work well done, while keeping after him about what he needed to improve. A number of the lawyers played squash for fast exercise, and Roger's athletic skills served him well in this new sport.

STAGE FOUR: REACTIVATION

Patients with ADHD who are having a life crisis, faced with a challenge or with a setback, can regress and become intensely symptomatic. Some patients fail to make the needed progress. The clinician then reactivates treatment, which may need to change in several areas.

> After he graduated, Roger joined the small firm. His mentor told him that staff lawyers had to pass the bar examination. Rationalizing that serving clients came first, he avoided studying and flunked the exam.

He was deeply worried that he would be fired, although he was working long hours. Once again, he drank heavily on weekends. He excori-
ated himself. "It's official. I am a loser. I'm working my ass off, but they
may fire me. Lauren and I are fighting a lot, especially because I've been
drinking more, again." His Clinical Global Impression–Improvement
scale score was 6, much worse. He needed reminding that his ADHD
was an ongoing problem and that he had strategies he could put back in
place.

Psychoeducation

In a crisis, the patient often reverts to former irrational self-criticism.
The clinician needs to help him or her regain emotional equilibrium.

Comorbid Conditions

In a crisis, prior comorbid symptoms can flare or new ones can appear.
These require assessment to see how destructive the symptoms are. The
comorbid conditions may require treatment.

> Roger was depressed and anxious again, but his energy level, appetite,
> and libido were unchanged. Although demoralized, he did not feel
> helpless or hopeless. We reconsidered medication for his symptoms. He
> agreed that he would take antidepressant medicine if he did not start
> feeling and doing better within a few weeks.
>   I directed him to stop drinking entirely and to go to Alcoholics
> Anonymous. Although resentful, he agreed to go, and what he heard
> there impressed him. He said, "Alcohol doesn't run my life—but I don't
> want to end up like the people at that meeting." He decided not to drink
> for at least 1 year.

Medication

Reactivating treatment calls for reassessing the patient's needs. Is part
of the reason for the setback a failure of the medication regimen? Does
it need to change?

> Roger felt that his poor performance on the bar examination had little to
> do with his drug regimen. However, he had stopped using supplemen-
> tary Adderall in the afternoon. When he restarted that, he could work
> better and still study in the evening. We discussed an alternate CNS
> stimulant, but he liked both forms of Adderall. He liked the option of
> taking the extra, shorter-acting form, if he chose. He resisted trying
> Strattera, because he did not like having to take medicine every day.
> Hearing that Strattera might dampen his sex drive or impair his potency
> sealed his opposition to it.

Psychotherapy

A setback causes old issues and old feelings to resurface. Patients may need active treatment to deal with cognitive avoidance and self-criticism. Key relationships suffer. Often the relationship with a significant other needs investigation.

> After Lauren threatened to leave Roger, I met with them both. She said, "The bar exam is important, but so am I." She had been reading about ADHD and its impact on couples. Reluctant to lose her, he agreed to invest more in the relationship.

Environmental Interventions

When the patient is in crisis, the clinician can intervene more effectively than usual. The patient may be more willing and able to implement changes.

> I pushed Roger to deal directly with his work problems. Reluctantly, he confided to his firm mentor that he had ADHD and proposed that he take 4 weeks off without pay to study. The partner told Roger the firm wanted him, but if he flunked the examination again he would get fired. Roger was granted the unpaid leave time to study. When he went back to the office, he had help from an assistant to keep him on track. With the new regimen in place, he passed the bar exam on his second attempt.

STAGE FIVE: ENDING TREATMENT (TERMINATION)

Some adults with ADHD may do stably well, so they do not need medication or other therapeutic measures. In finishing treatment, the patient and clinician review progress and plan for the future. The two consider what the patient will do if he or she becomes symptomatic again.

For many adults with ADHD, however, treatment is ongoing. Those whose regimen is stable and whose progress is steady only need brief meetings at 3-month intervals.

> Roger has now established himself, but other challenges lie ahead. Will Lauren stay with him? If they marry and have children, will one or more of them have ADHD? He still quarrels with his dad; how will Roger be as a father? He can predict problem points. "When I'm up for partner I may get down on myself, and then I may avoid doing work." If problems come up, however, Roger has skills to deal with his shortcomings. More important, he is in a field that plays to his strengths. His Clinical Global Impression–Improvement scale score is now 2, much improved.

SUMMARY

- Effectively treating adults with ADHD requires that the clinician do more than simply prescribe the right amount of the right medication. These patients profit by psychological treatment as well. Psychotherapeutic tasks vary with the stage of treatment: assessment and diagnosis, active treatment, maintenance, reactivation, and termination. In providing psychological treatment, psychiatrists differ in their interests, training, and practice patterns. Decide which therapeutic tasks you will do and which to refer to others.
- In working with adult ADHD patients, clinicians enhance patients' executive function. Identify patients' weaknesses and vulnerabilities. More important, help patients see and build on their strengths. CBT has many applications for adult ADHD patients. Other treatment approaches have much to offer.
- Rare is the adult patient who has only ADHD as a psychiatric disorder. Other conditions, such as affective and anxiety disorders, substance abuse, and personality disorders, have psychotherapeutic needs. At times individual treatment is best; at others, group, couples, or family treatment is indicated.

REFERENCES

American Psychiatric Association: Diagnostic and Statistical Manual of Mental Disorders, 4th Edition, Text Revision. Washington, DC, American Psychiatric Association, 2000

Beck AT, Freeman A: Cognitive Therapy of Personality Disorders. New York, Guilford, 1990

Biederman J, Chrisman AK, Dodson W, et al: Adult ADHD: spelling out the clinical strategies. Medical Crossfire 12:1–18, 2003

Charney D: The psychobiology of resilience to extreme stress. Grand rounds, Boston, MA, Massachusetts General Hospital, January 2006

Dulcan M: Practice parameters for the assessment and treatment of children, adolescents and adults with attention deficit hyperactivity disorder. J Am Acad Child Adolesc Psychiatry 36(suppl):85S–121S, 1997

Hartmann T: Beyond ADD. Grass Valley, CA, Underwood Books, 1996

Hesslinger B, Tebartz van Elst L, Nyberg E, et al: Psychotherapy of attention deficit hyperactivity disorder in adults: a pilot study using a structured skills training program. Eur Arch Psychiatry Clin Neurosci 252:177–184, 2002

Hinshaw S, Erhart D: Attention deficit hyperactivity disorder, in Child and Adolescent Therapy: Cognitive-Behavioral Procedures. Edited by Kendall P. New York, Guilford, 1991, pp 98–122

McDermott SP: Cognitive therapy of adults with attention-deficit/hyperactivity disorder, in Attention-Deficit Disorders and Comorbidities in Children, Adolescents, and Adults. Edited by Brown TE. Washington, DC, American Psychiatric Press, 2000, pp 569–606

Seligman MEP: Authentic Happiness. New York, Free Press, 2002

Solden S: Journeys Through ADDulthood. New York, Walker Publishing, 2002

Wilens TE, McDermott SP, Biederman J, et al: Cognitive therapy in the treatment of adults with ADHD: a systematic chart review of 26 cases. Journal of Cognitive Psychotherapy 3:48–53, 2002

Wishnie HA: Working in the Countertransference: Necessary Entanglements. Lanham, MD, Rowman & Littlefield, 2005

CHAPTER 9

COMORBID AND TREATMENT-REFRACTORY ADHD

ADHD AND COMORBIDITY

Discussing ADHD as a single entity helps define the disorder and delineate its characteristics. However, ADHD impairments typically co-occur with other disorders, with a frequency that greatly exceeds chance. Comorbid conditions worsen the life impact of one condition and darken treatment outcomes in adults who have ADHD (Brown 2000b). These conditions contribute to therapeutic failure (see "Refractory ADHD" later in the chapter).

Estimates of comorbidity come from comparing the incidence of two disorders in a population and then determining the incidence of one disorder among persons who have the other. With ADHD, comorbidity is the rule rather than the exception. That is what one would expect in adults who, marked and scarred by their life journey, have not yet been treated for their ADHD. The high level of comorbidity in patients suggests that rather than "one ADHD," we are dealing with a group of conditions with different etiologies, risk factors, and outcomes.

When the clinician considers comorbidities, the best tool is the patient's developmental history. How has the patient done, over a lifetime? ADHD typically begins in childhood, as do some of the comorbid conditions. Developmentally ADHD presents early, often by age 3 or 4 years. Conduct disorders and other psychiatric illnesses tend to present later. As expected, the rate of comorbidity increases with age. For example, in the Multimodal Treatment Study of Children With Attention Deficit Hyperactivity Disorder, only 31% of the participating children (ages 8–12 years) presented with ADHD alone. Most had one or more comorbid problems, including oppositional defiant disorder (40%), anxiety (34%), conduct disorder (14%), tics (11%), and mood disorders (4%) (MTA Cooperative Group 1999). ADHD, often the initial problem, is usually the continuous one. Comorbidities such as disorders of anxiety or mood may be present or recurrent, but they are less likely to be continuous.

Psychiatrists trained to treat only adults may lack the developmental perspective of child and adolescent psychiatrists. We may miss the ADHD in adults because we do not include it in our differential diagnosis. An estimated 20%–25% of adult outpatients—a substantial percentage—with depression, anxiety, or substance abuse have ADHD as well (Wilens et al. 2004). The disorder also occurs in patients who have Tourette's disorder, dissociative disorders, personality disorders, drug withdrawal (especially cocaine), and varied medical conditions and cognitive brain syndromes (Dulcan 1997). In effect, look for ADHD in any adult patient, especially those who are not responding well to treatment for other disorders.

Similarly, expect to find other psychiatric problems in adults who have ADHD. Over their lifetime, they are *two to five times* as likely to have anxiety, depression, or substance abuse as those without ADHD (Adesman et al. 2003; Mannuzza et al. 1991). About three-quarters of adults with ADHD report interpersonal problems, compared with about half of control subjects (G. Weiss and Hechtman 1993). In one clinic for adults with ADHD, only 12% of the patients had no other DSM-III-R (American Psychiatric Association 1987) Axis I diagnoses (Shekim et al. 1990).

Full and accurate documentation is important. Different disorders have symptoms in common. Most patients who have both ADHD and one or more comorbid diagnoses maintain their ADHD diagnosis even if the clinician subtracts their overlapping symptoms (Milberger et al. 1995). It is harder to keep treatment goals clear and priorities straight with these patients. Comorbidity darkens prognosis. The cardinal rule is "treat what's worst, first" (Wilens 2005).

Most adults with ADHD have other psychiatric disorders. Sometimes recognizing and treating the ADHD lights up the person's whole life. Anxiety and depression fade away. At other times, the coexisting problems require treatment before the clinician can address the ADHD. Does the patient have one disorder, or more than one? Sometimes the symptoms are not from another disorder; they are from inadequately treated ADHD. Has the patient had adequate trials of adequate amounts of representative medications from both classes of stimulants? Is the patient following treatment guidelines? Is the timing of his or her medication optimal? Does the patient have full treatment, including psychological and social interventions, or just medication? Are side effects causing irritation and rebound symptoms that he or she interprets as depression or anxiety?

Treatment regimens for patients with ADHD and comorbid psychiatric disorders often require the patient to take more than one medication. Although multiple medications may be necessary, remember that ADHD adults struggle with complex regimens. Each change in medication dosage or schedule can lead to fresh forgetting. Simpler is better.

ADHD AND AFFECTIVE DISORDERS

Major Depressive Disorder

The DSM-IV-TR (American Psychiatric Association 2000) diagnostic criteria for ADHD and disorders of mood overlap considerably. Of the nine items for major depressive disorder (MDD), several apply to ADHD as well: decreased interest, decreased appetite, insomnia, and psychomotor retardation or agitation. Difficulty concentrating, procrastination, and lack of motivation occur in both. Irritability, a common symptom of ADHD, is increasingly considered the "leading edge" of depression, especially in men. There is a difference between the low frustration tolerance that is characteristic of ADHD, however, and persistent rage attacks.

Given the burden of their symptoms, adults who have ADHD are more likely to be depressed than peers who do not have the disorder. Just less than half of adult ADHD patients present with mood symptoms. Often they are irritable and demoralized, constantly thinking the worst (Brown 1996). One of the most common symptoms is lability: quick, often intense changes of mood. Angry, inappropriate behavior characterizes many patients; they can antagonize other people. Treatment with stimulants sometimes causes irritability, anxiety, depression, insomnia, and somatic complaints.

Children, Depression, and ADHD

Prospective studies show that both boys and girls with ADHD have significantly more MDD than do age peers without ADHD (Biederman et al. 1996, 1999a). They have true depression, not simply demoralization secondary to their ADHD (Biederman et al. 1998b). Conversely, the rate of ADHD is significantly higher in children with MDD. In a study of 136 children diagnosed with depression, 103 (76%) had a comorbid diagnosis of ADHD. Of 66 severely depressed children in this study, 49 (74%) had comorbid ADHD (Biederman et al. 1995a). This finding is important, because having ADHD with depression may worsen outcome (Brent et al. 1988). Hyperactive young adults who were hyperactive children make more suicide attempts than do control subjects (G. Weiss et al. 1985).

Adults, Depression, and ADHD

One-quarter to one-third of adult men and women presenting for ADHD treatment qualify for a diagnosis of MDD (Biederman et al. 1993, 1994). About 30% of ADHD adults report problems with depression in childhood (Faraone and Biederman 1997). Depressed patients with ADHD may be severely ill. In one study, 10% of young adults with ADHD made a suicide attempt, and about 5% died either from suicide or accidental injury. These rates are far higher than in control subjects (G. Weiss and Hechtman 1993).

ADHD feels normal to persons who have it. They have "been this way" their whole life. Depressive symptoms are new and upsetting, or they are recurrent and upsetting, but they are practically never continuous for years to decades like ADHD symptoms. Many patients who seek treatment for depression may not refer to or complain about ADHD. In one study of adults with MDD, 16% had full or subthreshold criteria for ADHD. Depression in the adults with ADHD was as severe and as chronic as depression in those who did not have ADHD (Alpert et al. 1996).

Untangling depression and ADHD can be difficult. Having ADHD can be depressing, and depressed people are disorganized and inattentive. If the patient's disorganization and inattention came only after he or she started feeling depressed, it is unlikely that he or she has ADHD. If the patient has long struggled with those symptoms, ADHD is more likely (Brown 1995). To clarify the diagnosis, ask about symptoms over time. Are they situational? Have the problems with depression preceded those with attention and hyperactivity/impulsivity (Adler and Cohen 2004)?

Families, Depression, and ADHD

Family studies enrich our understanding of the interaction of ADHD and depression. In 9 of 11 family studies, relatives of children with ADHD had significantly higher rates of both ADHD and depression than did relatives of control subjects (Spencer 1995). Family members of children who had ADHD and MDD had higher rates of both disorders. A common genetic factor may occur in both.

Another study showed that relatives of children with ADHD are at greater risk for MDD than relatives of control subjects. Relatives of children in both ADHD subgroups had higher rates of ADHD and comorbid depression than did the relatives of control subjects. ADHD and MDD may be different expressions of the same genetic factors behind the appearance of ADHD (Biederman et al. 1991a, 1992). We do not know why some patients have one disorder, some the other, and still others have both.

Treatment of the Depressed Adult ADHD Patient

When an adult patient has ADHD and MDD, both disorders need vigorous treatment. If the patient wants treatment other than medication, try alternative treatments. If treating with medication, which should you choose? Is the patient intensely depressed, with symptoms a stimulant might worsen, such as irritability, decreased appetite, and poor sleep? If so, treat with an antidepressant. Choose one such as bupropion (Wellbutrin) that also treats ADHD, or select a selective serotonin reuptake inhibitor (SSRI) that you can later safely combine with ADHD medication. Once the patient has stabilized affectively, assess his or her ADHD. Is the antidepressant helping that? If not, add a central nervous system (CNS) stimulant. It is unclear whether a comorbid mood disorder significantly lessens the impact of CNS stimulants on ADHD (Spencer et al. 2000).

In other cases, begin pharmacological treatment with a stimulant alone. If both the ADHD and depression respond, continue treating with the stimulant only. If the ADHD improves but not the depression, try adding an SSRI antidepressant.

If the ADHD initially fails to yield to a stimulant, consider the depression as primary and treat it with an SSRI. If the depression lifts but the patient still has ADHD symptoms, consider trying other stimulants in turn. If that fails, a good strategy is supplementing the SSRI with bupropion (Wellbutrin) (Pliszka et al. 2000).

The SSRIs are the leading group for treating major depression. Although they do not provide relief for ADHD, they are safe to combine with the CNS stimulants and bupropion.

Mick was a sad-eyed youth of 19 who had been suspended from college for a year because of academic failure. His MDD responded to individual psychotherapy and sertraline (Zoloft), 100 mg/day. Although he returned to college in better spirits, he soon fell behind in his classes and started turning in papers late. It became clear that underlying his behavior was a long-standing pattern of inattention and distractibility. A daydreamer, he had never been mischievous or hyperactive, so he was never "in trouble" at school. Quick-witted, he wrote easily and well. At home, his mother despaired of his ever cleaning his room, doing his homework, or remembering domestic chores like taking out the trash on Tuesday nights. Whatever interested him held him, whether it was video games or the success of the Washington Redskins. What did not interest him, like algebra homework, went undone.

Mick had negotiated high school adequately. Highly intelligent, he did imaginative work when it interested him. He relied on his mother's nagging to get other assignments in on time. In college, when he faced higher academic demands without that structure, his grades plummeted and he became depressed.

Only after he was diagnosed and treated for ADHD as well as for depression did Mick reach solid ground, emotionally. His grades shot up. He reported, "I've turned into the kind of student I hate. I do the reading, ask questions in class, and I actually remember what the professor said in the lecture. I think the most I ever got before was, perhaps, 10% of what the guy was saying." After he had a successful college year, he and I agreed he could discontinue his antidepressant. He continued to thrive, taking Adderall 15 mg twice a day.

When considering an SSRI for the patient who is already taking atomoxetine (Strattera) for ADHD, use escitalopram (Lexapro) or sertraline (Zoloft) first. Neither inhibits the 2D6 isoenzyme of the P450 cytochrome system as paroxetine (Paxil) and fluoxetine (Prozac) do. When used with paroxetine or fluoxetine, Strattera dosages typically must be lowered to avoid higher blood levels and more side effects.

Options for the depressed patient whose illness does not respond to an SSRI include agents such as Effexor XR (venlafaxine). In a few open studies, venlafaxine has moderately improved ADHD symptoms in adults as well as relieved depressed mood (Reimherr et al. 1995). The serotonin-norepinephrine reuptake inhibitor antidepressant duloxetine (Cymbalta) is available, but there are few data about its use in ADHD patients. Tricyclic antidepressants such as desipramine (Norpramin) help. In one study, 68% of adult patients with ADHD had a positive response to Norpramin; no patients in the control group had a response to placebo. Patients in this study were not depressed at the time. The researchers concluded that desipramine effectively treats ADHD symptoms in adults with a lifetime history of depression (Wilens et al. 1996). Patients often find the tricyclics difficult to tolerate, however.

For patients with an atypical clinical picture, or who fail to respond to the usual agents, try a monoamine oxidase inhibitor (MAOI) antidepressant. Although MAOIs can help ADHD, they may combine with substances in food, other medicines, and alcoholic drinks to raise blood pressure. The usual recommendation is *not* to use MAOIs and CNS stimulants in combination. However, a stimulant may work in carefully selected cases in which a severely depressed patient with ADHD responds only to an MAOI (Feinberg 2004). A stimulant may even help relieve common side effects of the MAOIs such as hypotension or daytime somnolence (Schatzberg et al. 2003). If a transdermal preparation of selegiline becomes available, that may encourage clinicians to try the combination of an MAOI and a stimulant (Feinberg 2004). Although the MAOIs can help, many psychiatrists are reluctant to use them. These medications require the patient to be vigilant about what he or she eats and drinks, and MAOIs often interact dangerously with other medications.

Dysthymic Disorder

Most clinical studies of affective illness in ADHD deal not with dysthymic disorder but with MDD or bipolar disorder. However, dysthymic disorder commonly occurs in adults with ADHD. Sometimes it is the result of living for years with unrecognized, undiagnosed, and untreated ADHD. In other patients, the dysthymia may co-occur with but not be causally related to the ADHD (Adler and Cohen 2004).

Although less pressing clinically than other affective disorders, dysthymic disorder darkens many lives. Early studies of adults with ADHD found rates of dysthymia as high as 67%–81% (Wender et al. 1985). One researcher studying ADHD adults excluded patients with major affective disorder and still found significant dysthymia (25%) and cyclothymia (25%) (Shekim et al. 1990). Another study that compared adult women with ADHD and age peers without the disorder found that the ADHD group had greater rates of dysthymia (16% vs. 4%) as well as MDD (36% vs. 6%) (Biederman et al. 1994).

Although not as severe as MDD or bipolar disorder, dysthymic disorder can be difficult to treat. Some dysthymic patients are reluctant to try medication, asserting that if they "just lived right" they would not be depressed. Having dysthymic disorder, however, is like going surfing to have fun but instead finding yourself repeatedly dumped on shore, your knees and back scraped, with sand jammed under your bathing suit. Psychological therapies such as interpersonal psychotherapy (Weissman and Markowitz 1994) and cognitive-behavioral therapy (CBT) help (Dunner et al. 1996). The SSRIs and other antidepressants are effective, as they are for MDD (Dunner et al. 2002). Combined treatments may give the best results (Akiskal et al. 1995).

Treat the combination of dysthymic disorder and ADHD vigorously. Occasionally a patient taking only a stimulant shows improved mood as well as improved ADHD. Use the stimulants with the same dosage schedule as for ADHD patients with MDD. Generally a stimulant is a poor solo treatment for mood disorder. If it fails, then use adequate trials of full dosages of antidepressants, plus adequate trials of full courses of psychotherapy. Many, but not all, dysthymic patients respond. For many, psychotherapy is required. Both cognitive and behavioral treatments and psychodynamic psychotherapy can make significant contributions to the patient's well-being.

Bipolar Disorder

Patients with major or unipolar depression have only depressive episodes. Those with bipolar disorder have upward mood swings as well as downward. Patients with type I bipolar disorder have multiple high or manic episodes as well as depressive ones. Type II bipolar patients have at least one hypomanic episode and many depressive episodes (American Psychiatric Association 2000). Our view of bipolar disorder is changing rapidly. Once thought rare, it now appears to be much more common.

Especially when patients present clinically with depression, it is easy to miss type I bipolar disorder. Patients typically do not remember hypomanic or manic episodes. When they are depressed, mania or even hypomania seems normal or even desirable. When hypomanic, they are typically enjoying themselves too much to seek a psychiatrist, and their behavior may not cause substantial trouble. Being hypomanic is a little like being in love: the patient feels witty, energetic, and intensely alive. It is easy to dismiss other people's concerns. A manic episode, however, can be a nightmare of engulfing moods and uncontrolled behavior. The episodes are rarely purely pleasurable. Often the manic patient is labile and irritable; many have symptoms of depression mixed in. Even if they admit that their highs are pathological, bipolar patients often insist that the highs had benefits.

> "I sure miss all the great sex," mused one man, looking back on a manic episode.

It is increasingly common in clinical practice to screen patients with depressive symptoms with a standard rating scale such as the Hamilton Rating Scale for Depression. It is even more prudent to screen for bipolar symptoms as well in any patient with a depressed presentation. A useful screen is the Mood Disorder Questionnaire, which asks about manic or hypomanic symptoms now or in the past (Hirschfeld et al. 2000). During the initial evaluation it is important to do this exercise with a family member or significant other in the patient's life, because patients with bipolar symptoms may be unreliable reporters of their past. When a depressed patient fails to respond to treatment, look further into his or her history. Having history from a person close to the patient is often revealing. Such screening provides more accurate diagnosis and better treatment results. Clinicians also want to avoid triggering mania with medication they prescribe for depression.

The intractability of bipolar depression has pushed clinicians to treat it differently than unipolar depression. Instead of antidepressants, increasingly we turn to mood stabilizers, originally (and still) used as anticonvulsants, and to second-generation antipsychotic medications. Are the unipolar and bipolar disorders relatives on the same spectrum or are they separate entities? That question is still unsettled.

This controversy has practical consequences in treating ADHD patients. Children show a striking association between ADHD and bipolar disorder: remarkably, an estimated 90% of children and adolescents diagnosed with bipolar disorder also have ADHD (Geller et al. 2002). In community studies of children who had only ADHD, their relatives also had only ADHD. The relatives of children who had ADHD and bipolar disorder, however, had elevated rates of both ADHD and bipolar disorder. This combination may be a distinct familial disorder (Faraone et al. 1997).

Clinically, children who have both disorders are similar to chronically impaired, irritable adults with treatment-refractory bipolar disorder. The ADHD symptoms of children with both disorders are worse than those of age peers who only have ADHD. Children with bipolar disorder and ADHD require mood stabilization before their ADHD can be treated. In such children treated successfully with mood stabilizers, CNS stimulants were minimally effective for ADHD symptoms (Biederman et al. 1998a). Compared with adolescents who had only bipolar disorder, those with both the affective disorder and ADHD were more likely to have mixed mania, irritability, higher scores on mania rating scales, and sometimes lower serum thyroxine concentrations (West et al. 1996).

The natural history of depression in adults sheds some light on bipolar disorder and ADHD in children. One study examined the clinical course of 559 depressed adults over 11 years (Akiskal et al. 1995). Participants who became classic bipolar I disorder patients were indistinguishable from patients who continued to have only unipolar depression. Those who developed bipolar II disorder, however, were different. They developed varied symptoms early. They were daydreamers, with high energy and activity and labile mood. Substance abuse was frequent. Educational, marital, and occupational disruption were common. Often they committed minor antisocial acts. As a group, they were more sick: they had a prolonged course with shorter intervals of feeling well. They described themselves as "temperamentally unstable."

This combination of symptoms in adults with bipolar II disorder resembles that of children with ADHD and childhood-onset bipolar disorder. The study suggested that the combination correlates with the early onset of bipolar-like symptoms and with the persistence of ADHD into adulthood. The study by Akiskal et al. (1995) did not examine participants for the comorbid diagnosis of ADHD. We might see a higher-than-expected percentage, however, in study subjects who develop bipolar II disorder.

An association exists between ADHD and bipolar disorder in adults. An estimated 5%–10% of adult patients with ADHD have bipolar disorder (Spencer 2005a). It may be difficult to decide when adult symptoms are due to bipolar disorder and when they are due to ADHD. For example, patients with both disorders show dysfunctional behavior such as impulsive shopping and rapid driving.

Continuity of symptoms is key to the differential diagnosis. Manic persons may be highly productive and sociable, hard to tell from high-powered ADHD adults who rush from one project to another. Most of the time, the typical bipolar patient is mood neutral or depressed. Periods of hypomania or mania are fewer and shorter; it is during those periods that ADHD-like symptoms usually occur. The person who has ADHD alone is more or less "like this" all the time, for many years. Adults with ADHD may talk rapidly, but they usually know that they are shifting from topic to topic. Their talk has logical connections. Their symptoms improve when they take CNS stimulants and worsen when they are off the medication. Manic patients, also fast talkers, are unaware of the shifts in their flights of ideas. Stimulants can make those symptoms in manic patients worse, not better (Pierce 2003).

ADHD symptoms in persons who have only that disorder resemble those in persons who have both ADHD and bipolar disorder. In differentiating ADHD from bipolar disorder, consider the bipolar symptoms first. The adult who has both disorders typically has six bipolar symptoms, whereas the adult who only has ADHD typically has only one such symptom (Wilens et al. 2003a).

The relationship between ADHD and bipolar II disorder is confusing. Patients who have both disorders tend not to do well with the usual treatments for either. CNS stimulants may destabilize their moods. Impulsive, disorganized patients have trouble adhering to a complex regimen of medicines. Substance abuse often complicates the treatment of both (M. Weiss et al. 1999).

Among adults who present with bipolar disorder alone, those who had ADHD as children have an earlier onset of bipolar symptoms and do worse with treatment than bipolar adults who did not have ADHD in childhood. Among adults who acknowledged an early onset of depression or bipolar disorder, 15%–20% had ADHD. Data from the Systematic Treatment Enhancement Program for Bipolar Disorder suggest that such patients may have a specific form of ADHD associated with early development of these comorbidities (Simon et al. 2004).

Persons with bipolar disorder and ADHD need specialized psychiatric attention. Stabilizing the mood disorder takes precedence. ADHD and mania may be relatively refractory to lithium; other mood stabilizers such as lamotrigine may help (McElroy et al. 1992). In recent years, there has been movement away from using antidepressants such as the SSRIs to treat bipolar depression. Severely ill patients may require the use of antipsychotic medication, especially some of the newer second-generation agents such as risperidone (Risperdal), olanzapine (Zyprexa), or ziprasidone (Geodon). Some patients require combinations of a mood stabilizer and a second-generation antipsychotic (Patel and Sallee 2005).

Once the mood of the patient with bipolar disorder is stable, the clinician can focus on the ADHD. But what medication is safe? Clinicians do not want to precipitate an affective episode, especially a manic one. Will the CNS stimulants cause a manic episode or make one more likely? The answer, usually, is no. However, clinicians need to be watchful, and family members need to stay in close contact with the doctor.

In addition to medication, patients with bipolar disorder need psychotherapy to understand their illness and its effect on their life. Treating patients who have a combination of ADHD and bipolar disorder can tax the most resourceful clinician. Both disorders have emotional turbulence as a central symptom. A treatment team may be needed to work effectively with these patients. For best treatment results, a good working alliance with the family is essential.

ANXIETY DISORDERS

Anxiety is the brain's warning signal of potential danger. Anxious people have difficulty concentrating and attending. The anxiety disorders are clinical conditions with this symptom as a central feature. Clinically, patients rarely present with just one anxiety disorder. Instead, they typically present with a combination: other anxiety disorders, affective disorders, and abuse of alcohol or other substances. Far from being mild or transient, the anxiety disorders are chronic problems that markedly compromise quality of life (Mendlowicz and Stein 2000).

ADHD and one or more anxiety disorders co-occur in about 25% of cases in children (Biederman et al. 1991b). Youngsters with ADHD seem more likely to have overanxious disorder and separation anxiety than phobias. In one study, relatives of ADHD children who had anxiety disorders were twice as likely to have such a syndrome as the relatives of ADHD children who did not have any anxiety disorders.

ADHD patients cannot predict how they will function on a given day. That is a recipe for anxiety. Living with ADHD, patients may not realize that their anxiety is abnormal or that it is adding to their problems. In one review, 52% of the adults referred with ADHD met criteria for at least two anxiety disorders (Biederman et al. 1993). A later review estimated that 25%–50% of adults with ADHD have anxiety disorders (Adler and Cohen 2004). An added anxiety disorder compounds the poor self-esteem, bad stress management, and impaired function that mark ADHD. It may be difficult to tease apart the disorders in adults. Patients have had symptoms for so long that they regard them as "just the way I am" rather than as separate disorders.

Genetic studies show that the anxiety disorder and ADHD occur independently of each other. Family members are more likely to have one or the other than to have both together. The disorders are not genetically related (Biederman et al. 1991b).

During the initial evaluation of the patient for ADHD, it is useful to screen for current and past anxiety symptoms. Does the patient have panic attacks? Does he or she have irrational, upsetting thoughts or behavior patterns he or she cannot control? Has something traumatic happened that has caused new symptoms to flare? If, on questioning, patients have multiple symptoms, interview them with the Anxiety Disorders Interview Schedule (DiNardo et al. 1994). Patients are usually quick to discuss their ADHD symptoms, but they may be reticent about anxiety, especially obsessions and compulsions. It is important to identify and treat specific anxiety disorders when they are present. Although the disorders share common themes, each disorder has features that require specific treatments.

Panic Disorder

Panic attacks, the hallmark of panic disorder, are acute, overwhelming symptoms of both psychological and physical distress. Intensely real physical symptoms often make patients fear they have a potentially fatal illness. Although panic attacks are relatively common, for a patient to warrant a diagnosis of panic disorder, he or she must have lasting concern about the impact of the attacks or a constricted life, or both. Often the initial panic attacks have specific precipitants, such as when the person is in a situation he or she feels is inescapable. Spontaneous panic attacks follow and then anticipatory anxiety and phobic avoidance. Some patients become hypochondriacal. Major depression and suicidality are also common. Some patients, turning to alcohol and other substances for relief, develop substance abuse or dependence (American Psychiatric Association 2000). A familial disorder, panic disorder has a strong genetic component. The neurobiological model for panic disorder posits a fear network in the limbic system, with the amygdala at its center. Although the course of the illness varies, it is generally chronic, with relapses and remissions (American Psychiatric Association 1998).

Practice guidelines for treating panic disorder emphasize that many medications help, including the tricyclic antidepressants, benzodiazepines, and MAOIs, but the SSRIs are the agents of first choice (Bruce et al. 2003). CBT, especially systematic desensitization, and family and community support are also essential (American Psychiatric Association 1998). Even with good treatment, however, many patients remain symptomatic for years (Doyle and Pollack 2004).

Although patients with ADHD tend to overreact to situations, their lability is not the intensity and suddenness of a panic attack. In panic disorder, disturbing physical symptoms generally accompany acute anxiety. Patients with ADHD do not complain of such symptoms.

Generalized Anxiety Disorder

Persons with generalized anxiety disorder (GAD) have excessive worry, anxiety, and hypervigilance. The disorder is common, with a lifetime prevalence of 5%. Women have the disorder more often than men, and the rate rises over age 40 (American Psychiatric Association 2000). The impact of GAD on patients' lives is as severe as that of major depression and of chronic somatic diseases such as diabetes or arthritis. Patients with GAD have many somatic symptoms that drive them repeatedly to physicians. The disorder is highly comorbid with other anxiety disorders and with depression (Wittchen and Hoyer 2001).

CBT for GAD teaches patients to monitor their anxiety, to relax fully, and to change how they think about their symptoms. Patients who persist with CBT often have lasting clinical improvement (Borkovec and

Ruscio 2001). Among medications for GAD, SSRIs are the mainstay. The serotonin-norepinephrine reuptake inhibitor venlafaxine (Effexor XR) also has demonstrated efficacy. By and large, in GAD antidepressants are preferable to benzodiazepines or buspirone, especially with comorbid depression. Even with good treatment, symptoms may linger. Patients need full dosages of medications for remission. They should take them for at least 1 year, if not indefinitely (Davidson 2001).

Differentiating ADHD from GAD may be difficult. Are patients anxious because they cannot attend, or are they not paying attention because they are anxious? Patients with GAD can usually pay attention when they are relaxed, but their worries and physical distress override their ability to focus. The estimated range for the diagnosis of GAD among adults with ADHD is 24%–43% (Biederman et al. 1993). Clearly, there is a substantial clinical problem.

Social Anxiety Disorder

Patients with social anxiety disorder are intensely uncomfortable in social or other situations where they fear others will judge or look down on them. As a result they avoid interacting with other people, and both their work and social lives suffer. This disorder affects more than 10% of the population (American Psychiatric Association 2000). Public-speaking anxiety is so common that it seems more "normal" than a disorder. The generalized form of social anxiety may be crippling. Patients are highly vulnerable to comorbid depression and abuse of alcohol or other substances (Lepine and Pelissolo 2000).

Social anxiety disorder is a chronic neurodevelopmental illness, with both heritable and environmental stress factors. It may involve a dysfunction or hyperactivity of the amygdala's evaluative function (Amaral 2002). To date, however, neuroimaging and other studies have not shown demonstrable brain abnormalities (Bebchuk and Tancer 1999). There may be lowered dopamine receptor binding potential in the striatum of patients with generalized phobia compared with control subjects (Schneier et al. 2000). The "low dopamine" theory of social phobia is not proved (Mathew et al. 2001). However, it is of particular interest because researchers suspect that low CNS dopamine, especially in the striatum, is part of the neurobiology of ADHD. As with other anxiety disorders, patients with social phobia make good progress with CBT (Heimberg 2002). They respond to medications, especially the SSRI antidepressants and the benzodiazepines, with MAOI antidepressants and other agents also useful (Blanco et al. 2002). Successful cognitive-behavioral and medication interventions produce similar physiologic results (Furmark et al. 2002).

Some patients with ADHD avoid social gatherings because they feel distracted and overstimulated there. It is not as though they fear being scrutinized by others, as in social anxiety disorder. When both coexist, successful treatment of ADHD can ease many symptoms of social phobia.

> "I'm much less anxious in social situations now," said Derek, 42, describing the impact of treatment for his ADHD. "I used to be so focused on what was happening inside my head, trying to make sense of it, that there was little left of me to interact. Now that I can count on myself better, I'm more open to others."

Obsessive-Compulsive Disorder

Obsessive-compulsive disorder (OCD), once thought rare, now seems relatively common, with a lifetime prevalence of 1%–3%. Affected persons have *obsessions* (intrusive, upsetting, irrational thoughts, feelings, or impulses); *compulsions* (repetitive, irrational, intrusive behavior patterns); or both. They are usually aware of how irrational their concerns and behavior are—which keeps them from sharing information about their symptoms with others, including clinicians. A chronic disorder, OCD typically has remissions and flare-ups. It is highly comorbid with other anxiety disorders, with affective disorders, and with abuse of alcohol and other substances (American Psychiatric Association 2000). Patients with OCD have cognitive deficits associated with frontal or striatal function, or both. They have selective deficits in tasks involving controlled attentional processing and self-guided spontaneous behavior (Schmidtke et al. 1998). For assessing patients, the Yale-Brown Obsessive Compulsive Scale is standard (Taylor 1998).

Estimates of the overlap of OCD and ADHD in children are between 10% and 33% (Brown 2000a). Although there are individual cases, there does not seem to be a significant association between OCD and ADHD in adults. Only among adults with comorbid tic disorder and ADHD is OCD more common: 12% of these adults have OCD, versus 2% of ADHD adults without tics (Spencer et al. 1997).

Persons with comorbid ADHD and OCD may seek treatment without knowing that they have both. They may attribute their attentional problems to ADHD, not aware that their obsessional concerns or compulsive behaviors are due to another disorder. Even if they suspect something else is wrong, they may be reluctant to discuss it as such. Sometimes they hope that treatment for ADHD will make all their symptoms go away. Sometimes they defer talking about obsessions and compulsions until later, when they are more comfortable. Others present thinking that OCD is their problem. They may not realize their attentional problems relate to ADHD. If they have OCD, treat that first, then comorbid ADHD when it is present (Brown 2000a).

The range of effective somatic treatments for OCD is small. Only serotonergic agents, the SSRIs, and the tricyclic antidepressant clomipramine (Anafranil) consistently moderate symptoms. High dosages of medication for weeks to months are usually necessary. Improvement occurs in 55%–65% of cases and is usually partial rather than complete (Pigott and Seay 1998). OCD patients, especially those with compulsions such as checking or washing, respond to CBTs such as exposure therapy and response prevention (Foa et al. 1998). Deciding on treatment for OCD alone is complex. Most clinicians start with either CBT or a serotonergic antidepressant. In complex or more severe cases, a combination of approaches may help.

The SSRI medications do not help symptoms of ADHD; the stimulants atomoxetine and bupropion do not treat obsessions or compulsions. If anything, stimulants may transiently induce overfocused or compulsive behavior in patients and worsen those behaviors in patients with OCD. When that occurs, patients notice and complain about the effects (Solanto and Wender 1989).

Treatment guidelines for adults with OCD and ADHD recommend CBT plus an SSRI plus a psychostimulant as first-line treatment. Other treatment approaches include CBT plus clomipramine (Anafranil) plus a psychostimulant; CBT plus any serotonergic agent; and CBT alone (March et al. 1997). Some complicated patients will present with ADHD and OCD along with other anxiety disorders and depression. They require complex assessment and ongoing trials of treatment combinations: medications and other interventions.

Posttraumatic Stress Disorder

After exposure to a life-threatening experience, some persons develop new symptoms. They persistently reexperience the event; they may avoid stimuli associated with the trauma. They may display emotional numbing and estrangement from others, and they may have new symptoms of increased arousal. These are the hallmarks of posttraumatic stress disorder (PTSD) (American Psychiatric Association 2000). Persons who have acute dissociative symptoms such as emotional numbing and derealization are at particular risk. The disorder is common. In the National Comorbidity Survey, an estimated 8% of respondents—5% of men and 10.4% of women—had PTSD during their lifetime (Kessler et al. 1995).

The stressor initiates traumatic memories. In a period of "cognitive appraisal" that follows, the traumatized individual processes and reworks the experience. Reaching out to others, he or she tries to integrate what has happened. PTSD emerges when the person cannot modify the hyperarousal and neurobiological cascade that the traumatic memories precipitate. Through a process of neurological kindling, the patient reacts to reminders of the trauma, or even to neutral stimuli, with the same intensity as in the original event. Once established, the patient's pattern of overreaction can become chronic (McFarlane 2000).

Increased brain norepinephrine causes startle reactions, insomnia, and autonomic hyperarousal. Increased brain dopamine activity results in generalized anxiety, panic attacks, and hypervigilance. There is increased central corticotropin-releasing factor, but the ambient cortisol level is low (Charney et al. 1993). In PTSD there is an enhanced negative-feedback inhibition of the hypothalamic-pituitary-adrenal axis. Involved brain regions include the amygdala, locus coeruleus, hippocampus, and sensory cortex (Yehuda 2002). Some researchers find that patients with PTSD have a smaller hippocampus than do control subjects. Is the smaller hippocampus a result of stress-induced atrophy (Bremner et al. 2003) or a preexisting condition that predisposes to PTSD in extreme stress (Medina 2003)? That question remains unsettled.

Once established, PTSD can last for decades, shadowing every aspect of life (Kessler 2000). Patients commonly develop generalized anxiety and alcoholism, phobias, depression, and panic disorder. As many as one in five persons with PTSD attempts suicide (Bremner et al. 1996).

PTSD is not simply a static biological dysregulation; it is a "complex of conditional associations which the patient must overlearn" (Marshall 2000), as with a phobia. That understanding has practical consequences for treatment (Foa and Meadows 1997). In a safe environment, CBT systematically exposes the patient to his or her traumatic memories. Exposure therapy should continue for at least 6 months, with follow-up (Marks et al. 1998). Eye movement desensitization and reprocessing (EMDR) is a variant of CBT. The patient focuses on a disturbing image, thought, or sensation related to a traumatic memory. At the same time, the therapist induces in the patient a series of left-to-right eye movements or other form of bilateral stimulation. Treatment results may be faster than in conventional CBT, but EMDR remains controversial (Scheck et al. 1998).

Medication also helps. Once more the SSRIs are the agents of choice, with 10%–30% of patients having a full remission (Friedman 2003). Medication alone typically does not eliminate symptoms; a good response is a 30%–50% reduction. SSRIs reduce symptoms in all three

PTSD clusters: hyperarousal, reexperiencing, and avoidance. Patients who cannot tolerate the SSRIs or who do not improve may try MAOIs or tricyclics. With PTSD patients, clinicians often try adjuvant medication such as lithium or buspirone. Alpha-agonist agents such as clonidine may relieve nightmares. To date, there is insufficient evidence of the usefulness of carbamazepine, valproate, lamotrigine, or other anticonvulsants in PTSD. Benzodiazepines do not have efficacy for core symptoms of PTSD. Second-generation antipsychotics such as risperidone, quetiapine, and olanzapine may be useful, especially to augment first-line medications. For best results, patients should take medication for at least 1 year.

For most patients with PTSD, treatment that combines medication (especially an SSRI) and CBT gives the best results. While medication makes exposure treatment more tolerable, patients must still unlearn their fear through desensitization (Marshall 2000). Providing the right combination of treatments in the right sequence is the clinical art.

Persons with PTSD have symptoms that suggest ADHD. They can be inattentive or hypervigilant, intensely reactive, or agitated. With PTSD, a specific trauma or set of traumas sets off the symptoms. In contrast, ADHD symptoms are not situation specific. They often surface in the early school years and evolve as the youngster develops into an adult. Unless PTSD patients had a traumatic episode in childhood or cumulative traumas growing up (as many do), their symptoms will not be developmental like those of ADHD (Glod and Teicher 1996). Although persons can have both disorders, there is no evidence that ADHD predisposes to PTSD (Tzelepis et al. 1995). When present, both disorders need treatment.

Treating ADHD in the Anxious Patient

If a CNS stimulant is used to treat a patient's ADHD, what impact will it have on his or her anxiety? Anxious ADHD children do worse with stimulant medications than those who are not anxious (Tannock et al. 1996). Anxious adult ADHD patients may respond less well to the CNS stimulants than adult ADHD patients without anxiety disorders. For adult ADHD patients with anxiety disorders, increase the dosage of CNS stimulant slowly. These patients may need to experiment with dosages for some time before they get stable therapeutic results (Popper et al. 2003). Stimulants do not usually worsen mild anxiety in ADHD patients, and atomoxetine (Strattera) can help both problems.

Some patients with acute and chronic anxiety do well taking a benzodiazepine. However, these agents may not help patients with ADHD.

They may worsen confusion, forgetfulness, and lack of motivation (M. Weiss et al. 1999).

Anxious ADHD patients taking a stimulant can safely combine it with an SSRI. With patients taking Strattera, choose the SSRI carefully. You may need to lower the dosage of Strattera in patients taking paroxetine (Paxil IR, Paxil CR) or fluoxetine (Prozac). Using escitalopram (Lexapro) or sertraline (Zoloft) avoids this interaction.

ADHD AND ABUSE OF ALCOHOL AND OTHER SUBSTANCES

An adult presenting for outpatient evaluation for ADHD has about a 10% chance of currently abusing substances and a 50% chance of having abused substances in the past. The risk of developing a substance disorder over a lifetime among ADHD individuals (55%) is twice that among adults without ADHD (27%). Conversely, ADHD is more prevalent in individuals with substance abuse disorders (Biederman et al. 1995b).

ADHD is an independent risk factor for the development of drug abuse. In a recent study of children from age 5 to midadolescence, researchers compared 363 youths who had ADHD with 726 matched control subjects. The youths with ADHD had a threefold risk of developing substance abuse disorder compared with the control subjects (Katusic et al. 2003). Adolescents who abuse drugs other than alcohol have higher rates of ADHD than those who abuse alcohol. In a study of 57 adolescent inpatients with substance abuse disorder, conduct disorder, and mood disorder, one-quarter had current ADHD (DeMilio 1989). As expected, teenagers with combined ADHD and substance abuse have higher rates of mood disorders and conduct disorder (Wilens et al. 2000). Although the stereotypical teenage drug abuser is a boy, girls are involved as well. Because they typically socialize with older boys, ADHD girls are more at risk of abusing drugs at an earlier age than their male ADHD peers (Disney et al. 1999).

There are similar patterns of comorbidity in adults. Persons with ADHD are more at risk for substance abuse disorder, and for developing it earlier, than age peers without ADHD. The increase is especially striking in those who have comorbid conduct or bipolar disorder (Biederman et al. 1998c). Overall, studies of adults with ADHD consistently show higher rates of substance abuse disorders than in the general population. The risk of ADHD adults developing alcohol abuse is 32%–53%. The risk of abuse of other substances such as cocaine and marijuana is 8%–32%, and the risk of polydrug abuse is 17%–21% (Adler and Cohen 2004). The percentages are higher in patients who have antisocial personality disorder as well. Marijuana is by far the most common drug of abuse other than alcohol, with stimulants, cocaine, and hallucinogens following. Adults with ADHD who also have substance abuse disorder have an earlier onset of symptoms, have more severe symptoms, and do worse in substance abuse treatment (Carroll and Rounsaville 1993). Such patients are significantly more likely to have comorbid depression and anxiety than control subjects, adults who only have ADHD, or adults who only have substance abuse (Wilens et al. 2004).

ADHD as a Risk Factor for Developing Substance Abuse

Children with ADHD are more likely to smoke cigarettes than their age peers, and they start at an earlier age. Adults with ADHD are three times more likely to smoke than other persons in the general population. They smoke for longer periods of time and have more difficulty discontinuing cigarettes than do peers who do not have ADHD (Pomerleau et al. 1995). Many clinicians regard smoking cigarettes as a gateway to using, abusing, and becoming dependent on other substances (Milberger et al. 1997).

Caffeine is another drug heavily used by those with ADHD (Adler and Cohen 2004). Although clinicians can overlook the excessive use of caffeine, it is often present. Many untreated ADHD patients rely on caffeine, but after an initial lift, the effect rapidly tapers. Some people develop tolerance. In large amounts, caffeine irritates the gastrointestinal tract, causing discomfort or diarrhea or both. Once ADHD patients are treated effectively with medication such as a CNS stimulant, they usually need less caffeine. Their gut settles down. The more stable blood levels of the stimulants, especially the long-acting stimulants, give relief from the roller-coaster effect of caffeine. With treatment, many ADHD patients drastically reduce their caffeine intake, with fewer side effects.

> Before getting treated for ADHD, 42-year-old Jack recalled, "I had a full pot of coffee every morning just to wake me up. Then all day long, I used to drink Jolt Cola, that high-caffeine stuff. I must have drunk 2 or 3 liters a day. My gut was all torn up, but I still had to have it to function. On top of that, some days I took caffeine tablets as well."

Having ADHD predisposes adolescent boys and girls to develop substance abuse. This may be a particular risk among youth who are aggressive, hyperactive, or impulsive. Adolescents with ADHD who also have conduct disorder or bipolar disorder are most likely to develop substance abuse or another major psychiatric problem. ADHD accelerates the transition from drug experimentation to abuse and dependence. When young adults with ADHD move from home to college or independent living, they need special warning about substance abuse disorders (Wilens et al. 2000).

Adults with ADHD who abuse drugs express *no* preference for stimulants, cocaine, or the amphetamines. They tend to abuse what is available, such as alcohol or marijuana. Adults with ADHD who develop substance abuse do so earlier and have a worse course than substance-abusing age peers who do not have ADHD (Carroll and Rounsaville 1993). Compared with age peers without ADHD, ADHD adults who abuse drugs abuse substances longer and take more than twice as long to achieve remission (Wilens et al. 1998).

In adult women with ADHD, abuse of alcohol or other substances has far-reaching consequences. Women with ADHD are already at risk for having children with ADHD. If they abuse alcohol or other substances in pregnancy, their children will more likely have fetal alcohol or other neurobiological syndromes. This combination of factors can result in a chaotic family life, with impaired parents unable to care for their special-needs children (Barkley 1998a).

Family Factors in ADHD and Substance Abuse

If ADHD and substance abuse are related in a familial/genetic way, then family members who have one disorder should be at higher risk for the other. Children of parents who abuse alcohol or other drugs are at greater risk for ADHD relative to control subjects (Earls et al. 1988). Studies of youths with ADHD show elevated rates of alcoholism in their parents, relative to control subjects (Cantwell 1972).

What Propels the Person With ADHD Toward Substance Abuse?

Is it the urge to self-medicate that leads an individual with ADHD to use and abuse substances? That seems a sensible theory, given the stress and demoralization of many ADHD patients. Despite popular opinion to the contrary, cocaine and the stimulants are *not* the favored substances of abuse in ADHD; marijuana is preferred (Biederman et al. 1995b).

Is the tendency for substance abuse a genetic predisposition? The controversy is not settled. ADHD adults are most at risk for substance abuse when there are conduct, bipolar, or antisocial disorders in the individual and the family (Biederman et al. 1990). A family history of substance use disorder largely accounts for its presence in ADHD youths

(Milberger et al. 1998). A polygenic mechanism may be operating (Wilens et al. 2000).

Clinical Significance of Comorbid ADHD and Substance Abuse

The symptoms of one disorder can worsen those of the other. Treatment results for substance abuse are worse when there is concurrent ADHD, and vice versa.

> Carlo, age 31, sought treatment for his depression and anxiety. He was abusing alcohol and dependent on benzodiazepines. A former rock guitarist, Carlo had never completed college. Now he was trying to earn his degree and start a new career. He had repeated relapses, however, requiring inpatient detoxification and treatment. An alert clinician in Carlo's chemical dependency treatment program diagnosed ADHD for the first time as well. When Carlo started taking Strattera and learned how to structure his life better, he made lasting progress. He still needed his SSRI, as well as active participation in Alcoholics Anonymous, to maintain his equilibrium.

Evaluating the Patient Who Has Substance Abuse and ADHD

Clinical evaluation of the patient who has both ADHD and substance abuse needs to be thorough (Table 9–1). Accurately assessing the nature and extent of ADHD symptoms is usually possible once the patient has a documented month of abstinence (Wilens et al. 2004). Such patients need psychiatric, dependence, social, cognitive, educational, and family evaluations. It is always useful, when diagnosing ADHD, to have an informant other than the patient. An informant is even more important when assessing patients who abuse alcohol or other drugs. These patients are also at risk for other psychiatric problems, such as mood and anxiety disorders.

Naturally, it is risky to use medication to treat ADHD in a person who has abused drugs or continues to do so. However, using stimulants (such as methylphenidate) and antidepressants (such as bupropion) to treat adolescents and adults with both disorders reduces the symptoms of the ADHD while *reducing*, not exacerbating, substance abuse or craving (Levin et al. 1998a, 1998b). Persons actively abusing alcohol or other substances often cannot effectively use psychoeducation or other interventions such as CBT. They have problems adhering to treatment, including taking medicine on schedule. The clinician is always concerned when he or she does not know what a patient is ingesting other than prescribed medication.

TABLE 9–1. Clinical evaluation of the patient with comorbid substance abuse and ADHD

Assessment	Components
Psychiatric evaluation	Personal interviews Consider cognitive screen for learning disorders
Addiction history	Interview Questionnaire Urine toxicology screen
Sources of information	Patient, parents, significant others, other caregivers
Psychosocial issues	Ask about current stressors and supports
Family issues	Family history of psychiatric disorders, especially substance abuse, and learning problems
Differential diagnosis	Dependence issues (e.g., detoxification, withdrawal) Medical concerns (e.g., endocrinopathies) Neurological concerns (e.g., seizures, infections) Psychiatric comorbidity (e.g., mood, anxiety, personality disorders)
Treatment strategies	Review expectations Propose multimodal treatment Psychotherapy (group or individual or both) for differing needs, including affiliation with 12-step program (e.g., Alcoholics Anonymous) Pharmacotherapy for ADHD, substance abuse, and other psychiatric disorders Social and community supports

Source. Adapted from Wilens TE, Spencer TJ, Biederman J: "Attention-Deficit/Hyperactivity Disorder With Substance Use Disorders," in *Attention-Deficit Disorders and Comorbidities in Children, Adolescents, and Adults.* Edited by Brown TE. Washington, DC, American Psychiatric Press, 2000, pp 319–339. Used with permission.

Any substance abuse, whether of alcohol, marijuana, or other substances, takes priority when affected persons seek treatment for ADHD (Riggs 1998). Patients with a current or past history of substance abuse should demonstrate that they have abstained from those substances for at least 3 months before receiving medication for ADHD. The current consensus is that after such a period of abstinence, it is possible to use any of the effective medications to treat ADHD. That includes the CNS stimulants or the nonstimulants (Wilens 2005). Sometimes treatment for the substance abuse must be aggressive, such as inpatient detoxification. Substance abuse treatment centers are grappling with this thorny combination of disorders (Horner and Scheibe 1997).

One open-label, prospective study followed adults with ADHD who had cocaine dependence in remission (Castaneda et al. 1999). The 19 adults, whose mean age was 37, had a wide range of comorbid diagnoses. The study used medications in a sequence that moved from less to more stimulating agents: fluoxetine (starting at 20 mg/day), bupropion (initial dosage 100 mg twice a day), pemoline (initial dosage 37.5 mg/day), methylphenidate (initial dosage 20 mg/day), dextroamphetamine (initial dosage 10 mg/day), and methamphetamine (initial dosage 15 mg/day). To be fully effective, treatments had to suppress 80% of the initial symptoms, as rated by the Utah criteria, for at least 1 full year (Wender et al. 1981). Eleven of the 19 patients received single-drug regimens that were fully effective for 36–52 weeks.

Whether in inpatient or outpatient settings, when a patient has ADHD and substance abuse, the primary focus should be on the drug problems. Treating the ADHD alone results in only minor improvement in that disorder and does not cause the substance abuse to abate (Wilens 2005). Once the patient is abstinent for at least 3 months, he or she may do well in treatment for ADHD, including using CNS stimulants or other medications as part of a full range of interventions.

Starting treatment of ADHD with medication in a patient who is abusing drugs may encourage the futile hope that treating the ADHD will eliminate the substance abuse (Riggs 1998). For such patients, nonstimulant agents such as atomoxetine (Strattera) or the antidepressant bupropion are preferable. Even when these patients have been abstinent from substance abuse, the extended-release CNS stimulant agents are preferable because they are less subject to abuse and diversion. Typically, persons who abuse stimulants crush and sniff them or inject them intravenously, but these tactics do not work with some extended-release CNS stimulant medications. Some individuals with substance abuse take oral, repeated high dosages of the extended-release stimulants. Another reason to consider stimulants as second-line agents in ADHD patients with comorbid substance abuse is that these medications may worsen their anxiety level. It is sensible to use a nonstimulant first in ADHD patients with a history of amphetamine or cocaine abuse. A CNS stimulant may rekindle past intense experiences with those substances. Patients who became psychotic on an amphetamine in the past should not be treated with a CNS stimulant for their ADHD. Even years after such an experience, taking a CNS stimulant can precipitate another psychotic reaction.

When family members are available and sympathetic, educating and involving them helps treatment succeed. Some patients, however, have burned through their family's stock of goodwill. Friends or members of an alternate social network can help. Although there are few formal data about the usefulness of psychotherapy in this population, this approach is often needed. Effective therapeutic interventions should include structured and goal-directed sessions, an interactive therapist, and treatment staff knowledgeable about both conditions. Participation in a 12-step program such as Alcoholics Anonymous or Rational Recovery is usually essential (McDermott 2000).

Dual-diagnosis patients need frequent monitoring, with random toxicology screenings and coordination of care with addiction counselors and other caregivers. These patients may require searches of their homes and cars for drugs and alcohol. Some clinicians advocate written contracts with their dual-diagnosis patients that make treatment expectations explicit and that lay out consequences of noncompliance (Croft 2005). Follow-up programs need to include contingency plans. For example, a positive urine sample means that the patient will attend Alcoholics Anonymous/Narcotics Anonymous meetings if not already doing so. Another positive urine sample triggers outpatient substance abuse treatment. If abuse is severe, treatment may need to be on an inpatient basis. Still, a high proportion of patients in such programs fail to reach or sustain abstinence (Wilens et al. 2004).

Patients with a history of substance abuse may be wary of medication, such as the stimulants, which have a potential for dependency. Table 9–2 lists guidelines for using CNS stimulants in such ADHD patients. While these patients may prefer another option, such as atomoxetine, current expert opinion is that they can safely be treated with any of the available agents (Wilens et al. 2004).

> Faith, age 55 years, had a long history of recurrent depression and alcohol dependence. Through steady participation in Alcoholics Anonymous, she had 14 years of sobriety. Despite success in some areas of life, she had persistent problems at work, where she was disorganized, distractible, and inefficient. Her impulsivity and outspokenness antagonized others.
>
> Reviewing her history showed that her problems with attention and organization started in grammar school and persisted. The diagnosis of ADHD, combined type, explained many of Faith's difficulties. With her history, she was afraid of taking any medicine that might produce dependency. She was already taking 300 mg/day of extended-release bupropion for depression, but it did not improve her ADHD symptoms. She agreed to try a low dosage of osmotic-release oral system methylphenidate (Concerta). After careful increases, she found that 36 mg/

TABLE 9–2.   Guidelines for using central nervous system stimulants in ADHD patients with a substance abuse history

1.   Patient has used stimulants to improve function rather than to get high (induce euphoria).
2.   Clinician has a good therapeutic alliance with the patient.
3.   Clinician can monitor the medication closely, perhaps in an inpatient setting.
4.   Patient's problems seriously interfere with his or her life functions.
5.   Other approaches have failed.

Source.   Adapted from Schatzberg AF, Cole JO, DeBattista C: *Manual of Clinical Psychopharmacology,* 4th Edition. Washington, DC, American Psychiatric Publishing, 2003, p. 422. Used with permission.

day of Concerta helped her stay focused and concentrate. She rounded out her ADHD regimen with reading about the disorder in books and on the Internet and with help from a job coach.

Does Treating ADHD Make Later Substance Abuse Less Likely?

Naturally, clinicians worry that treating ADHD patients with stimulants will make substance abuse more likely. The stimulants are themselves substances of abuse. Methylphenidate is the third most often abused prescribed substance in the United States. Among teenagers, it is not the ones who have ADHD who are abusing methylphenidate, however (Drug Enforcement Administration 1995). The short-acting stimulants are more likely substances of abuse than the long-acting preparations (Wilens et al. 2004). We have little information about the prevalence of abuse of CNS stimulants by patients who take them for ADHD. In one small study, 3 (8%) out of 37 ADHD patients abused prescribed stimulants (Higgins 2002).

Treating ADHD with stimulant medication reduces the likelihood of later substance abuse. One 5-year study traced ADHD adolescents and young adults after such treatment. By the end of the study period, subjects who had not been treated with stimulants, and those who responded poorly to them, were more likely to have illegal substance abuse (Loney et al. 1981). Another study followed youths for 4 years, starting in mid-adolescence. Again, medicated ADHD youths were less likely to abuse alcohol, cocaine, stimulants, and other illicit drugs than their unmedicated age-peers who had ADHD. Rates of substance abuse were similar between the medicated ADHD group and the non-ADHD control group (Biederman et al. 1999b).

The most recent study of the impact of stimulant treatment during childhood and high school found "no compelling evidence that such treatment of children with ADHD leads to an increased risk for substance experimentation, use, dependence, or abuse by adulthood" (Barkley et al. 2003, p. 107). In a recent meta-analysis of studies involving 674 medicated ADHD patients and 360 unmedicated patients, stimulant therapy lowered the risk of later substance abuse by nearly twofold. The effect on adolescents was more marked than it was on adults. Their 50% reduction in risk indicates that the ultimate risk of substance abuse in individuals treated for ADHD with CNS stimulants may approach that of the general population (Wilens et al. 2003b).

ADHD, LEARNING DISORDERS, AND LEARNING DISABILITIES

Learning disorders are difficulties in acquiring and using one or more cognitive skills. Affected persons have problems processing information. Having a learning disorder means that a person has a significant discrepancy (at least 1.5 standard deviations) between his or her cognitive abilities (IQ) and achievement scores on psychometric testing. Other signs include reversing letters or having difficulties in sequencing, reading, doing mathematics, or learning language.

In DSM-IV-TR, the diagnoses in children with these problems are on Axis I as learning disorders and communication disorders (American Psychiatric Association 2000). For the diagnosis to apply, patients must have a significant discrepancy between their potential and actual levels of achievement. As with other disorders, this diagnosis requires determining that the disturbance is not due primarily to other disorders such as physical or neurological disorders, pervasive developmental disorders, and so on. Neither is the learning disorder due to inadequate educational opportunities.

Learning disabilities is a legal term that refers to a federal law disability category that determines eligibility for special education services. Strictly speaking, *learning disabled* refers only to persons who have met the legal definition of the term. In this book, however, the term *learning disability* applies to a child or an adult with one or more learning disorders.

Persons with a learning disability have circumscribed impairments in a minority of the cognitive modules in the mental status domain. In contrast, mentally retarded persons are impaired in a majority of these cognitive modules (Denckla 2000). Learning-disabled individuals typically have problems such as poor short-term memory, letter reversals, sequencing problems, and spatial confusion. Often psychological testing reveals a pattern of strengths and weaknesses.

Children with learning disorders are sometimes labeled "dyslexic." Strictly speaking, the term *dyslexia* refers to language-related deficits in naming, repetition, syntax, and verbal memory. The classic hallmark of dyslexia is slow, effortful reading.

Having learning disabilities does not mean that someone is stupid. Many learning-disabled persons are gifted and talented. They are, however, frustrated when they feel that they cannot consistently make full use of their abilities. Learning-disabled students may take longer than others to process information. They have strong preferences in their learning style. They often need accommodations such as sitting near the teacher, getting tutors and note-taking services, and having additional time on tests.

Learning Disorders and ADHD in Children

Where there are learning disabilities there is also often ADHD. Both are typically diagnosed in childhood and persist. Both are associated with academic problems. Compensating for learning disabilities requires sustained attention, which the ADHD child (or adult) lacks.

ADHD and learning disorders, however, are not two names for the same problem. They usually exist independently of each other (DuPaul and Stoner 1994). Studies consistently show that ADHD and, for example, reading disorders are genetically independent (Biederman et al. 1993). Clinicians define ADHD solely in terms of behavior. We define learning disorders as measured deficits in one or more basic psychological processes, independent of behavior (Tannock and Brown 2000).

As a conservative estimate, one in four children with ADHD also has specific learning disabilities. Conversely, of the 5%–10% of children who have a learning disorder, about one in three also has ADHD. Children with both ADHD and learning disabilities frequently have difficulty understanding and following directions. They may miss interpersonal social cues (Tannock and Brown 2000).

Researchers attribute both learning disabilities and ADHD to abnormalities of the brain, but questions linger about the nature of the lesions. Learning disabilities are associated with left-hemisphere structural and functional abnormalities and with a larger corpus callosum. The findings in ADHD differ: here, there are frontal-striatal abnormalities, especially in the right hemisphere; cerebellar abnormalities; and a smaller corpus callosum (Seidman et al. 2004).

An ADHD child suspected of having learning disorders needs specialized testing. Treating the ADHD with CNS stimulants typically produces academic improvement but does not relieve the learning problems. Supportive psychotherapy often helps. Children having both disorders need treatment for both (Tannock and Brown 2000).

Learning Disabilities, Executive Dysfunction, and Adult ADHD

Only a small portion of learning-disabled persons are diagnosed and treated effectively when they are in school. Many learning-disabled adults continue to be dyslexic. Not only do they struggle to read, but they also have spelling errors, make grammatical mistakes, and use words improperly. Many adults never realize they have learning disabilities. It is often difficult to find skilled assessment and treatment. Problems persist even after a good evaluation, because the adult may need workplace accommodations. Is getting special treatment worth the stigma? An estimated 20% of adults with ADHD have learning disabilities, especially visual processing problems such as dyslexia and auditory processing deficits (Barkley and Murphy 1998).

Executive dysfunction is the "zone of overlap between ADHD and learning disabilities" (Denckla 2000, p. 307). Think of ADHD as the clinical symptom and executive dysfunction as the neuropsychological sign of the same disorder. Adults with executive dysfunction may be highly intelligent but inefficient; they underachieve. They show consistent response patterns on neuropsychological tests. The combination of executive dysfunction and dyslexia makes it hard for them to meet the demands of adulthood (Denckla 2000).

Some adults have nonverbal learning disabilities, sometimes called "learning disabilities of the right hemisphere" (Tranel et al. 1987). These impairments in tactile and visual perceptual domains can cause socioemotional problems. Affected individuals are often described as "spacey" or "in a fog." They may be able to do academic tasks but fail in vocational and social settings. As a result, they are particularly vulnerable to depression and suicide (Voeller 1991).

Making the diagnosis of nonverbal learning disabilities may require specialized testing by a behavioral neurologist. Such patients often need social skills and other kinds of specific training, especially in group settings. Obviously, the symptoms of nonverbal learning disabilities overlap with those of ADHD.

Clearly, learning-disabled persons are at risk for ADHD. Having one difficulty makes the other worse. Problems with learning interfere with paying attention and completing tasks. Inattention and distractibility make it harder to learn. Among persons with ADHD, those with the predominantly inattentive subtype may be more at risk for learning disabilities (Lahey et al. 1994).

Conventional wisdom is that learning disabilities per se do not respond to CNS stimulants (Nadeau 1995). However, when a patient has both ADHD and learning disabilities, treatment with a CNS stimulant or other medication may enhance educational interventions for the learning disabilities. Those with the inattentive subtype may respond particularly well to the stimulants (Barkley et al. 1991).

> After Dirk flunked out of college, he started his own business. Energetic and resourceful, he struggled with being distractible and disorganized, and he finally sought evaluation for ADHD. The clinician diagnosed the disorder on the basis of Dirk's long-standing academic and social issues and his responses to standard rating scales. In addition, formal educational testing showed that although highly intelligent, Dirk had specific learning disabilities in mathematics and reading. This additional diagnosis explained his academic difficulties more fully. It allowed Dirk to develop strategies for his learning problems, while confirming his view that he was smart. Treatment for his ADHD dramatically boosted his productivity. His business thrived, and those close to him noticed his greater maturity and responsiveness.

CONDUCT DISORDERS

Conduct problems—oppositional behavior, defiance, aggression, and delinquency—account for most of the reported comorbidity in children with ADHD (Newcorn and Halperin 2000). The two DSM-IV-TR diagnoses covering this range of behavior are oppositional defiant disorder (ODD) and conduct disorder. Children with ODD defy authority, fail to comply with adult requests, and bully and blame others. They have minor violations of age-appropriate norms. Children with conduct disorder, on the other hand, show major violations of these norms. They commit nonaggressive acts such as truancy or running away. They also commit aggressive acts such as starting fights, carrying weapons, or assaulting others. Many young children with ODD warrant a conduct disorder diagnosis as they get older (American Psychiatric Association 2000).

ADHD is a risk factor for developing conduct disorder. ODD and conduct disorder are present in 40%–70% of children with ADHD. ODD and conduct disorder are not simply variations of the same clinical disorder. Children with ADHD and conduct disorder present with the symptoms of both disorders and have the poorest clinical outcome within each group. Children with this double diagnosis, typically active and impulsive, show symptoms early. Vigorous treatment of each disorder is important, not just for better quality of life in the present but to lessen future trouble.

In a study by Spencer et al. (2004), children who had ODD took mixed amphetamine salts, extended release, or placebo. The 308 children, ages 6–17 years, received 10, 20, 30, or 40 mg/day of active medicine or placebo. Of the sample given the extended-release formulation, 21% had ODD alone and 79% had comorbid ADHD. By the end of the 4-week study, children with comorbid ADHD and ODD who were taking active medication had significantly fewer symptoms than matched peers taking placebo. The improvement was significantly greater for youngsters taking 30 or 40 mg/day. Study participants generally tolerated the medication well. This study, interesting in itself, has implications for treating conduct disorders in adults.

A small population of children has a combination of ADHD, bipolar disorder, and conduct disorder. This combination is strongly genetic; when present, it transmits itself in families. This combination is not "just the same disorder." It is an underlying severe mood dysregulation that may express itself as bipolar disorder, conduct disorder, or ADHD (Sklar 2005).

Children with early, severe, and lasting ADHD symptoms and early, persistent disturbed behavior often develop substance abuse problems later. Many children who have conduct problems mature out of them by the end of adolescence, but some do not. Severe behavioral problems persisting past age 18 years warrant a diagnosis of antisocial personality disorder.

PERSONALITY DISORDERS

Everyone has a personality, a characteristic way of interacting with others. The term *personality disorder* fits people whose awkward or destructive interactions with others keep them from living productively and happily. Dysfunctional personality traits occur in recognizable clusters, as reflected in common descriptive phrases: "He's so full of himself," "She's a hopeless flirt," or "He's such a user." Although personality disorder diagnoses reflect consistent patterns of maladaptive traits, they are controversial. There is less interrater reliability with them than with Axis I diagnoses. However, these maladaptive behavior patterns exist. They complicate life, and they worsen the outcome of treatment for conditions such as ADHD. Now that clinicians are treating patients with personality disorders more fully with medication as well as psychotherapy, outcomes are better than before. Still, patients with personality disorders tend to interact poorly with others, including the clinicians who treat them (American Psychiatric Association 2000).

How many ADHD patients qualify for personality disorder diagnoses? Estimates have been as high as 20% (Roy-Byrne et al. 1997). In one study, 12% of adolescents and adults with ADHD were inappropriately dramatic and were diagnosed with histrionic personality disorder. Eighteen percent missed deadlines, botched assigned tasks, and otherwise failed to follow through; they had passive-aggressive personality disorder. Twenty-one percent had antisocial personality disorder, showing exploitative, abusive, or criminal behavior (Fischer et al. 2002).

Antisocial Personality Disorder

Children with ADHD who have ODD or other conduct disorders can act out impulsively with dangerous or antisocial behavior. Continued rebelliousness in young adulthood, often coupled with substance abuse, gets them into trouble (Mannuzza et al. 1989). In studies of hyperactive children grown up, antisocial behavior occurs in 18%–45% (Dulcan 1997). Persons over age 18 years who commit illegal, aggressive acts may have antisocial personality disorder. Although many ADHD patients have problems conforming to social norms, most do not want to violate them the way persons with antisocial personality do (Wender 1995).

In one study that followed children into young adulthood (G. Weiss and Hechtman 1993), 20% of hyperactive subjects committed acts of physical aggression in the 3 years before the study, compared with 5% of control subjects. Hyperactive youngsters were more likely to have contact with the police and courts (18% who were hyperactive vs. 5% who were not). Another study comparing young adults with ADHD versus matched control subjects (Barkley 1998b) showed a similar pattern: disorderly conduct (68% vs. 54%), carrying a weapon (39% vs. 11%), assault with a weapon (22% vs. 7%), intentionally setting fires (16% vs. 5%), and breaking and entering (20% vs. 8%). Overall, 22% of the formerly hyperactive group had been arrested for a felony, whereas the percentage for control subjects was 3%.

The great majority of individuals with ADHD are not antisocial as adults. About 18%–25% show consistently aberrant behavior and warrant an antisocial personality disorder diagnosis. As expected, hyperactive/impulsive symptoms predispose to antisocial behavior. Inattention does not appear to play a significant role (Babinski et al. 1999).

Cases of antisocial conduct likely overlap with the 10%–20% of ADHD adults who abuse alcohol or other substances (Mannuzza et al.

1993). Many common criminals likely have undiagnosed and untreated ADHD. One study showed that 25.5% of a random sample of inmates in the Utah state prison warranted the diagnosis of ADHD. The prevalence of major depression in this population was also 25.5% (Eyestone and Howell 1994). Such figures are likely underestimates. One study of new inmates at one of the largest prisons in California found that 75% had a childhood history of ADHD or learning disabilities, or both (Dizmang 1997). These studies support what seems obvious—but what, to date, has received little formal study—that persons who cannot regulate their behavior in socially acceptable ways are likely to have ADHD.

Conduct or behavior problems can be resistant to treatment. One approach to troubled children who have ADHD, which may also help adults with the disorder, comes from the protocol of the Texas Consensus Conference on ADHD (Pliszka et al. 2000). With such patients, the first decision is whether to try treatment other than medication, such as CBT. If you decide to try medication, start with stimulant monotherapy. The medication often reduces overt aggressive behavior in children, and it may do so in adults (Murphy et al. 1992). If both the ADHD symptoms and the aggressive outbursts subside, continue treatment with the stimulant alone. If the ADHD symptoms respond poorly or not at all to stimulant monotherapy, use the other medication options in the ADHD treatment algorithm. If aggression fails to respond or responds poorly, try a mood stabilizer such as lithium carbonate or divalproex sodium. If the mood stabilizer fails, try an alpha-agonist, such as clonidine (Catapres) or guanfacine (Tenex). In severe or unresponsive cases, try a second-generation antipsychotic such as risperidone (Risperdal). Start with as low as 0.5 mg/day of Risperdal and increase to as much as 6 mg/day (Pliszka et al. 2000).

If a patient has antisocial personality disorder, it is harder to treat his or her ADHD successfully. Families need support to deal with the destructive impact of the patient's behavior. Clinicians should never prescribe stimulant medications for these patients when there is the risk of abuse, overdose, diversion, or illegal sale. ADHD is easier to treat than the personality disorder. Treating antisocial persons for ADHD may help them focus and concentrate, but it does *not* help control antisocial behavior. Patients and family members need to know this fact so they can have realistic expectations.

Borderline Personality Disorder

The diagnostic criteria for ADHD and borderline personality disorder (BPD) overlap. In both conditions, patients have long-standing difficulties, often with unsatisfying school and work experiences. In both disorders, patients are moody and impulsive and prone to substance abuse. Often these patients have good reason to feel that they have not achieved what they would like in life.

Patients with BPD live intensely, often with outbursts of anger. They swing between idealizing and devaluing others. Needy and afraid that they will not be gratified, they reject others before they can be spurned. Often their distrust springs from physical, sexual, and emotional abuse that started in childhood and continues. Their work history is turbulent. Impulsive and emotional, they can become suicidal. Many cut themselves or overdose on prescription or other medications when life feels intolerable. Treatment for patients with BPD is more effective than in the past. An interactive form of psychotherapy often helps. Varied medications, including antidepressants, mood stabilizers, and antipsychotic medications, lessen their mood swings and extreme reactivity (American Psychiatric Association 2000).

Differentiating BPD and ADHD can be difficult. Some patients come to be evaluated for ADHD, citing work problems, scattered concentration, and erratic emotional life. Initially they may seem emotionally healthier than they are, and the psychiatrist may underestimate their problems. In some patients, the extent of their borderline psychopathology becomes clear only later in treatment.

Although formal research provides little help in distinguishing the two disorders, there are some important differences, clinically (Barkley 1998a). ADHD typically begins in childhood, but borderline symptoms flare in adolescence. Patients with ADHD are irritable and impulsive but rarely show the affect storms or rages that characterize BPD. ADHD adults often have good relationships; unlike the hostile-dependent borderline patients, ADHD individuals are willing to strike out on their own in life.

Persons with ADHD often have a strong sense of identity, unlike the profound uncertainty of borderline patients. People close to ADHD patients find them exasperating because they are unreliable, inconsistent, and "oblivious"; however, people dealing with borderline persons describe them as manipulative and overly sensitive. Although ADHD adults can perform poorly under stress, they do not transiently lose contact with reality as those with BPD do. ADHD adults are less likely to be suicidal or to act out emotionally or manipulatively. Patients with BPD lash out actively, fueled by inner rage; ADHD adults are impulsive without meaning harm.

Depressed borderline patients who feel empty, angry, and frightened can become intensely and repetitively suicidal. In contrast, ADHD patients feel depressed when they fail to meet their life goals or when they disappoint others, but they are rarely suicidal.

Both ADHD and BPD patients complain of boredom. The patient with BPD seeks out intensely emotional relationships, because outside of them life seems flat. For many borderline patients, sex is a refuge from emotional boredom. They feel more real when they are in intimate physical contact with another person (M. Weiss et al. 1999). In contrast, the adult with ADHD craves excitement: sex, intense athletics, or a stimulating business environment—anything to get into a "charged state of hyperfocus" (Barkley 1998a).

Some borderline patients also meet the diagnostic criteria for ADHD; in one study, 14% of adolescents and adults had both disorders (Fischer et al. 2002). In patients with BPD who also have ADHD, the severity of the personality disorder controls the clinical outcome. Treating the personality disorder comes first, and that may be challenging (M. Weiss et al. 1999). Some clinicians feel that borderline patients do not do well with the stimulants and develop problems with them in the long term. Clinicians must also be vigilant about possible abuse of alcohol or other substances (Barkley 1998a).

When evaluating patients, keep in mind the possibility of personality disorder, especially borderline personality. That awareness may save considerable trouble later.

TIC DISORDER/TOURETTE'S DISORDER

Tics are repetitive behaviors that are only partially under voluntary control. They occur in muscles or muscle groups, presenting as eye blinking, facial twitching, and neck jerking. They can also be vocal, such as making grunting, snorting, or sniffing noises. Typically tics start in early childhood, peaking between the ages of 8 and 12, and subside over time. By 18 years of age, one-half of a group of children who had had tics were free of them (Leckman et al. 1998).

Children who have multiple motor tics and at least one vocal tic have Tourette's disorder. Such children risk being teased or having other social problems. The disorder, which runs in families, often occurs in children with ADHD (American Psychiatric Association 2000). Estimates of children with Tourette's disorder who have ADHD range from 31% to 86% (M. Weiss et al. 1999). Most ADHD children who have tics respond to stimulant treatment without increasing their tics (Gadow et al. 1999). However, stimulants sometimes worsen tics; clinicians need to warn patients and family members about this possibility (Zametkin and Ernst 1999).

In one study of adults with ADHD, 11% of 309 patients reported tics. More than 90% of the patients dated the onset of their tics to childhood. The presence of the tic did not adversely affect the treatment of the adult's ADHD (Spencer et al. 1997). In such cases, a CNS stimulant is still the medication of first choice. If the ADHD symptoms respond, and the tics stay the same or lessen, continue with stimulant monotherapy. If the tics worsen when the patient tries a stimulant, use an alternate ADHD medication. If tics continue, adding an alpha-agonist such as clonidine or guanfacine may help. That measure failing, the clinician may try a second-generation antipsychotic such as risperidone (Pliszka et al. 2000).

There is an added benefit to investigating tics and explaining them to patients. When children who have tics grow up and become parents, they often have youngsters who also have ADHD and tics. Knowledgeable adults can explain these tics to their children as neurological symptoms, not as "bad" or sick behavior. That empathetic explanation may spare the next generation some of the suffering that their parents endured (M. Weiss et al. 1999).

PSYCHOTIC DISORDERS

It is rare for ADHD to be comorbid with a psychotic condition in an adult. Making an accurate diagnosis of psychotic agitation is important, because treatment with a psychostimulant or an antidepressant can worsen psychotic symptoms.

> At age 30, Nikki sought treatment for ADHD. She was wary, demoralized by her life experiences. With good reason, she felt that others had exploited her good nature and generosity. On evaluation, she had ADHD, not otherwise specified. After taking a CNS stimulant for a few days, she became overtly paranoid. She asserted that a huge "secret society" existed, whose purpose was to do her harm. After she discontinued the stimulant and took antipsychotic medication instead, her paranoia subsided. She was able to try alternative treatment for ADHD, with moderate success.

ADHD patients do not have hallucinations, delusions, or breakthrough primary process thinking. However, they may have loose thought patterns, engage in dangerous behavior, and show little awareness of their environment. The motor activity of hyperactive ADHD patients seems continuous, and the tempo of their impulsivity seems fairly constant. This symptom pattern contrasts with the irregular, less predictable affective and body tempo of psychotic adults. The cognitive distortions of psychotic adults can produce anger and emotional over-reactions that last for hours. The overreactions of adults with ADHD typically come from misunderstandings and disagreements. Their angry outbursts typically resolve quickly. Although psychotic disorders tend to worsen over time, ADHD symptoms gradually improve (Popper et al. 2003).

ADHD AND MULTIPLE COMORBIDITIES

Patients with ADHD and multiple comorbid diagnoses are the ones who make us stretch. With every additional diagnosis, the problems multiply and the prognosis darkens.

> At 28, Jodi had a long-standing history of abuse of alcohol and other substances plus recurrent anxiety and depression, including suicide attempts. In high school, panic attacks paralyzed her in social situations. She found that cocaine calmed her down and helped her to concentrate. She flunked out of college. She impulsively married a heroin-addicted man who was a drug dealer. Although she managed to stay off heroin, she abused other drugs.
>
> When Jodi was in an outpatient drug treatment program, her psychiatrist diagnosed her with ADHD as well as depression and abuse of alcohol and cocaine. While Jodi was abstinent from substances, her doctor tried medication for ADHD; Adderall XR helped. However, Jodi could not maintain her sobriety, and she dropped out of treatment.
>
> Her adoptive parents maintained their faith in her and urged her to get help. When we started working together, Jodi was a day laborer and was managing to be abstinent from drugs. As well as having depression and ADHD, she had severe abdominal pain and diarrhea. She became suicidally depressed and required hospitalization. Medical workup showed that she had iron-deficiency anemia and Crohn's disease. Medically stabilized and treated for depression, she started vocational rehabilitation. After her release, psychotherapy with a fine therapist helped her. Maintaining her sobriety, she began taking a therapeutic dosage of Wellbutrin XL. She got a job working in a nursery, which she enjoyed.
>
> Then she started having episodes in which she talked a lot and slept little. Further investigation showed that she had had symptoms like these before. Treatment that had focused on her ADHD had missed her history of hypomanic episodes. In addition to her other problems, she had type I bipolar disorder.
>
> Jodi's mood stabilized after starting to take Depakote with her other medication. She started functioning better at work and in her social life. She got divorced, and she found a new boyfriend. He was co-parenting twins with his ex-girlfriend, but at least he was not abusing or dealing drugs.

REFRACTORY ADHD

What Is Treatment-Refractory ADHD?

One of the great pleasures of working with adult ADHD patients is seeing their life prospects brighten when treatment works well. However, as with any psychiatric disorder, despite sustained and comprehensive treatment, some patients do not thrive. Among the many unanswered questions about ADHD in adults is how to define when the disorder is treatment refractory (Johnston 2002). The state of clinical practice concerning ADHD in adults is less advanced than, for example, the affective disorders. Although ADHD rating scales are useful, none has the general acceptance as a clinical research instrument that the Hamilton Rating Scale for Depression has for major depression (and even that scale has its detractors). We do not yet have an accepted way to quantify response and remission for adults who have ADHD. There is no agreement about what decrements are necessary on a rating scale such as the Adult ADHD Self-Report Scale to define treatment remission, response, or failure. In clinical trials, "improvement" is a 30% reduction in symptoms (Adler et al. 2005).

Without clear standards, we cannot quantify the patients we regard as having illness that is refractory to treatment. For now, it may help to use the Clinical Global Impression (CGI) Scale (Table 9–3). For decades, this scale has proven its utility in clinical research. The scale conveys how sick or how well a patient is and how well the patient is or is not responding to treatment. Researchers record their initial assessment of a patient using the CGI-Severity scale and then note their later observations of his or her course using the CGI-Improvement scale.

Using this scale, perhaps a useful definition of treatment-refractory ADHD would be the persistence of a CGI-Improvement rating of 4–7 for a period of 6 months despite sustained treatment with medication and psychotherapeutic components. The CGI Scale is simple, and judgments can be rapid. Although using the CGI Scale is a good way to track any patient's clinical progress, it is not part of the standard practice of all clinicians.

Factors Involved in Treatment-Refractory ADHD

There are multiple biological, psychological, and social reasons for ADHD to be refractory to treatment. Biological problems include the estimated 30%–40% of patients who do not respond to repeated trials of suitable medications, including the CNS stimulants and other agents.

TABLE 9–3. Clinical Global Impression Scale

Write the appropriate number on the line next to the item (only one response).

1. **Severity (CGI-S):** _____
Considering your total clinical experience with this particular population, how
mentally ill is the patient at this time?
    1=Normal, not at all ill
    2=Borderline, mentally ill
    3=Mildly ill
    4=Moderately ill
    5=Markedly ill
    6=Severely ill
    7=Among the most extremely ill of patients

2. **Improvement (CGI-I):** _____
Compared with the patient's condition on initial presentation, how much has
the patient changed?
Rate total improvement whether or not, in your judgment, it is due entirely to
drug treatment.
    1=Very much improved
    2=Much improved
    3=Minimally improved
    4=No change
    5=Minimally worse
    6=Much worse
    7=Very much worse

There are numerous stratagems to enhance the impact of medications, and these approaches are discussed in more detail later in this section. At the same time, other medical or neurological disorders and their treatments may make addressing the ADHD difficult to impossible.

Among the psychological factors for treatment failure is the demoralization of patients for whom intervention is too little or too late. Often patients are undone by the magnitude and severity of their other psychiatric disorders, especially affective disorders and substance abuse. Not all patients like to do the work in psychotherapeutic approaches, whether in CBT or in psychodynamic psychotherapy. Finding a skilled clinician to deliver treatment may be difficult. Not all patients want to make the life changes that seem called for. Some, in a power struggle with a family member or a significant other, "win" by failing to comply with treatment. Other negative personality factors may come into play. Unresolved or unaddressed transference issues, such as unrealistic expectations, unconsciously casting the psychiatrist in a negative light, or acting out unacknowledged and unaddressed feelings, can disrupt treatment. Clinicians need to be aware of the potential of such issues and deal with them when they arise. Unaddressed countertransference in the psychiatrist can cause problems as well (see Chapter 4, "Allies in Treatment").

Social and economic issues also burden patients. Family forces, such as disapproving relatives or critical, unsupportive significant others, can undermine the most thoughtful treatment. Building a better alliance with hostile or disbelieving family members may be necessary. On occasion, referral for couples or family therapy will be useful. Lack of a sustaining social network contributes to treatment failure in patients who feel isolated and unsupported.

Another example of the social and economic issues that affect treatment is the gulf between those patients who have access to the Internet and those who do not. Computer-literate patients can readily access abundant information about their disorder and its treatment (see Appendix). They can link up with a global community of people with similar issues and problems, getting support as well as information. Adults with ADHD may be disproportionately among those who do not have access to the resources of the World Wide Web. Directing patients and families to community libraries or courses about computers may help them bridge the technology gap.

Economically, not having enough money or insurance coverage for medication or other treatment can waylay even the best-motivated patient. Clinicians may need to make recommendations to low-cost or sliding-scale treatment sources in the community, when those exist.

Medication-Resistant ADHD

Among the reasons for the failure of ADHD treatment in adults, problems with medication rank high. Successful treatment rarely results from trying one medication for a few weeks. What if the patient is not responding to the usual medication? Although there is no formal protocol for ADHD medication, the flowchart in Figure 9–1 may be a useful clinical summary.

Worsened or Unchanged ADHD Symptoms

If the patient is taking a CNS stimulant, try increasing the dosage of the stimulant. However, if improvement is only temporary, do not continue increasing the dosage. Change the timing of administration, change the preparation, or try another stimulant. Consider an alternative medica-

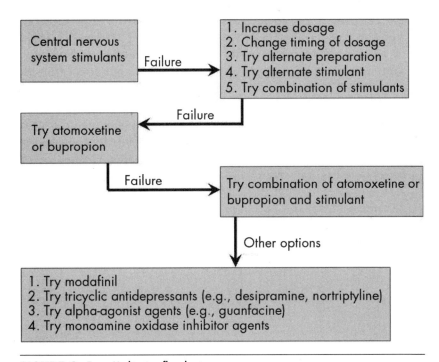

FIGURE 9–1. Medication flowchart.

tion (such as atomoxetine or bupropion). Because of different mechanisms of action of methylphenidate and amphetamine, a clinician can even consider combining these drugs to use in patients with refractory illness (Prince and Wilens 2002).

Partial Response

Treatment of ADHD with a stimulant medication can ease symptoms dramatically in one part of a patient's life but leave other symptoms untouched. With a collaborative patient, the clinician may try different medications to see what works for which symptoms. Sometimes a methylphenidate formulation may help at one time of day and an amphetamine at another. To make this adjustment, the patient needs to document the specific changes that the different formulations offer. Only a small minority of adult ADHD patients are willing and able to do that extra work.

Increasingly, clinicians are combining medications for patients who respond partially. The following combinations have proven useful (Spencer 2005b):

1. Atomoxetine and a CNS stimulant—there are no drug–drug interactions.
2. A tricyclic antidepressant, with either atomoxetine or a CNS stimulant, alone or together—this combination does not affect tricyclic blood levels.
3. Bupropion with a stimulant—this combination does not usually have adverse effects. When using this combination, monitor the patient's blood pressure particularly carefully, because both agents can raise it. Avoid this combination in a patient who has a history of seizures or of tics.

Despite sophisticated and thoughtful efforts, some patients will not respond to treatment. A patient who fails to respond to treatment needs reevaluation of all the biological, psychological, and social elements involved.

SUMMARY

- Comorbidity is usually present in the adult ADHD patient. Screen for other disorders, especially ones that are "hidden," such as a history of bipolar symptoms. Sometimes, when treatment "just for ADHD" succeeds, secondary anxiety and depression decrease. Sometimes affective and other disorders need specific and skilled interventions. Manic patients in particular require mood stabilization before trying CNS stimulants for ADHD. Patients with substance abuse must have a period of abstinence before being treated for their ADHD. A history of drug abuse, per se, should not keep clinicians from treating ADHD, but such persons bear particularly close watching.
- Patients with ADHD do not all respond to treatment as hoped. A possible definition of treatment-refractory ADHD is the persistence of a CGI-Improvement scale rating of 4–7 for 6 months despite sustained treatment that includes medication as well as psychotherapy and environmental intervention. Several strategies address medication-resistant or treatment-refractory ADHD. These strategies include maximizing dosage, switching medication, and combining medications known to be effective. Comorbid conditions, especially if unaddressed or unsuccessfully treated, are a major cause of refractory adult ADHD. Numerous other biological, psychological, and social factors play into a patient's failure to respond. These factors need to be reevaluated in the case of the patient with treatment-refractory ADHD.

- With treatment-refractory ADHD patients, it is important to document both the treatment course taken and the reasons for doing so. Often it is useful to consult colleagues, a clinical supervisor, or both. They may provide different interventions and alternate strategies. Sometimes, however, their best contribution is to assure you that you have done what there is to do, regardless of whether you succeed. "We have considered all the options for now. We will continue to think about the patient as his clinical situation changes, and then we will see how he looks tomorrow" (J. Sabin, personal communication, Massachusetts Mental Health Center, Boston, MA, 1967).

REFERENCES

Adesman A, Brown TE, Faraone SV, et al: Optimizing ADHD outcomes. ADHD Podium 2:1–11, 2003

Adler LA, Cohen J: Diagnosis and evaluation of adults with attention-deficit hyperactivity disorder. Psychiatr Clin North Am 27:187–201, 2004

Adler LA, Dodson WW, Spencer T, et al: Diagnostic strategies for adult ADHD. Medical Crossfire 6:1–13, 2005

Akiskal HS, Maser JD, Zeller PJ, et al: Switching from 'unipolar' to bipolar II: an 11-year prospective study of clinical and temperamental predictors in 559 patients. Arch Gen Psychiatry 52:114–123, 1995

Alpert JE, Maddocks A, Nierenberg AA, et al: attention deficit hyperactivity disorder in childhood among adults with major depression. Psychiatry Res 62:213–219, 1996

Amaral DG: The primate amygdala and the neurobiology of social behavior: implications for understanding social anxiety. Biol Psychiatry 51:11–17, 2002

American Psychiatric Association: Diagnostic and Statistical Manual of Mental Disorders, 3rd Edition, Revised. Washington, DC, American Psychiatric Association, 1987

American Psychiatric Association: Practice Guideline for the Treatment of Patients With Panic Disorder. Washington, DC, American Psychiatric Association, 1998

American Psychiatric Association: Diagnostic and Statistical Manual of Mental Disorders, 4th Edition, Text Revision. Washington, DC, American Psychiatric Association, 2000

Babinski LM, Hartsough CS, Lambert NM: Childhood conduct problems, hyperactivity-impulsivity, and inattention as predictors of adult criminal activity. J Child Psychol Psychiatry 40:347–355, 1999

Barkley RA: Comorbid disorders, social relations, and subtyping, in Attention Deficit Hyperactivity Disorder, 2nd Edition. Edited by Barkley RA. New York, Guilford, 1998a, pp 139–163

Barkley RA: Developmental course, adult outcome and clinic-referred attention deficit hyperactivity disorder in adults, in Attention Deficit Hyperactivity Disorder, 2nd Edition. Edited by Barkley RA. New York, Guilford, 1998b, pp 186–224

Barkley RA, Murphy K: Attention-Deficit Hyperactivity Disorder: A Clinical Workbook, 2nd Edition. New York, Guilford, 1998

Barkley RA, DuPaul GJ, McMurray MB: Attention deficit disorder with and without hyperactivity: clinical response to three dose levels of methylphenidate. Pediatrics 87:519–531, 1991

Barkley RA, Fischer M, Smallish L, et al: Does the treatment of attention-deficit/ hyperactivity disorder with stimulants contribute to drug abuse? a 13-year prospective study. Pediatrics 111:97–109, 2003

Bebchuk JM, Tancer ME: Neurobiology of social phobia. CNS Spectr 4:42–48, 1999

Biederman J, Faraone SV, Keenan K, et al: Family genetic and psychosocial risk factors in DSM III attention deficit disorder. J Am Acad Child Adolesc Psychiatry 29:526–533, 1990

Biederman J, Faraone SV, Keenan K, et al: Evidence of familial association between attention deficit disorder and major affective disorders. Arch Gen Psychiatry 148:633–642, 1991a

Biederman J, Faraone SV, Keenan K, et al: Familial association between attention deficit disorder and anxiety disorders. Am J Psychiatry 148:251–256 1991b

Biederman J, Faraone SV, Keenan K, et al: Further evidence for family genetic risk factors in attention deficit hyperactivity disorder: patterns of comorbidity in probands and relatives in psychiatrically and pediatrically referred samples. Arch Gen Psychiatry 149:728–738, 1992

Biederman J, Faraone SV, Spencer T, et al: Patterns of psychiatric comorbidity, cognition and psychosocial function in adults with attention deficit hyperactivity disorder. Am J Psychiatry 150:1792–1798, 1993

Biederman J, Faraone SV, Spencer T, et al: Gender differences in a sample of adults with ADHD. Psychiatry Res 53:13–29, 1994

Biederman J, Faraone SV, Mick E, et al: Psychiatric comorbidity among referred juveniles with major depression: fact or artifact? J Am Acad Child Adolesc Psychiatry 4:579–590, 1995a

Biederman J, Faraone SV, Mick EA, et al: Psychoactive substance use disorders in adults with attention deficit hyperactivity disorder (ADHD): effects of ADHD and comorbidity. Am J Psychiatry 152:1652–1658, 1995b

Biederman J, Faraone S, Milberger S, et al: A prospective 4-year follow-up study of attention-deficit hyperactivity and related disorders. Arch Gen Psychiatry 53:437–446, 1996

Biederman J, Mick E, Bostic JQ, et al: The naturalistic course of pharmacologic treatment of children with maniclike symptoms: a systematic chart review. J Clin Psychiatry 59:628–637, 1998a

Biederman J, Mick E, Faraone SV: Depression in attention deficit hyperactivity disorder children: true depression or demoralization? J Affect Disord 47:113–122, 1998b

Biederman J, Wilens T, Mick E, et al: Does attention-deficit hyperactivity disorder impact the developmental course of drug and alcohol abuse and dependence? Biol Psychiatry 44:269–273, 1998c

Biederman J, Faraone SV, Mick E, et al: Clinical correlates of attention deficit hyperactivity disorder in females: findings from a large group of pediatrically and psychiatrically referred girls. J Am Acad Child Adolesc Psychiatry 38:966–975, 1999a

Biederman J, Wilens T, Mick E, et al: Pharmacotherapy of attention-deficit/hyperactivity disorder reduces risk for substance use disorder. Pediatrics 104:e20, 1999b

Blanco C, Antia SX, Liebowitz MR: Pharmacotherapy of social anxiety disorder. Biol Psychiatry 51:109–120, 2002

Borkovec TD, Ruscio AM: Psychotherapy for generalized anxiety disorder. J Clin Psychiatry 62(suppl):37–42, 2001

Bremner JD, Southwick SM, Darnell A, et al: Chronic PTSD in Vietnam combat veterans: course of illness and substance abuse. Am J Psychiatry 153:369–375, 1996

Bremner JD, Vythilingam M, Vermetten E, et al: MRI and PET study of deficits in hippocampal structure and function in women with childhood sexual abuse and posttraumatic stress disorder. Am J Psychiatry 160:924–932, 2003

Brent DA, Perper JA, Goldstein CE, et al: Risk factors for adolescent suicide: a comparison of adolescent suicide victims with suicidal inpatients. Arch Gen Psychiatry 45:581–588, 1988

Brown TE: Differential diagnosis of ADD versus ADHD in adults, in A Comprehensive Guide to ADD in Adults. Edited by Nadeau KG. New York, Brunner/Mazel, 1995, pp 93–108

Brown TE: Assessment methods for ADHD in children, adolescents, and adults. Paper presented at the annual meeting of the American Academy of Adolescent Psychiatry, Philadelphia, PA, October 1996

Brown TE: Attention-deficit disorders with obsessive-compulsive disorder, in Attention-Deficit Disorders and Comorbidities in Children, Adolescents, and Adults. Edited by Brown TE. Washington, DC, American Psychiatric Press, 2000a, pp 209–230

Brown TE: Emerging understandings of attention-deficit disorders and comorbidities, in Attention-Deficit Disorders and Comorbidities in Children, Adolescents, and Adults. Edited by Brown TE. Washington DC, American Psychiatric Press, 2000b, pp 3–54

Bruce SE, Vasile RG, Goisman RM: Are benzodiazepines still the agents of choice for patients with panic disorder with or without agoraphobia? Am J Psychiatry 160:1432–1438, 2003

Cantwell D: Psychiatric illness in the families of hyperactive children. Arch Gen Psychiatry 27:414–417, 1972

Carroll KM, Rounsaville BJ: History and significance of childhood attention deficit disorder in treatment-seeking cocaine abusers. Compr Psychiatry 34:75–82, 1993

Castaneda R, Sussman N, Levy R, et al: A treatment algorithm for attention deficit hyperactivity disorder in cocaine-dependent adults: a one-year private practice study with long-acting stimulants, fluoxetine, and bupropion. Subst Abus 20:59–71, 1999

Charney DS, Deutch AY, Krystal JH, et al: Psychobiologic mechanisms of post-traumatic stress disorder. Arch Gen Psychiatry 50:294–305, 1993

Croft HA: Physician handling of prescription stimulants. Psychiatr Ann 35:221–226, 2005

Davidson JRT: Pharmacotherapy of generalized anxiety disorder. J Clin Psychiatry 62(suppl):46–50, 2001

DeMilio L: Psychiatric syndromes in adolescent substance abusers. Am J Psychiatry 146:1212–1214, 1989

Denckla MB: Learning disabilities and attention-deficit/hyperactivity disorder in adults: overlap with executive dysfunction, in Attention-Deficit Disorders and Comorbidities in Children, Adolescents, and Adults. Edited by Brown TE. Washington, DC, American Psychiatric Press, 2000, pp 297–318

DiNardo P, Brown TA, Barlow DH: Anxiety Disorders Interview Schedule for DSM-IV. San Antonio, TX, Psychological Corporation, 1994

Disney ER, Elkins IJ, McGue M, et al: Effects of ADHD, conduct disorder, and gender on substance use and abuse in adolescence. Am J Psychiatry 156:1515–1521, 1999

Dizmang L: Attention deficit disorder/learning disorder at the California Medical Facility in Vacaville, CA. Paper presented at the Kitty Petty Institute Symposium, Vacaville, CA, May 1997

Doyle A, Pollack MH: Long-term management of panic disorder. J Clin Psychiatry 65(suppl):24–28, 2004

Drug Enforcement Administration: Methylphenidate Review Document No. 20537. Washington, DC, Office of Diversion Control, Drug and Chemical Evaluation Section, Drug Enforcement Administration, 1995

Dulcan M: Practice parameters for the assessment and treatment of children, adolescents, and adults with ADHD. J Am Acad Child Adolesc Psychiatry 36(suppl):85S–118S, 1997

Dunner DL, Schmaling KB, Hendricksen H, et al: Cognitive therapy versus fluoxetine in the treatment of dysthymic disorder. Depression 4:34–41, 1996

Dunner DL, Hendricksen HE, Bea C, et al: Dysthymic disorder: treatment with citalopram. Depress Anxiety 15:18–22, 2002

DuPaul GJ, Stoner G: ADHD in the Schools: Assessment and Treatment Strategies. New York, Guilford, 1994

Earls F, Reich W, Jung KG, et al: Psychopathology in children of alcoholic and antisocial parents. Alcohol Clin Exp Res 12:481–487, 1988

Eyestone LL, Howell RJ: An epidemiological study of attention-deficit hyperactivity disorder and major depression in a male prison population. Bull Am Acad Psychiatry Law 22:181–193, 1994

Faraone SV, Biederman J: Do attention deficit hyperactivity disorder and major depression share familial risk factors? J Nerv Ment Dis 185:533–541, 1997

Faraone SV, Biederman J, Mennin D, et al: Attention deficit hyperactivity disorder with bipolar disorder: a familial subtype? J Am Acad Child Adolesc Psychiatry 36:1378–1387, 1997

Feinberg SS: Combining stimulants with MAOIs: a review of uses and a possible indication. J Clin Psychiatry 65:1520–1524, 2004

Fischer M, Barkley RA, Smallish L, et al: Young adult follow-up of hyperactive children: self-reported psychiatric disorders, comorbidity, and the role of childhood conduct problems and teen CD. J Abnorm Child Psychol 30:463–475, 2002

Foa EB, Meadows EA: Psychosocial treatments for posttraumatic stress disorder: a critical review. Annu Rev Psychol 48:449–480, 1997

Foa EB, Franklin ME, Kozak MJ: Psychosocial treatments for obsessive-compulsive disorder: literature review, in Obsessive-Compulsive Disorder: Theory, Research and Treatment. Edited by Swinson RP, Antony MM, Rachman S, et al. New York, Guilford, 1998, pp 258–276

Friedman MJ: Pharmacologic management of posttraumatic stress disorder. Primary Psychiatry 10:66–68, 71–73, 2003

Furmark T, Tillfors M, Marteinsdottir, et al: Common changes in cerebral blood flow in patients with social phobia treated with citalopram or cognitive-behavioral therapy. Arch Gen Psychiatry 59:425–433, 2002

Gadow KD, Sverd J, Sprafkin J, et al: Long term methylphenidate therapy in children with comorbid ADHD and chronic multiple tic disorder. Arch Gen Psychiatry 56:330–336, 1999

Geller B, Zimmerman B, Williams M, et al: DSM-IV mania symptoms in a prepubertal and early adolescent bipolar disorder phenotype compared with attention-deficit/hyperactive and normal controls. J Child Adolesc Psychopharmacol 12:11–15, 2002

Glod CA, Teicher MH: Relationship between early abuse, posttraumatic stress disorder, and activity levels in prepubertal children. J Am Acad Child Adolesc Psychiatry 35:1384–1393, 1996

Heimberg RG: Cognitive-behavioral therapy for social anxiety disorder: current status and future directions. Biol Psychiatry 51:101–108, 2002

Higgins ES: ADHD and substance abuse. Current Psychiatry 1:59–65, 2002

Hirschfeld RM, Williams JB, Spitzer RL, et al: Development and validation of a screening instrument for bipolar spectrum disorder: the Mood Disorder Questionnaire. Am J Psychiatry 157:1873–1875, 2000

Horner BR, Scheibe KE: Prevalence and implications of attention-deficit hyperactivity disorder among adolescents in treatment for substance abuse. J Am Acad Child Adolesc Psychiatry 36:30–36, 1997

Johnston C: The impact of attention deficit hyperactivity disorder on social and vocational functioning in adults, in Attention Deficit Hyperactivity Disorder: State of the Science, Best Practices. Edited by Jensen PS, Cooper JR. Kingston, NJ, Civic Research Institute, 2002, pp 6–16 to 6–18

Katusic SK, Barbaresi WJ, Colligan RC, et al: Substance abuse among ADHD cases: a population-based birth study. Paper presented at the Pediatric Academic Society, Seattle, WA, April 2003

Kessler RC: Posttraumatic stress disorder: the burden to the individual and to society. J Clin Psychiatry 61(suppl):4–12, 2000

Kessler RC, Sonnega A, Bromet E, et al: Posttraumatic stress disorder in the National Comorbidity Survey. Arch Gen Psychiatry 52:1048–1060, 1995

Lahey BB, Applegate B, McBurnett K, et al: DSM-IV field trials for attention deficit hyperactivity disorder in children and adolescents. Am J Psychiatry 151:1673–1685, 1994

Leckman JF, Zhang H, Vitale A, et al: Course of tic severity: the first two decades. Pediatrics 102:14–19, 1998

Lepine JP, Pelissolo A: Why take social anxiety disorder seriously? Depress Anxiety 11:87–92, 2000

Levin F, Evans S, McDowell D, et al: Bupropion treatment for adult ADHD and cocaine abuse. Paper presented at the annual meeting of the College of Problems in Drug Dependence, Scottsdale, AZ, September 1998a

Levin FR, Evans SM, McDowell DM, et al: Methylphenidate treatment of cocaine abusers with adult attention-deficit/hyperactivity disorder: a pilot study. J Clin Psychiatry 59:300–305, 1998b

Loney J, Klahn M, Kosier T, et al: Hyperactive boys and their brothers at 21: predictors of aggressive and antisocial outcomes. Paper presented at the Society of Life History Research, Monterey CA, March 1981

Mannuzza S, Gittelman-Klein R, Konig PH, et al: Hyperactive boys almost grown up, IV: criminality and its relationship to psychiatric status. Arch Gen Psychiatry 46:1073–1079, 1989

Mannuzza S, Klein RG, Bonagura N, et al: Hyperactive boys almost grown up, V: replication of psychiatric status. Arch Gen Psychiatry 48:77–83, 1991

Mannuzza S, Klein RG, Bessler A, et al: Adult outcome of hyperactive boys: educational achievement, occupational rank, and psychiatric status. Arch Gen Psychiatry 50:565–576, 1993

March JS, Frances A, Carpenter D, et al: Treatment of obsessive-compulsive disorder: the expert consensus guidelines. J Clin Psychiatry 58(suppl):1–72, 1997

Marks I, Lovell K, Noshirvani H, et al: Treatment of posttraumatic stress disorder by exposure and/or cognitive restructuring. Arch Gen Psychiatry 55:317–325, 1998

Marshall R: Clinical review of post traumatic stress disorder. Currents in Affective Illness 19:5–10, 2000

Mathew SJ, Coplan JD, Gorman JM: Neurobiological mechanisms of social anxiety disorder. Am J Psychiatry 158:1558–1567, 2001

McDermott SP: Cognitive therapy for adults with attention-deficit/hyperactivity disorder, in Attention-Deficit Disorders and Comorbidities in Children, Adolescents, and Adults. Edited by Brown TE. Washington, DC, American Psychiatric Press, 2000, pp 569–606

McElroy SL, Keck PE, Pope HG Jr, et al: Clinical and research implications of the diagnosis of dysphoric or mixed mania or hypomania. Am J Psychiatry 149:1633–1644, 1992

McFarlane AC: Posttraumatic stress disorder: a model of the longitudinal course and the role of risk factors. J Clin Psychiatry 61(suppl):15–20, 2000

Medina J: Hippocampal volume and predicting PTSD. Psychiatric Times, February 2003, p 8–11

Mendlowicz MV, Stein MB: Quality of life in individuals with anxiety disorders. Am J Psychiatry 157:669–682, 2000

Milberger S, Biederman J, Faraone SV, et al: Attention-deficit hyperactivity disorder and comorbid disorders: issues of overlapping symptoms. Am J Psychiatry 152:1793–1799, 1995

Milberger S, Biederman J, Faraone SV, et al: ADHD is associated with early initiation of cigarette smoking in children and adolescents. J Am Acad Child Adolesc Psychiatry 36:37–44, 1997

Milberger S, Faraone S, Biederman J, et al: Familial risk analysis of the association between attention deficit/hyperactivity disorder and psychoactive substance use disorders. Arch Pediatric Adolesc Med 152:945–951, 1998

MTA Cooperative Group: A 14-month randomized clinical trial of treatment strategies for ADHD. Multimodal Treatment Study of Children With ADHD. Arch Gen Psychiatry 56:1073–1086, 1999

Murphy DA, Pelham WE, Lang AR: Aggression in boys with ADHD: methylphenidate effects on naturalistically observed aggression, response to provocation, and social information processing. J Abnorm Child Psychol 20:451–466, 1992

Nadeau K: A Comprehensive Guide to Attention Deficit Disorder in Adults. New York, Brunner/Mazel, 1995

Newcorn JH, Halperin JM: Attention-deficit disorders with oppositionality and aggression, in Attention-Deficit Disorders and Comorbidities in Children, Adolescents, and Adults. Edited by Brown TE. Washington, DC, American Psychiatric Press, 2000, pp 171–208

Patel NC, Salle FR: What's the best treatment for comorbid ADHD/bipolar mania? Current Psychiatry 4:27–37, 2005

Pierce K: ADHD and comorbidity. Primary Psychiatry 10:69–76, 2003

Pigott TA, Seay S: Biological treatments for obsessive-compulsive disorder: literature review, in Obsessive-Compulsive Disorder: Theory, Research, and Treatment. Edited by Swinson RP, Antony MM, Rachman S, et al. New York, Guilford, 1998, pp 298–326

Pliszka SR, Greenhill LL, Crismon ML, et al: The Texas Children's Medication Algorithm Project. Report of the Texas Consensus Conference Panel on Medication Treatment of Childhood ADHD, part II: tactics. J Am Acad Child Adolesc Psychiatry 39:920–927, 2000

Pomerleau O, Downey K, Stetson F, et al: Cigarette smoking in adults diagnosed with attention deficit hyperactivity disorder. J Subst Abuse 7:373–378, 1995

Popper CW, Gammon GD, West SA, et al: Disorders usually first diagnosed in infancy, childhood, or adolescence, in The American Psychiatric Publishing Textbook of Clinical Psychiatry, 4th Edition. Edited by Hales RE, Yudofsky SC. Washington, DC, American Psychiatric Publishing, 2003, pp 833–974

Prince JB, Wilens TE: Pharmacotherapy of adult ADHD, in Clinician's Guide to Adult ADHD: Assessment and Intervention. New York, Elsevier Science, 2002, pp 165–186

Reimherr FW, Hedges D, Strong R: An open trial of venlafaxine in adult patients with attention-deficit hyperactivity disorder. Paper presented at the New Clinical Drug Evaluation Unit Program, Orlando, FL, June 1995

Riggs P: Clinical approach to treatment of ADHD in adolescents with substance abuse and conduct disorder. J Am Acad Child Adolesc Psychiatry 37:331–332, 1998

Roy-Byrne P, Scheele L, Brinkley J, et al: Adult ADHD: assessment guidelines based on clinical presentation to a specialty clinic. Compr Psychiatry 38:133–140, 1997

Schatzberg AF, Cole JO, DeBattista C: Manual of Clinical Psychopharmacology, 4th Edition. Washington, DC, American Psychiatric Publishing, 2003, pp 423–435

Scheck MM, Schaeffer JA, Gillette C: Brief psychological intervention with traumatized young women: the efficacy of eye movement desensitization and reprocessing. J Trauma Stress 11:25–44, 1998

Schmidtke K, Schorb A, Winkelmann G, et al: Cognitive frontal lobe dysfunction in obsessive compulsive disorder. Biol Psychiatry 43:666–673, 1998

Schneier FR, Liebowitz MD, Abi-Dargham A, et al: Low dopamine D_2 receptor binding potential in social phobia. Am J Psychiatry 157:457–459, 2000

Seidman LJ, Valera EM, Bush G: Brain function and structure in adults with attention-deficit/hyperactivity disorder. Psychiatr Clin North Am 27:323–347, 2004

Shekim WO, Asarnow RF, Hess E, et al: A clinical and demographic profile of a sample of adults with attention deficit hyperactivity disorder, residual state. Compr Psychiatry 31:416–425, 1990

Simon NM, Otto MW, Weiss RD, et al: Pharmacotherapy for bipolar disorder and comorbid conditions: baseline data from STEP-BD. J Clin Psychopharmacol 24:512–520, 2004

Sklar M: The genetics of attention deficit hyperactivity disorder. Paper presented at ADHD Across the Life Span, Boston, MA, March 2005

Solanto MV, Wender PH: Does methylphenidate constrict cognitive functioning? J Am Acad Child Adolesc Psychiatry 28:897–902, 1989

Spencer T: Adult ADHD. Paper presented at the annual meeting of the American Academy of Child and Adolescent Psychiatry, New Orleans, LA, October 1995

Spencer T: Adult ADHD. Presented at ADHD Across the Life Span, Boston, MA, March 2005a

Spencer T: Nonstimulant pharmacotherapy of ADHD. Presented at ADHD Across the Life Span, Boston, MA, March 2005b

Spencer T, Coffey B, Biederman J: Chronic tics in adults with ADHD, in Scientific Proceedings of the annual meeting of the American Academy of Child and Adolescent Psychiatry. Washington, DC, American Academy of Child and Adolescent Psychiatry, 1997, pp 76–77

Spencer T, Wilens T, Biederman J, et al: Attention-deficit/hyperactivity disorder with mood disorders, in Attention-Deficit Disorders and Comorbidities in Children, Adolescents, and Adults. Edited by Brown TE. Washington, DC, American Psychiatric Press, 2000, pp 79–124

Spencer T, Wilens T, Biederman J: Mixed amphetamine salts XR may improve ODD symptoms in children. Poster 69 at the 17th Annual U.S. Psychiatric and Mental Health Congress, San Diego, CA, November 2004

Tannock R, Brown TE: Attention-deficit disorders with learning disorders in children and adolescents, in Attention-Deficit Disorders and Comorbidities in Children, Adolescents, and Adults. Edited by Brown TE. Washington, DC, American Psychiatric Press, 2000, pp 231–295

Tannock R, Ickowicz A, Schachar R: Effects of comorbid anxiety disorder on stimulant response in children with ADHD. The ADHD Report 3:13–14, 1996

Taylor S: Assessment of obsessive-compulsive disorder, in Obsessive-Compulsive Disorder: Theory, Research and Treatment. Edited by Swinson RP, Anthony MM, Rachman S, et al. New York, Guilford, 1998, pp 229–257

Tranel D, Hall LE, Olson S, et al: Evidence for a right-hemisphere developmental learning disability. Dev Neuropsychol 3:113–127, 1987

Tzelepis A, Schlubinger H, Warbasse LH: Differential diagnosis and psychiatric comorbidity patterns in adult ADD, in A Comprehensive Guide to Attention Deficit Disorder in Adults. Edited by Nadeau K. New York, Brunner/Mazel, 1995, pp 35–48

Voeller KKS: Social-emotional learning disabilities. Psychiatr Ann 21:735–741, 1991

Weiss G, Hechtman L: Hyperactive Children Grown Up, 2nd Edition. New York, Guilford, 1993

Weiss G, Hechtman T, Milroy T, et al: Psychiatric status of hyperactives as adults: a controlled 15-year prospective follow up of 63 hyperactive children. J Am Acad Child Psychiatry 211–220, 1985

Weiss M, Hechtman L, Weiss G: ADHD in Adults. Baltimore, MD, Johns Hopkins University Press, 1999

Weissman MM, Markowitz JC: Interpersonal psychotherapy. Arch Gen Psychiatry 51:599–606, 1994

Wender PH: Attention-Deficit Hyperactivity Disorder in Adults. New York, Oxford University Press, 1995

Wender PH, Reimherr FW, Wood DR: Attention deficit disorder ('minimal brain dysfunction') in adults: a replication study of diagnosis and drug treatment. Arch Gen Psychiatry 38:449–456, 1981

Wender PH, Reimherr FW, Wood D, et al: A controlled study of methylphenidate in the treatment of attention deficit disorder, residual type, in adults. Am J Psychiatry 142:547–552, 1985

West SA, Sax KW, Stanton P, et al: Differences in thyroid function studies in acutely manic adolescents with and without attention deficit hyperactivity disorder (ADHD). Psychopharmacol Bull 32:63–66, 1996

Wilens T: Comorbidity of ADHD and substance abuse. Paper presented at ADHD Across the Life Span, Boston, MA, March 2005

Wilens TE, Biederman J, Prince J, et al: Six-week, double-blind, placebo-controlled study of desipramine for adult attention deficit disorder. Am J Psychiatry 153:1147–1153, 1996

Wilens TE, Biederman J, Mick E: Does ADHD affect the course of substance abuse? findings from a sample of adults with and without ADHD. Am J Addict 7:156–163, 1998

Wilens TE, Spencer TJ, Biederman J: Attention deficit hyperactivity disorder with substance use disorders, in Attention-Deficit Disorders and Comorbidities in Children, Adolescents, and Adults. Edited by Brown TE. Washington, DC, American Psychiatric Press, 2000, pp 319–339

Wilens TE, Biederman J, Wozniak J, et al: Can adults with attention-deficit/hyperactivity disorder be distinguished from those with comorbid bipolar disorder? findings from a sample of clinically referred adults. Biol Psychiatry 54:1–8, 2003a

Wilens TE, Faraone SV, Biederman J, et al: Does stimulant therapy of attention-deficit/hyperactivity disorder beget later substance abuse? a meta-analytic review of the literature. Pediatrics 111:179–185, 2003b

Wilens TE, Faraone SV, Biederman J: Attention-deficit hyperactivity disorder in adults. JAMA 292:619–623, 2004

Wittchen HU, Hoyer J: Generalized anxiety disorder: nature and course. J Clin Psychiatry 62(suppl):15–19, 2001

Yehuda R: Neuroendocrine alterations in posttraumatic stress disorder. Primary Psychiatry 9:30–34, 2002

Zametkin AJ, Ernst M: Problems in the management of ADHD. N Engl J Med 340:40–46, 1999

C H A P T E R   1 0

ADHD ISSUES

Work, Women, and Family

ADHD AND WORK

Work is one of the great domains of life. We tend to define ourselves by what we do and how we do it. For many people, work is what they do to survive. For a lucky few, work expresses who they are: "I like what I do, and I'm lucky that I get paid to do it." The better our work fits us, the happier we tend to be. Work has its limitations, however. In Semrad's memorable words, "Nobody likes to work. It's a substitute activity for loving" (quoted in Rako and Mazer 1980, p. 63).

Many adults with ADHD find work frustrating and disappointing. Successful work requires good executive function: organizing, planning, and following through. All of these tasks are hard for persons with ADHD. Work, especially white-collar and professional jobs, often requires formal preparation such as advanced education or special training. These prerequisites are just the credentials that ADHD persons have trouble earning.

> Leah said, "My brain works part-time; I just can't predict when, so I have to work like a madwoman when I can. Before treatment, I used the pressure of deadlines to force my brain to come through for me." Despite some stunning successes as a lobbyist, she could not think of herself as smart. She had mixed feelings about her work, which she started when she could not progress beyond the master's level in her academic field. The disciplined, steady labor of writing a Ph.D. thesis on public policy was beyond her.

A recent study documents the impact of ADHD on work performance. Affected persons lost an average of 35 workdays a year, a total that included 13.6 days of absenteeism and 21.6 days of diminished performance on the job. Only 16% of those with ADHD in this survey had received any professional treatment for their disorder in the previous 12 months (Kessler et al. 2005).

Occupational problems often drive adults with ADHD to seek treatment. They may persistently struggle to retain jobs because they perform below their level of competence. Crucial questions about work for the ADHD adult are interpersonal rather than cognitive: How often have you changed jobs? Why did you change? Did you have trouble getting along with your boss (Wender 1995)? On the job, ADHD adults have problems monitoring their performance and self-correcting. They have difficulties prioritizing tasks and steadily completing them. They may compensate for their limited organizational skills by enlisting the help of support staff and other colleagues. Successful ADHD adults do so in masterly fashion, but many others flounder (Weiss et al. 1999).

Some adults with ADHD find jobs that suit their strengths. Others struggle in work that fits them poorly. When treating ADHD adults, clinicians need to be sensitive to the place that work has in the patient's life. Does it suit him or her? If not, how can the patient find new work or make the job situation better fit his or her personality and abilities?

In the following discussion, patients' experiences suggest that some occupations are more ADHD friendly than others. Beyond the specifics, however, is a general truth. Persons who best use their strengths, while compensating for their vulnerabilities, can make even unlikely settings work well for them.

ADHD-Friendly Work

No one job is going to be right for all persons with ADHD, because, when taken together, the range of ADHD symptoms is so great. Persons with what may be termed "classical" ADHD, who crave intensity and variety and engagement, enjoy high-stimulus jobs with frequent changes of focus and specific tasks and goals. Examples follow.

Journalist

With its variety, demands for work in intense bursts, and production on deadline, journalism appeals to many ADHD adults.

Eve was a young journalist reluctant to think that she might have ADHD. People from her blue-collar background did not see psychiatrists and were skeptical about "ADD." Because she had abused many drugs as a teenager and was now "clean," she did not want to take any medication, especially a central nervous system (CNS) stimulant.

Shortly after being evaluated for ADHD, she e-mailed the following (edited to conceal her identity): "I've gotten absolutely no work done today. I did an interview, then checked my e-mail and went to the office. I talked to a source of mine (not about work), then checked my e-mail. Then decided to eat lunch. I got sidetracked by checking the paper's Web site to see how I'm doing in the NCAA tournament office pool, and then noticed their job postings, which I clicked on. I read about some of the interns and then reminisced about when I was an intern and what I should have done differently about my career. Then I saw that an intern who left the paper to be treated for bipolar disorder had written about it. So naturally I looked up the story and read it, but I'm not anything like him. Then I went to WebMD, where I looked up information on the drug you gave me. Somewhere in between I called my boyfriend. And now I'm writing you. This is how my days go. I'm going to try to get some work done now."

It is hard for patients to decide whether to share information about the diagnosis and treatment of ADHD. Many worry that others will use the information against them. Psychiatric disorders and treatment still bear a stigma. However, some supervisors and coworkers are supportive and understanding. Increasingly, people personally know children and adults treated for ADHD. Generally, people are more tolerant, especially when they see that treatment means better productivity.

When Eve finally tried medication, she could think systematically, stay on task, and produce copy on time. After considerable thought, she told her editor about her ADHD. "His two teenagers have it, and he already assumed I did, too. He's just glad I'm getting treated."

Entrepreneur

Being a successful entrepreneur requires autonomous function, bold action, and, often, unconventional thinking. For some adults with ADHD, this type of work is just the thing. James Carville, the successful political consultant, regards his ADHD as an asset. His willingness to think outside conventional lines has made him a highly paid and original political entrepreneur. The case examples below highlight two executives who have ADHD: one who chose not to treat his ADHD and one who did.

David Neeleman, the owner and developer of the successful airline Jet-Blue Airways, attributes his success to his ADHD. In an interview in the *New York Times* (June 1, 2003), he attributed his creative thinking to his

ADHD. "My assistant helps me write letters and keeps my calendar. I have no idea what I'm doing from one day to the next. I don't write anything down; if I did, I'd lose the piece of paper."

Alex, a real estate developer who has ADHD, described his modus operandi: "I'm spontaneous. When I want to do a deal, I go to the guy's office and go in there. I don't check with a secretary or anything like that. I say to the guy, 'Are we going to do this deal or aren't we?' If he is, then let's get going. If he's not, then the deal's not going to happen anyway, so why dillydally? My friends can't believe what I say and do. Whenever they do something bold or unusual they say, 'I did an Alex.' My wife says, 'Why can't you be like other men and have a job?' I tell her I have a job, just not the usual 9 to 5 one. What is she complaining about, anyway? I make a load of money."

   However, when his ADHD was treated, he was much happier. "My wife says I'm actually listening to her, not just acting like I'm listening." He continued his "spontaneous" ways, making successful real estate deals but feeling more in charge of himself and better organized.

Physician

With its demand for protracted, steady application, medicine seems an unlikely work choice for adults with ADHD. Yet among the medical specialties, emergency medicine offers compelling, varied, and intensely focused work. This work is appealing to an ADHD adult, if he or she can surmount the hurdles of training.

Abe loved working in a busy, big-city emergency department. Fully engaged, he made good clinical decisions fast. Who cared if the administrators complained that he was always behind on his charts? His apartment was a mess and his finances were a disaster, but he had his priorities straight: he was saving lives.

   He came for treatment when a frosty note from the head of his service warned him that his university-affiliated hospital expected staff physicians to be board certified. Abe could not imagine studying for the exam and passing. He barely survived the first years of medical school, where only clinical work ignited his interest. His girlfriend told him that he reminded her of her brother, who had ADHD. Abe wondered if that disorder was part of his problem. On investigation, Abe proved to have a long history of learning problems starting in grammar school: English? History? Spanish? Forget them! He loved science, however, immersing himself in doing experiments and winning prizes in science fairs.

   Only when he was diagnosed and treated for ADHD was Abe able to study in a sustained way and pass his board examination. "I can even read journals!" he exulted. He continued his high-quality clinical work, with an unexpected bonus: he even caught up on dictating patient charts.

Professor

The academic life offers flexibility about work hours and, when a career goes well, control over how professors can spend their time.

> Carl, a professor, described himself: "I was born absentminded. My family told me to go into academic life, saying, 'They know how to take care of people like you.' I couldn't survive without my secretary to run my office and my wife to run my life." An African American, he specialized in the history of the black experience in this country. With his department chair's repeated urging and his editor's continual hammering, he had written several books. He admitted, however, "I've never read a book from cover to cover, not even one of my own. I've always turned away from the big challenges. I've been trying to write a comprehensive textbook for 15 years."
>
> When his ADHD was diagnosed and treated, the professor became more efficient and more productive. He said, "For the first time in my life, I finished a chapter and sent it in before it was due. My editor was flabbergasted. My wife was astonished that I was around to help pack for vacation instead of being up all night making last-minute edits." He has fresh hope about tackling and completing his comprehensive text.

Salesperson

Sales jobs seem natural to adults with ADHD, especially to those who are high-energy, engaging, and resourceful. They use their personal qualities to compensate for their weaknesses, such as neglected details or projects done at the last minute.

> Duncan was number one in his company, nationwide, for selling information technology packages. He was hyperfocused, relentlessly pushing deals to close during the critical time of year when his clients had money to spend. He was his own best advertisement for technology, practically fusing with his BlackBerry. Duncan was continually in touch, and he loved it that way. He engaged his clients fully—but his home life suffered. Only after his wife left him did he realize how absent he had been, both emotionally and literally. Even during the separation, distraught about less contact with his wife and three sons, he still had his best two work quarters ever.

ADHD-Unfriendly Work

Given their proclivities, persons with ADHD do well to avoid particular types of work. Like anyone, ADHD adults can get into jobs that do not suit them. Many end up unhappy at work because they did not get treatment for their ADHD earlier in life. That lack of treatment constricts their choices. The clinician has the challenge of helping these patients change or adapt.

Accountant

Accounting jobs require precise attention to multiple details and steady, organized work—both of which are particularly difficult for many ADHD patients.

> As a youngster, Sam was "all over the place." He was fascinated with law and politics, but his accountant father wanted him to join the family business. He barely scraped into college. His major was accounting, but he spent most of his time immersed in campus politics. He also partied, drank, and smoked marijuana. Although his political science grades were straight As, it took him 7 years to accumulate the credits for his accounting major.
>
> After graduation, he dutifully went into business with his dad. They continually quarreled about his disinterest in the meticulous, detailed work. After a long search, he found a law school that allowed him into a night program. Once in, he stopped his binge drinking and marijuana use, but it still took him 6 years to graduate. He liked the work better than accounting, but his law career was a struggle. A poor listener, he tended to blurt out his own thoughts and alienate clients. He bounced from firm to firm.
>
> When his son was diagnosed with ADHD, Sam was surprised at how well the diagnostic criteria fit himself. Even more surprising to Sam was the change made when he took the right amount of the right CNS stimulant. Now that his work is steadier and his manner less impulsive, Sam hopes that his career will stabilize.

Bureaucrat

Requiring uniformity and meticulous attention to detail, administrative work puts stress on adults who have ADHD.

> "Oooooh! All these little details are driving me crazy," said Helen, shaking her hands in exasperation. "I admit that I am lazy and immature, but something else is wrong. I'm getting desperate. Could it be ADHD?
>
> "I was an only child, my parents' little precious. They didn't care if I zoned out all the time or my room was a mess. I did zero work through high school. In college I was surprised and angry when the teachers expected me to hand in papers, and on time. I lasted exactly one semester. I drifted into work for the feds. Typing. Filing. Entry-level stuff. Sooooo boring! I hated it, and often I just didn't show up, but somehow I got promoted. My last boss, though, made it her mission in life to get me fired, and that takes some doing in the government. She almost succeeded, but then, thank God, she got promoted and left the agency.

That was a wake-up call. I'm single, I'm 47, my education is zip, and my work history stinks. My job is awful. I have to scroll through several computer screens and make dozens of little keystrokes in just the right order. Paper! Paper just propagates itself. Thank God for the computer, because without it I'd drown in paper and never be able to find anything. My office is choked with clutter, and my supervisor is bugging me about it."

Learning that she had ADHD relieved some of Helen's shame and guilt. Taking medicine for it, however, was problematic. Obese and hypertensive, she had escalating health problems. She was already taking pills for diabetes, arthritis, esophageal reflux, hypertension, and gout. "More pills? No way," she said. Instead, she hired helpers at the office and at home. Still struggling, Helen is looking for a job that will let her use her verbal skills. She's "thinking about" taking a writing course, but will she be able to produce prose for class?

Helping Patients Maximize Their Work Life

The work life of adults with ADHD responds to many commonsense recommendations: When possible, ADHD adults should have a quiet, small office space with no office mates. They should have a minimum of visitors and avoid chatting or visual contact with passersby. They should have few telephone interruptions. The work environment should be uncluttered and undistracting, with few or no windows and no nearby sound-making machinery (Popper et al. 2003).

The following psychotherapeutic process can help the ADHD adult make the most of his or her work life. The first step is looking for the patient's strengths and weaknesses, now and in the past. Although the natural focus is on work life, other successful experiences can be useful. With this information, the patient can then develop a "life mission statement" of goals that fit. Some patients like to write this out, in specifics. Others prefer to have it more as a general framework. Finally, looking at the patient's wishes in the context of his or her resources and abilities, the patient makes the changes needed to enhance his or her work life.

Evaluating the Patient's Strengths and Weaknesses

As with any patient, the evaluation of adults with ADHD starts with an assessment of their current life situation. Work that is not going well typically has several hallmarks: patients keep avoiding tasks and excusing poor performance. As a result, they persistently feel worse. Persons in ill-suited jobs operate "by the steps." Dancers start learning a dance as combinations of steps that, with practice, become a seamless whole.

Similarly, for most people, work sequences soon become smooth and automatic, but adults with ADHD feel that they never progress to mastery. Patients working in an area of weakness go through the motions just to be done. They cannot keep their eyes on a higher goal because they do not have one.

> Sandy, 58, said, "I'm sick of feeling like a loser. My Web designs are great, but I take too long. I do everything at work except what I'm supposed to do. My coworkers are all excited about new ways to use computers and do things faster. I used to think, 'What is *wrong* with you people?' but I realize now it's my problem. Some days I turn on the computer and then I look at it like I've never seen one before. I know perfectly well what to do and I do it, but every day I start all over. Retirement seems so far away. When I first came to Washington I saw these gray people on the bus, dragging themselves to work. I promised myself I wouldn't become one of them. And here I am."

After the assessment of the patient's current work situation, start reviewing the past. Sitting down with paper and pen helps to review life experiences in detail. Some patients resist, feeling that their work life has been a sorry list of failures and disappointments. Among the signs of work trouble are failure to progress, not improving on suitable skills, and feeling incompetent. Are there consistent themes or repetitive reasons for failure? Are there specific problems related to ADHD, such as failing to plan, focus, and implement steadily? Not having professional or other formal qualifications in place for a desired job? Isolation? Issues with alcohol or other substances of abuse?

> Sandy had academic problems from early on. "I was never a 'behavior problem,' but my grades through college—I majored in art history—were spotty. After I graduated, I worked in art galleries at low-paid, boring jobs." In her 40s, divorced and pressed for money, she took computer classes that led to better-paid work. She was still unproductive and unhappy.
>   Disorganization and the inability to stay on task, at home or at work, were Sandy's biggest problems. Alcohol or other drugs had no appeal to her, but burnout was a big issue. Despite her best intentions, with each new job she fell behind. "I was jumping from ice floe to ice floe, like little Eva in *Uncle Tom's Cabin*." Twice in 15 years, she sought help for depression. Treatment enabled her to get back to work but did not solve her underlying problem.

ADHD adults need help identifying strengths in their past life experiences, not just in work. One signal is being in a situation where they learn quickly and easily. Another is being in a new situation and sensing, "This feels right." People working from strength are proud of their work and pleased with themselves. When they practice, they get better. Other people respond enthusiastically to their efforts. Often, but not always, successful work is financially profitable. When people are operating out of strength, they are fully engaged and unself-conscious, "in the flow" (Csikszentmihaly 1990). Athletes describe being "in the zone"; for actors, it's being "in the moment." Flow experiences can occur in the most mundane of daily activities. Recommending that ADHD adults look for "flow" may backfire, however. They struggle with being zoned out, with being unfocused, elsewhere, or absent. They should look to activities where they hyperfocus: they get absorbed and cannot disengage. Someone operating in an area of strength can happily do the activity for hours. Good work energizes people; it does not exhaust them.

Patients need to be as specific as possible about their flow experiences. In reviewing these events, they should look for themes in their successes. What or who made those experiences possible? Was the patient on his or her own or part of a team? Was the situation highly structured or free-form? Did it call on the patient to think creatively? Was it intensely interpersonal or was it isolated? How important was money in the person's sense of success?

> Sandy was happiest when she was drawing and painting. In college, on her own, she put together a portfolio of drawings and paintings. One of her teachers encouraged her to enter two paintings in an exhibition. When they each sold for $25, she felt rich.

Building the Patient's Life Mission

Reviewing patients' present and past helps them find their mission in life. Many people stumble through life without a role or purpose. Especially if they are sabotaging themselves with substance abuse or if they struggle repetitively with depression, the life mission of many ADHD adults is simple: survive. Even these unfortunate individuals may be selling themselves short. Rare is the person who has no special interests or abilities.

Finding interests and abilities is the purpose of the life review. Factual achievements and real successes are important, certainly, but so are the patients' yearnings. Is there something they have long wanted to do but have not let themselves consider? Something they care about intensely that they have not been able to pursue? What appeals to them? Is it doing the job? The status or the income that comes from doing it? If they could control their destiny, how would they spend every day?

Patients review their strengths and decide what is central. Ideally, a life mission has a larger framework or purpose than the patient's own individual concerns and well-being. Some people ally themselves with the goals of an organization or institution, such as an educational unit, a religious group, or the military. Physicians are fortunate because a career in medicine provides many such opportunities. Others find transcendent value in tasks that seem lowly, such as the maid who knows that her well-cleaned rooms lift the spirits of hotel guests. The patient's mission is more than a longed-for ideal; it is a plan for effective action. Once patients have a better grasp of their life mission, they can begin making the most of their work. Will they stay in a current job, making it finance what they really want to do, or will they change their work entirely?

> "I'm an artist," said Sandy. "I love everything about it. The feel of the brush. The smell of the paints. Turning a blank canvas into a blaze of color. Yes, and praise, too. I'm starving for it." She paused, and then admitted, "I want to do art, but surviving comes first." On a medication regimen that allowed her to focus and to concentrate, Sandy solidified her job. More efficient, she met deadlines. She got a raise, maintained her medical benefits, and started accumulating money toward retirement.

Managing Weaknesses

More than just recognizing areas of weakness, patients need to manage and change these weaknesses. If patients are overwhelmed with multiple tasks, for example, they should cut down on the nonessential ones. They may need to ask for and get help. More than contracting out work, patients need partners to complement them. Many adults with ADHD are far-reaching, restless, and visionary—"hunters" in a world full of "farmers," sober types who do steady, mundane work (Hartmann 2002). Hunters need to launch their missions boldly, but they need farmers who follow through and attend to details they miss.

> Sandy reviewed her job description with her supervisor. They agreed she could stop some routine tasks she particularly disliked. Even so, she sneaked an organizer into her office on weekends, saying, "She costs a lot, but without her I'd lose my job."
>
> Sandy befriended a coworker, Nell, over their common interest in cross-stitching. Sandy loved designing canvases but rarely finished them. Her friend always did. When they collaborated, the resulting piece was a such a success that office friends offered to pay well for others. Excited, Sandy proposed that she and Nell start an online business. However, that idea required more work than Nell could do.

Making the Most of Strengths

In a study that followed gifted children into adulthood, researchers found that success in adulthood was not related to IQ. The high achievers showed "prudence and forethought, willpower, perseverance, and desire. They chose among their many talents and concentrated their efforts" (Clifton and Nelson 1992, p. 60). In other words, good executive functions lead to success. Because adults with ADHD generally have poor executive functions, they are more likely than others to fail. They have to identify their strengths and operate from them.

Once the patient has decided on an area of strength, he or she needs to work in it consistently. Adults with ADHD will need to use their creative thinking.

> On the job, Sandy used her artistic skills to make Web sites glow with color and imaginative design. Clients were delighted. In her free time, she took up her oils again and painted little still lifes. At Nell's urging, she took digital pictures of her paintings and uploaded them onto an online auction and trade site. Internet buyers snatched up her paintings as fast as she could make them. She found an accountant to set up a business system. Several months later, she said, "I'm no van Gogh, but I have repeat buyers, and I charge more for each painting. I can do larger pieces, which are higher priced. I'm supplementing my income and having fun."

Some patients, burdened from early life with poor academic records, end up in jobs that bore and depress them. Treatment for ADHD can help give them hope and other work options.

> Early in life, Jack had been a shy, easily bullied misfit. In school he did not, or could not, pay attention, and he felt endlessly humiliated and ashamed. His father compared him with his three older student-athlete brothers. As a teenager he finally filled out physically, but his academic problems and poor self-esteem continued. He barely scraped into community college. There, four or more beers eased his paralyzing shyness. His good looks got him dates, but his drinking and impulsivity resulted in his getting three girls pregnant in one semester. Unable to keep up the academic pace, he flunked out.
>
> Caught in a cycle of binge drinking, Jack repetitively lost jobs, relationships, and places to live. He tried working as a gardener, as a maintenance man, and as a handyman, doing anything to survive. At a big family reunion, he drank too much and passed out. Afterward no one would tell him what he said or did, and his brothers swore they would never talk to him again. That incident was finally the stimulus he needed to stop drinking and stay sober, through Alcoholics Anonymous.

> After more than a year of sobriety, Jack sought evaluation for ADHD. With his dramatic history, and with severe symptoms of inattention and hyperactivity on the rating scales, there was no question about the diagnosis. After trying a number of agents, we found that 10 mg of Dexedrine twice a day helped him to concentrate and be calm. He said, "It's always been so *noisy* in my head. I'm not accustomed to the quiet. I can actually hear the air conditioning now." Jack successfully stayed with a tough job for a year that led to another that doubled his base pay and offered bonuses as well.

Adults with ADHD may come to recognize that however hard they try, they cannot make their current job satisfying. That calls for finding a new direction, which may require career counseling or more education. Treatment for ADHD can help them reach their goals.

> Lance was an unruly boy in grammar school, diagnosed as having ADHD, combined type. Resisting taking medication, he stayed a "smart underachiever" through high school and college. After graduation, he spurned the office grind to work as a wildcatter in the oil fields of Texas. By his early 40s, when he tried to get a master's in business administration and move into management, "ADD came back to bite my butt." He sought treatment and found that medication helped. He was able to get his M.B.A., and that opened new career options.

ADHD AND WOMEN

The Changing View of ADHD in Girls and Women

In the past, girls and women received comparatively little attention with regard to ADHD. At first the disorder was all about rambunctious boys, and then about disorganized men. Who focuses on the dreamy little girl, just as inattentive but not as disruptive as the boy she sits next to? Girls, diagnosed with the primarily inattentive form of the disorder more often than boys, are less likely to be detected with ADHD and to be treated for it. Girls with ADHD have fewer behavior problems than affected boys, but they have the *same* prototypical symptoms, comorbid psychopathology, social dysfunction, cognitive impairment, school failure, and social problems. Girls are at the same relative risk as boys for adverse clinical outcomes, but they have a different clinical presentation. One surprising finding is that adolescent girls with ADHD are at greater risk than affected boys of developing substance use disorders (Biederman et al. 1999).

Formerly, there were 5–10 boys for every girl who was referred for diagnosis and treatment of ADHD (American Psychiatric Association

1994). The lower rate of conduct and oppositional disorders in girls may account for much of the disparity (Wilens et al. 2002). As clinics for adults with ADHD developed, more women than expected sought evaluation and treatment for the disorder. Certainly the percentage of women self-referring for treatment was higher than in previous reported estimates (Biederman et al. 1994). More recent studies support the impression that the disparity of ADHD between men and women is less than that between boys and girls (Faraone et al. 2000). In some community samples, the ratio of men with ADHD to women with the disorder is as low as 1.5 to 1 (Biederman 1998). If we look at the parents of children diagnosed with ADHD, as many mothers as fathers have the disorder. There, the ratio is 1 to 1 (Faraone et al. 2000). Although we still do not know the true prevalence of ADHD in girls and women, many more have the disorder than we used to think (Nadeau 2002).

Sex, the Brain, and ADHD

The biological differences between human males and females begin early in fetal development. The basic "default" organization of the human embryo is female. Even with a Y chromosome, if the right amount of testosterone is not in the uterus from the sixth to the twenty-fourth week of gestation, the fetus will not develop male genitals.

Abnormalities of sex chromosomes affect the entire life of the affected person. The most common of these is Klinefelter's syndrome, characterized by an extra X chromosome, or XXY. Physically, boys with Klinefelter's syndrome tend to have many bodily characteristics we regard as female. Typically they have multiple problems, including speech and language delays, learning disabilities, social awkwardness, and short-term memory deficits. Even more striking, an estimated 80% of children with the syndrome have ADHD. Their brains have features similar to those found in ADHD: smaller frontal lobes, basal ganglia, and cerebellum (Giedd et al. 2002). We do not know whether these differences reflect a link to the same genetic underpinnings as for regular ADHD, or if the chromosomal anomalies lead to altered brain circuits and symptoms of ADHD.

Do Girls and Women With ADHD Have Different Neurobiology?

Positron emission tomography (PET) scanning measures the amount of energy, as glucose, used by different parts of the brain during different tasks. A PET scan of children showed that related to control girls and to boys with ADHD, the girls with ADHD had lower global cerebral metabolism (Ernst et al. 1994). One PET scan study of adults compared men and women with ADHD and age peers without the disorder. Compared with control women, the ADHD women used 13% less brain glucose. For male ADHD patients, the percentage was 6% less than the age-matched control group. The small number of patients involved makes it hard to draw any definitive conclusions (Zametkin et al. 1990).

Magnetic resonance imaging (MRI) studies raise the possibility of structural differences in the brains of persons with ADHD. For example, the caudate nucleus may be smaller in ADHD patients, especially in girls and women. In one study, brain size differences correlated significantly with several indices of the severity of the ADHD (Castellanos et al. 2001). Although there are few studies, brain regions are reduced in girls with ADHD as they are in boys.

Intriguing as this finding is, to date we cannot rely on MRI to diagnose ADHD in children and, by extension, in adults. There is too much overlap in the sizes of brain structures in persons with or without ADHD to provide reliable guidance (Giedd 2001).

Social and Cultural Forces Affecting Women With ADHD

Women face different social and cultural expectations than men. Research shows that women with ADHD have a much more negative self-image than men with the disorder (Arcia and Connors 1998). A disorganized man is absentminded; a woman with similar problems is a flake (Solden 1995). Negative attitudes toward girls start early. Mothers are harsher critics of daughters with ADHD than they are of sons who have the disorder (Langner 2002).

ADHD and a "False Self"

Understandably, girls and women hide unacceptable parts of themselves. Worse, some girls develop a "false self," a cobbled-together identity that pleases key people in their life (Miller 1991). Parents and others may not accept who she genuinely is. This false self can develop in girls regardless of whether they have ADHD, but having that disorder predisposes them to a negative self-image. The false self is a temporary, unsuccessful solution. Maintaining it is costly emotionally, predisposing a woman to depression and other ills.

> One female patient said, "I've always had this perky personality. You know, Little Mary Sunshine. I used to take naps every day, because being upbeat all the time was exhausting. I felt like a hypocrite. This wasn't me; it was just a person I thought people would like. But it was

just so much *work.*" She paused, took a deep breath and sat right up. "Now that I've started treatment, I have much more energy. I don't have to work so hard at being someone else. The most surprising thing is, I've discovered that being upbeat and cheerful is my real personality!"

Sociocultural Expectations

In our society, girls are expected to be attractive, pleasing, and unselfish. We socialize them to acquire a false self: "they learn to sacrifice their wholeness in order to be loved" (Pipher 1994, p. 112). The resulting silent suffering often expresses itself as depression. Because girls and women tend to internalize, they criticize themselves for being stupid or incompetent. Even if a woman succeeds in maintaining the false self, and others approve of her, she may not feel loved.

Women also are expected to define themselves primarily in terms of their relationships, their human connectedness (Gilligan 1982). Being poised, organized, and well behaved is hard for girls and women with ADHD. Many contend with low self-esteem, self-criticism, underachievement, and, often, depression (Grossman and Grossman 1994).

> "A good girl! A good girl! That's all my parents wanted," protested Marie-Claire, age 37. Desperately trying not to cry, she jammed her clenched fists into her eyes, but her tears spilled through between her fingers. "Why didn't they believe me when I said I couldn't learn? All I want is to be normal, to do my job well, and get a promotion every year. To have a husband and a baby. Why does it have to be so hard for me?"

Despite difficulties, many resourceful girls and women learn how to function well. Often, however, they do that by maintaining controlled behavior and keeping their struggles hidden. The "mask of competency" costs them dearly (Solden 1995).

Women in our society are expected to be good communicators who listen to others and then respond. However, this role is particularly hard for the woman with ADHD. Listening is difficult if she is distracted, which often happens, or if the conversation does not especially interest her. Instead, she may interrupt or blurt out something that misses the point. Poor at reading interpersonal signals, she may not realize how others view her. Of course, men with ADHD also have these difficulties, but we expect less of them as communicators.

Women in our society are expected to be good friends. Maintaining friendships, however, means planning, remembering, contacting, and regularly staying in touch. These executive functions challenge the woman with ADHD, who is often restlessly on the move and forgetful. When others get annoyed with her and withdraw, she is hurt and isolated.

Women in our society also are expected to be mothers and home-makers. Despite some advances, with men sharing more tasks, women are still the center of family life. There is little difference if the family is blue-collar or a marriage between two professionals. As well as providing warmth, the woman is expected to ensure that everyone is clean, well fed, and clothed. She has to keep track of multiple tasks, maintain routines, make appointments, prioritize family needs, and plan, plan, plan. When a husband does not understand why his wife who has ADHD finds everyday tasks so hard, she feels worse. Her frustration interferes with her intimate relationships (Solden 1995).

Between household tasks and a job outside the home, the typical American woman works about 25 hours more a week than men (Hochschild 1990). Often the woman with ADHD lacks the executive functions she needs to do that double job well. Many women with ADHD feel this deficiency keenly (Brown 2000).

> In an initial interview, one woman suddenly jumped up, saying, "I forgot to put out Billy's ADD medicine. He'll never remember it. Can I phone him?" That done, she said, "This is what it's like. I can barely keep my own commitments straight, and then I have to keep track of Billy and his two sisters? Ooooh!" She slapped her forehead, exasperated.

If Mom has untreated ADHD, then typically the family has poor organization, loose scheduling, and irregular performance. This circumstance is difficult for everyone, but particularly for children who have ADHD. Needing structure, they turn to a mother who is particularly bad at providing it (Hochschild 1990).

> "It's the blind leading the blind in my house," sighed one woman.

If the woman with ADHD has children, typically one or more of them has the disorder. This circumstance makes her tasks exponentially more difficult.

> Leah, a lobbyist, has ADHD. So does her lobbyist husband. They are adoptive parents of fraternal twin boys, now 7 years old, who both have learning disabilities and the combined type of ADHD. Leah and Ned's biological daughter, Rachel, 15, has never accepted her adopted brothers. When the boys misbehave, which they often do, Rachel screams, "Send the little monsters back!" She locks herself in her bedroom and spends hours on the cell phone complaining about her "wacko" family. Leah often feels inadequate to maintain a stable emotional center for her family.

Many modern husbands share what was considered "women's work" in earlier generations. In most American families, however, the mother is still responsible for the emotional and logistical life of the family.

> Leah's husband, Ned, also worked full-time out of the house. She appreciated his greater patience with the children. Somehow, though, Leah was responsible for the family's well-being. "How did I buy into this?" she asked. "How is it that I'm supposed to ensure that everyone in the family is happy?"

Doing all of this caretaking with equanimity and good humor is another expectation for women in our society. In addition to organizing the daily household logistics, Mom is supposed to control the emotional climate in the home, which should be sunny and mild all the time. Society is far more accepting of men being openly angry than it is of women being so. Many women swallow their resentment or express it indirectly; but either choice may lead to them feeling more isolated and depressed.

> Leah said, "When I scold Rachel for some thoughtless teenage thing, she calls me 'a total bitch.' Ned doesn't scold Rachel; he agrees with her opinion of me, but he's not going to come out and actually say it. So what happens on the rare occasion that "The Master" gets ticked off at her? It's, 'Oh Daddy, I'm so sorry.'"

Women With ADHD Who Work Outside the Home

The woman working outside the home is supposed to work effectively and fast. With instant messaging, e-mail, cell phones, and pagers everywhere, she is to be instantly, continuously available. Between multiple demands and ever-present technology, women struggle to maintain an effective boundary between home and work.

Women in the professions ostensibly have more autonomy than those who have support or service jobs. They may have a harder time leaving work in the office, however. They can feel out of control in both sectors. Professional duties intrude on family time. Family duties such as responding to unexpected calls from school and children needing medicine or having other crises threaten scheduled meetings with clients or other professional responsibilities.

> Leah was still up at 2:30 one morning, preparing a PowerPoint presentation. The time she had scheduled for the task the previous day had been preempted by an emergency school conference. One of the twins had had a meltdown in class and hit another boy over the head with a book.

What should be weekend downtime becomes an even higher stress period for the woman professional. At least she has a support system at the office. At home, too often she *is* the support system, even if she is resourceful. It is hard to find helpers sensitive to the special needs of children with ADHD. Even if there is money available for domestic help, hiring and maintaining the schedule and relationship with these workers is an executive task, precisely the kind that is hard for the woman who has ADHD.

> Leah dreaded the weekends. It was hard enough getting help during the week. Family time on weekends was worse because it was precious, and everyone expected it to be wonderful. Rachel simply camped out at her best friend's house. Leah envied her. She longed for Monday morning: "My office is a zoo, but it is an island of peace and tranquility compared to my house."

In summary, ADHD symptoms are "more discordant with social expectations for women" than they are for men (Nadeau 2002).

Clinical Pictures of Women With ADHD

In general, girls present with ADHD later than boys do. The common assumption is that boys act out and get attention earlier. Girls tend to become symptomatic in middle school, at puberty (Huessy 1990). The DSM-IV-TR (American Psychiatric Association 2000) criteria include onset before the age of 7. Some have argued that this criterion for diagnosis is uncalled for and unproductive (Barkley 1997). Because of the clinical pattern in girls and women, the age-specific cutoff is particularly inappropriate (Weiss and Jain 2000).

Is there a clinical picture of ADHD that is specific to women? One study of adults with ADHD, 78 men and 50 women, found similarities in impaired psychosocial, cognitive, and academic functioning. ADHD adults of both genders were more disturbed and impaired, suffering much more with depression and anxiety than control subjects of the same gender. Women with ADHD had a lower occurrence of substance abuse and conduct disorder than did men with ADHD (Biederman et al. 1994). In another study comparing the ADHD symptoms of women and men, the women most often reported dysphoria, inattention, problems with organization, and impulsive conduct. In contrast, the men had prominent conduct problems, learning problems, stress intolerance, attentional problems, and poor social skills (Stein et al. 1995). In the current psychiatric diagnostic criteria, among "associated features and disorders" related to ADHD are mood lability, dysphoria, rejection by peers, demoralization, and poor self-esteem. All are prominent in women with the disorder (Solden 1995). Girls and women are more prone to the inattentive form of the disorder. Although they have symptoms of hyperactivity as well, these symptoms are generally less prominent than in boys and men with the disorder (Gershon 2002).

Part of the difficulty in knowing the true prevalence of ADHD in women is that we may be looking for the wrong clinical symptoms. Developed for the diagnosis of boys, our criteria have been adapted for use with girls, and now adult men and women. Our diagnostic criteria do not yet have a "gender-based threshold" (Barkley 1995).

Developmental Issues

Different developmental issues can cause girls and women with ADHD to seek treatment. The following case examples of women lawyers who have ADHD illustrate the challenges such patients face at different developmental stages.

> Naomi sought treatment because she was floundering in her first year of law school. She said, "I could bluff my way through college without doing the reading, but there's no way I can do that in law school."

Other patients manage to survive law school only to encounter worse problems in the conduct of their professional life.

> "In law school, I was the 'little airhead.' It was cute 10 years ago," said Fiona. "People think that because you work for the government you don't have to work hard. That's not the way it is in my office. They expect results. 'Cute' isn't cutting it any more. I'm sick of the 'flaky lady lawyer' label, especially since I deserve it."
>
> Fiona was fighting her ex-husband, another lawyer, over custody of their son, Ian, who also had severe ADHD. Her ex-husband claimed that her disorganization and inefficiency made her a bad mother. "The bastard admits I love Ian, but he claims that I just 'can't care for the boy.'" She rolled her eyes in mock concern. Terrified of losing both her son and her job, Fiona dug in. When, most days, she remembered to take her medication, she was far more productive at home and at work. She did not get promoted, but she also did not get fired. She proved to her husband and the court that she was a functioning adult, well able to parent her son.

Other women put off getting professional help for themselves because the needs of other family members come first.

> Robin only sought treatment for her ADHD in her 50s, delaying help for herself because her husband and four sons had been so needy. "Every

single person in the family has ADHD. Compared to them my ADHD is nothing. But the boys grew up and left, and my marriage collapsed. Now, though, I have to be a full-time lawyer. Before I was married, I only went to law school because my parents wouldn't support my art history interests. Somehow, I got through law school—then I got married and had the boys."

Full-time law work was a struggle for Robin. "I constantly dread being fired. Even though I read and reread documents, I overlook typos and other details. I miss deadlines. I'm continually in motion, picking my nails, getting out of my seat at meetings. The other day a senior partner was on the verge of shouting at me to sit down and stay put. I don't blame him. I'm frustrated that I can't sit and work for more than 5 minutes at a time."

When Robin started taking a CNS stimulant, her hyperactivity "just stopped." Although still somewhat distractible, she was more productive. She learned to be better organized. Her fears about her professional future eased.

Diagnosis Later in Life

ADHD goes unrecognized and untreated in many girls who have the disorder. For some women who are first diagnosed and treated as adults, the years of unrecognized symptoms have consequences in diminished self-esteem and lack of progress in life.

One study compared 51 women ages 26–59 years who had ADHD with 51 women in the same age range without the disorder (Rucklidge and Kaplan 1997). The women diagnosed later in life grew up feeling defective. At a loss to explain their difficulties, they usually felt they caused all their troubles, and they felt powerless to control their lives. Feeling helpless and struggling to cope, they were three times as likely to have depression and anxiety as their age peers without the disorder.

> Cindy battled for decades with recurrent depression that stabilized with medication and psychotherapy. Unmarried and alienated from her successful sisters, she felt stagnant and ineffective. Only in her early 50s did she discover that she had ADHD. "No wonder I've been depressed. My brain doesn't work right. I can't even take care of myself. What would it have been like if I'd married and had children? I shudder to think."

Although the diagnosis of ADHD provides relief after long unhappiness, many women grieve for what might have been. Newly diagnosed women hope to learn new strategies to deal with life better. Mothers with ADHD strongly want to spare their children the struggles they had.

Hormones, Pregnancy, and Breast-feeding

Many women report that their ADHD symptoms fluctuate with their hormones. They have the fewest symptoms when their estrogen levels are highest, during pregnancy, and the most symptoms when their estrogen levels are low, when they are premenstrual or perimenopausal (Quinn 2002). Medications for ADHD also seem to lose their effectiveness in women in these situations. Preliminary studies suggest that estrogen enhances the effect of stimulants, whereas progesterone dampens it. It may be useful to adjust the dosage of ADHD medications for women with the phase of their menstrual cycle (Justice and de Wit 2000). For menopausal women, just increasing the dosage of the ADHD medications may not help. The clinician may need to increase the amount of estrogen the woman has access to (Quinn 2002). Studies show that estrogen replacement therapy improves the verbal memory, vigilance, and reasoning of menopausal women. Such patients do better than those without supplementary estrogen on nearly all neuropsychological tests, especially those involving conceptualization, attention, and visual practical skills (Schmidt et al. 1996).

As a practical consequence, women with ADHD may require a more sophisticated medication regimen than men. Hormone replacement therapy, however, carries its own risks. Each woman needs to discuss it in detail with her obstetrician/gynecologist as well as with her psychiatrist before deciding.

Women with ADHD wonder what to do when they become pregnant. Doctors and patients alike shy away from medication during pregnancy and in the postnatal period. Apparently the CNS stimulants, when used to treat medical conditions, do not pose a significant risk for congenital abnormalities in the fetus. Newborns of mothers who have taken amphetamines may have mild withdrawal symptoms, but they show no long-term adverse effects. The U.S. Food and Drug Administration, however, still categorizes these medications in category C, which means that they are not recommended for use during pregnancy and breast-feeding.

Medical opinion is changing toward greater use of medication during pregnancy, especially to treat depression. Increasingly, the selective serotonin reuptake inhibitors and tricyclic antidepressants seem safe for women to take during pregnancy. The risks to mother and infant and to the parent–child bond may be less if a depressed woman takes antidepressant medication than if she stops or does not start it during pregnancy or postpartum. However, this usage is still a controversial area.

Some women are on complex medication regimens that require thorough discussion with their physicians. These women and their spouse or partner are making decisions that affect their children as well as themselves (Goodman and Quinn 2002).

All psychotropic medications that nursing mothers take are excreted into breast milk. Nursing babies therefore are exposed to them. The clinical impact is unclear. However, the American Academy of Pediatrics recommends against breast-feeding for women using CNS stimulants (American Academy of Pediatrics Committee on Drugs 2001).

Comorbidity

Are there gender differences in comorbid conditions between women and men who have ADHD? Women tend to internalize their distress and to have affective, anxiety, and eating disorders. On the other hand, men more often have higher rates of conduct disorder, antisocial or criminal behavior, and dependence on alcohol and other drugs (Gaub and Carlson 1997). Alert clinicians need to look for all these possibilities, however, in ADHD patients of both sexes. In diagnosing and treating women who have depression or substance abuse or both, it can be easy to overlook ADHD (Katz et al. 1998).

> At 55, Faith had been stably abstinent from alcohol for 10 years. Her depression responded well to psychotherapy and medication, but her finances were a muddle, her work was unsatisfying, and her apartment chaotic. She raised the question of ADHD. When we reviewed her history, she had a lifelong pattern of poor academic performance, inattention at school, and disorganization at home and work.
>
> Faith had mixed feelings about the diagnosis of ADHD. "Ugh, something else wrong with me. My family already thinks I'm nuts! But you know, it's a relief. It validates my feeling that there was something that we were missing, that I couldn't put my finger on. This is it."

Comprehensive Treatment Issues

Treatment for women with ADHD includes the same elements as for men with the disorder. However, the best treatment programs keep women's preferences and strengths in mind. Whether by temperament or by cultural training, women in our society have a greater capacity for and interest in interpersonal connections. The best treatment for their ADHD uses their natural interests, emphasizing interconnectedness.

For example, findings from the Multimodal Treatment Study of Children With Attention Deficit Hyperactivity Disorder suggested that boys with ADHD do best with medication alone. Girls, however, thrive with a treatment program that includes psychosocial treatments as well as medication (MTA Cooperative Group 1999). Although we do not yet have data about a similar difference in treating adult men and women with ADHD, women's response to combined treatment seems highly likely.

Psychoeducation

Like men, women with ADHD need to know about the disorder and its manifestations so they know what they are up against.

> Leah said, "It was like stumbling around in the dark, banging my shins against things. Now the light's on. The obstacles are still there, but I can see them, knowing where they are and how big they are. That's a relief."

Dealing with the facts about ADHD is not enough, however. The patient's feeling state also needs attention. Women in our society tend to blame themselves for problems and subordinate their needs to those of others. They need help in learning to say no. That's hard for the perfectionistic woman with ADHD, who has to lower her expectations.

> Although exhausted, Leah hurled herself at her tasks. "Somebody has to be the grown-up and do what needs doing," she said. It was a revelation that "what needs doing" was saying "No."

Comorbid Conditions

The clinician needs to be alert to comorbid conditions in the adult woman with ADHD. Women are more likely to have complicating anxiety or affective disorders that can obscure underlying or comorbid ADHD. If either or both of those conditions are diagnosed and treated, the clinician may have to reassess and recalibrate the patient's ADHD regimen.

Although less likely than men to abuse alcohol or other substances, women can still have these disorders. The true incidence of alcoholism in women is hard to find because of lingering shame and secrecy about drinking. If the woman patient has a problem with abuse of alcohol or other substances, like men she must demonstrate at least 3 months' abstinence before trying medication to treat ADHD.

Medications

Medication is an important part of treating women as well as men with ADHD. The CNS stimulants are the medications of first choice for women as well as men; they are equally effective, well tolerated, and safe (Prince and Wilens 2002). If the CNS stimulants fail, then next in line are agents such as atomoxetine (Strattera) or bupropion (Wellbutrin). Some women, like some men, find a combination of medications helpful.

Psychotherapy

Women with ADHD share the psychological and developmental concerns of women without the disorder. These concerns may be heightened by the burden of the ADHD symptoms. Failure in the key dimensions of life, as wife and mother and worker outside the home, is more likely. Women patients may profit by varied forms of psychotherapy, whether individual or group, cognitive-behavioral or insight-oriented.

Environmental Interventions

Technology such as electronic calendars, reminder systems, personal digital assistants, and computers can help women with ADHD get organized. E-mail, instant messaging, and online chat rooms make it easier for the computer-literate person to stay connected.

Several good books cover the issues for women with ADHD. Particularly helpful are the works of Sari Solden, L.C.S.W. (e.g., *Journeys through ADDulthood*) and of Patricia Quinn, M.D., and Kathleen Nadeau, Ph.D. (e.g., *Gender Issues and AD/HD*). For computer-literate women, there are resources online. One fine example is ADDvance (http://www.ADDvance.com), developed by Drs. Quinn and Nadeau with the needs of girls and women in mind.

Developing Strengths

The woman patient can profit from an active approach to ADHD. How can she put her strengths to use? Does she think creatively?

> In her spare time, Faith loved taking pictures of people, and she slowly acquired a reputation as a portraitist. She learned to modify her digital photographs on the computer so that the finished picture expressed her view of her subjects more vividly.

Exercise

In the past, exercise was rarely a regular part of women's life, but in recent decades this trend has changed. More women have been exercising regularly, finding the camaraderie in sports that men have long enjoyed. Among the many good reasons to recommend exercise to women with ADHD is that exercise helps manage their symptoms. Vigorous exercise helps them maintain their internal organization and is good for their health as well.

Spiritual Life

A healthy spiritual or religious life correlates well with mental health in both men and women. For many women with ADHD, an active religious life provides strength and solace. Thus, inquiring about the spiritual aspect of life with every patient is important. If patients have particular religious traditions, they may reconsider those freshly. If the tradition or affiliation from childhood or family has failed them, they can look into others. Some patients, of course, do not regard spiritual or religious views of life as meaningful. Without prescribing religion, clinicians can encourage patients to develop a larger framework for life than their own individual concerns.

Getting Help From Others

Today's woman with ADHD has access to different types of helpers. Who is best for her? Personal organizer? Coach? Individual psychotherapist? Couples therapist? Clinicians can usefully link such women to others who can help out. Knowing resources and making recommendations is an important part of our job.

Personal organizers help women declutter their life at home or in the workplace. Although digging out is a relief to the patient, more important for the clinician is providing an ongoing system so that the patient does not become overwhelmed again. Even so, some ADHD patients need return visits.

ADHD coaches, which are becoming increasingly popular, provide support, energy, and a clear sense of direction (Rumberg 1999).

Some women have problems that structure and coaching will not solve. For such patients, other treatments, such as psychotherapy, may need to be considered. Individual clinicians vary greatly in what they offer, depending on their background, training, and interests. Therapists who provide cognitive-behavioral treatments have much to offer many women with ADHD.

ADHD affects marriage and family life as well as individuals. It is often useful to include spouses and significant others in meetings with individual women patients. Then important others may learn more about ADHD, and they appreciate voicing their concerns. Their support is important to the woman patient. If issues in the couple or family are pressing, patients may need referral to clinicians who are expert in these areas.

ADHD AND FAMILY ISSUES

Adult patients presenting with ADHD rarely exist in isolation. They may have spouses and children, have a significant other, or be an important person in a network of friends and relatives. These other people may not be in the clinician's office with the individual, but they feel the impact of his or her symptoms. Adults with ADHD often have interpersonal problems. They may not be able to regulate their emotional reactions well, and they may not have good social "radar." The result is a high rate of divorce (Wender 1995).

ADHD is a family affair. When one or more parents have ADHD, the chances are at least 50% that one or more of their children have it also. In families with one or more children with ADHD, the chances are at least 50% that one or both of the parents also have it (Adler and Cohen 2004). If the affected parent fails to get medication or other effective treatment, that can have a major impact on the child's treatment, course of illness, and prognosis.

When more than one person in the family has ADHD, complications multiply (Hechtman 1996). A child's ADHD can influence parental satisfaction, marital harmony, and sibling development. Parents tend to be more anxious and controlling toward children with ADHD (Barkley 1990). Adults with ADHD have problems with executive function that impact their ability to run their household and raise their children. As parents, they can display impulsive caregiving, inattentiveness to child-rearing logistics, and disorganization. It is unreasonable to assume that adults with ADHD know how to manage a child with the disorder just because they are familiar with its symptoms. They may identify with the child's ADHD, they may project their own symptoms on their offspring, and they may feel guilty because they genetically transmitted the disorder (Popper et al. 2003). If you effectively treat either the parent or child, when both have ADHD, the other can improve. Alternatively, failing to treat either affected parents or affected children can hinder the clinical improvement of both.

A large recent study investigated the psychiatric comorbidity patterns of nonclinically referred adults with ADHD. Researchers compared 152 parents of children with ADHD who themselves had the disorder with 283 parents who did not. Affected parents, as anticipated, had higher lifetime rates of other psychiatric disorders, especially affective and substance abuse disorders. They had also had lower educational and occupational achievement. All of these factors may contribute to problems in parenting and family life—underscoring the fact that ADHD is truly a family affair (McGough et al. 2005).

Treatment Practices and Satisfaction in Families With ADHD

In a recent survey, investigators sent a direct-mail questionnaire about many aspects of ADHD and the family to 532,415 households with at least one member who had the disorder. The response rate was 13% (69,214 households). Using cluster analysis, researchers identified five clusters of families affected by ADHD: "successful kids," "successful adults," "complicated, marginally successful," "resigned," and "overwhelmed."

Nearly all (99%) of the families in the "successful kids" cluster had at least one child with ADHD, of whom most were 9–15 years old. Of these children, 75% were boys, and few had comorbid conditions; and 80% of the children were taking once-daily stimulant medication. The majority of the families were satisfied with treatment.

Families in the "successful adults" cluster typically had at least one adult with ADHD, with 53% of the children also having the disorder. Most patients in this cluster took immediate-release stimulants, with 39% satisfied with treatment.

In the "complicated, marginally successful" cluster, 37% of the families had at least one child with ADHD, of whom 69% were boys. In this cluster, 6% of families had at least one adult with ADHD; 80% were women, and most of them were college educated. The adult patients in this cluster had high rates of depression (46%) and of anxiety (28%).

The "resigned" cluster consisted primarily of families with at least one child with ADHD (97%), most 12–23 years old, of whom 75% were male. Only 63% of the affected children were taking medication for ADHD, with 26% taking once-daily medication. The children in this cluster had the highest rate of comorbidity.

Families in the "overwhelmed" cluster had a low utilization rate of once-daily medications (3% of children). Only 3% of the families were satisfied with treatment. The adults in this cluster had high rates of comorbid depression, anxiety, substance abuse, sleep disorders, and obsessive-compulsive disorder. Not surprisingly, these respondents least understood ADHD (Manos et al. 2004).

Common Family Problems With ADHD

The Uncooperative Spouse

When the spouse objects to the diagnosis or the treatment plan, the clinician should try to secure his or her cooperation.

> Ed, a 42-year-old lobbyist, presented because his 10-year-old son had been diagnosed with ADHD and he saw his son's symptoms in himself. His wife, Patty, believed in "natural" remedies only, not medicine. Young Eddie was not responding to her attempts to structure his life.
>
> Ed had long-standing symptoms of inattention and impulsivity. "I went to three different colleges over 6 years before finally getting my bachelor's. My colleagues resent my presentations—they're creative but last-minute. My boss says he will fire me if I ever interrupt him again in a meeting." He reported, "Patty says that I never sit down long enough to listen to her, and when I sit, I fidget. She had a fit when the power company shut off the electricity right before Christmas. It wasn't the first time. I'm often behind with the bills. She has taken over the finances, and she's angry about it."
>
> Ed had ADHD, combined type. Patty refused to participate in Ed's evaluation and objected to his taking medication. However, Ed found that a long-acting methylphenidate helped him be timelier at work and more patient at home. He put his BlackBerry to work to structure his life. Unwilling to divorce and be separated from his children, he said, "This would all be easier if my wife cooperated. Someday she'll admit that I'm doing much better."

The Overburdened or Resentful Spouse

Other spouses actively support the diagnosis and treatment of the ADHD. In some cases they are the ones pressuring the affected person to get treatment. However, they resent the burdens the patient's symptoms put on the marriage and family life. Husbands get angry at wives who cannot manage the household effectively or who do poorly in the workplace. Wives bristle at husbands who are unreliable about making money and doing their part of the child care.

Family situations may worsen when there are children. Youngsters, whether or not they have ADHD, feel the negative impact of the disorder in a parent. When a husband or a wife has ADHD, there is an increased likelihood that one or more of the children will have it. Given this challenge, the failings of the ADHD adult may come into bolder relief.

> "I have three children to look after, and two of them have ADHD," said one wife. "I'm sick of my husband being the fourth child. It's easier to help the kids; I resent his ADHD."

Although the initial focus may be on the child's dysfunctional behavior, poor parenting can worsen the situation and predispose to more negative outcomes, including aggressive behavior (Campbell et al. 1996). Negative family interactions are common correlates of ADHD. The load of symptoms in multiple family members can result in major distress and even abuse (Johnston and Mash 2001).

Clinicians have several options to help in this situation. The central concept is helping the couple maintain a healthy balance in their relationship. Contending with a spouse who has ADHD often makes the other partner resentful. It is never healthy for one partner to be identified as the sick or damaged one. Unless both husband and wife take steps, this imbalance threatens the marriage.

Psychoeducation is important not just for the patient but for the spouse. Clinicians can recommend appropriate books and pamphlets and refer the non-ADHD spouse to Children and Adults With Attention-Deficit/Hyperactivity Disorder (CHADD). Informational meetings or discussions may help partners see that others struggle as they do and that there are ways to cope.

Psychotherapy can be productive, if both spouses are willing to work. The therapist needs to know the special needs and issues in couples in which one member has ADHD. Group therapy for couples can be particularly powerful. By interacting with group members, the ADHD spouse gets information that is otherwise unavailable about his or her impact on others. The non-ADHD spouse realizes that others share his or her problems and know, truly, "what it's like." The non-ADHD spouse learns better what contribution he or she is making to the couple's difficulties. Both husband and wife can profit by the support of other participants. Unfortunately, few clinicians do group therapy for couples, much less where ADHD is a specific issue.

Some spouses forget that the partner with ADHD has assets that contribute substantially to the family's life. The clinician may usefully point this out.

> Ginny objected to Hugh's immersion in the stock market. However, his financial success funded family midwinter vacations in the Caribbean. For Ginny, who had seasonal affective disorder, these were emotional lifesavers. Although Ginny accused Hugh of "still being a kid himself," she admitted that he was a more understanding parent, partly because of his long struggle with ADHD.

Clinicians can remind patients and spouses that there is more to life than ADHD. In the daily grind, couples may forget what first attracted them to each other. Although domestic life has its demands, the clinician can encourage the couple to invest in their relationship, to find occasions for fun and for respite. A marriage can better withstand the chronic stress of adult ADHD if it is fulfilling emotionally and sexually. Many couples deal better with stress if they have a vigorous religious or spiritual life.

Spouses need support in their work with the adult with ADHD. Although the clinician's encouragement is helpful, on occasion a spouse may need referral for individual treatment.

The Chip Off the Old Block: When Parent and Child Have ADHD

The most typical situation is when father and son both have the disorder. There is danger of triangulation, with the non-ADHD parent resenting the other two members of the family. Alternatively, the father can use his knowledge of ADHD to help his son and to relieve the mother's burdens.

A child who does not have ADHD, but whose sibling does, faces additional challenges. Such a youngster may choose, or be forced into, precocious maturity. Although that seems adaptive, the child may struggle later because he or she never learned to acknowledge his or her needs and have them met. Other children who do not have ADHD sense that acting up is a way to get attention. That conclusion can evolve into a dysfunctional way of life. Parents can foster the development of the child who does not have ADHD by spending individual time with the youngster and by recognizing and supporting his or her strengths. Parents may usefully point out that there may well be things to learn and personal qualities to admire in the sibling who does have ADHD.

When "Everyone" Has ADHD

Having multiple persons in the family with ADHD presents multiple scenarios. In some instances, resourceful and loving parents can acknowledge each other's strengths and support each other. At times, the complexity and severity of problems overwhelm the most resilient and thoughtful patients and clinicians. Such parents, feeling stressed and incompetent, are particularly subject to depression (Donenberg and Baker 1993). Mothers, whether they do or do not have ADHD, often suffer the most from the multiple demands generated by ADHD (Anderson et al. 1994). Although each family is different, and the children may be challenging, it is important to maximize the function of the adults.

> Leah became depressed. She, her husband, and their adopted twin sons all took medication for their ADHD. No two regimens were identical. Each child saw a different psychiatrist, and Leah regularly consulted a behavioral psychologist about family functioning. Also, she and her husband were each in individual treatment with different therapists. Coordinating the children's psychiatric appointments, differing medication regimens, and multiple educational and other meetings was overwhelming. The cost of multiple treatments was daunting. Hard-pressed, Leah persuaded one child psychiatrist to treat the twins. He saw them together every other week to evaluate their progress and observe their interaction. On alternate weeks, that psychiatrist met with the parents, and they worked as a team to set reasonable family goals. Leah and Ned stopped their individual psychotherapy to focus on the issues between them in couples treatment.

No one recipe fits the many configurations of families where ADHD is an issue. What counts is that the adults find a process that works for them (Weiss et al. 1999). That task entails helping them to keep a sense of perspective. There are, after all, far worse problems than ADHD that some families must share. There is much more to each individual and to the family than the ADHD. Encouraging a sense of humor is vital. So is each person's appreciating the good things and special qualities about the others in the family unit. Some of the best things about the family's life can spring from the gifts and qualities of the person(s) with ADHD.

The simple strengths of any family are particularly important in families in which ADHD is an issue. Every family has rituals that mark life. Although these may be elaborate, such as at major holidays like Thanksgiving, these rituals also may be simple, such as a regular family outing for ice-cream cones or a tradition of reading together at night before bedtime.

There is more to life than ADHD. Everyone has difficulties to work on. Everyone has gifts to use and share. Family members who have ADHD often have strengths and abilities that nonaffected siblings, parents, and spouses can learn from and enjoy.

SUMMARY

- Work is one of the most common areas of difficulty for adults with ADHD. Some jobs seem better suited than others to ADHD adults. Suitable jobs often provide stimulation and rapid change. Ill-fitting jobs tend to be those that require steady, detailed attention. Adults with ADHD can maximize their work satisfaction using a three-step process: 1) exploring their current and past experiences for strengths and weaknesses; 2) using that information to develop a "mission statement" for their life; and 3) after reality testing their wishes against their resources and limitations, implementing the necessary changes in work.

- More likely to have the inattentive form of ADHD, girls and women are less likely to be diagnosed and treated for the disorder. Because of social and cultural factors, women with ADHD are at risk for developing a "false self" as a public persona. This fabricated self makes them more vulnerable to anxiety and to depression. Women with ADHD who are mothers have special problems running their household. Typically one or more of their children also have the disorder, further complicating life. ADHD symptoms in women are least severe when estrogen is high, as in pregnancy. The symptoms are their worst when estrogen is low, such as premenstrually or perimenopausally.

- For women as well as men with ADHD, the CNS stimulants are the medications of choice. Women respond best to comprehensive treatment for ADHD, which attends to psychosocial issues as well as providing medication. Psychiatrists can help women ADHD patients structure their lives more effectively and link them to specialized help.

- ADHD affects families, especially because it is likely that more than one family member has the disorder. Common family problems include a spouse who is uncooperative or overwhelmed and resentful. The clinician can help the couple maintain their emotional equilibrium. At times, varied forms of psychotherapy will be helpful. In some families in which several members have ADHD, a team approach to treatment may be necessary. Patients and family members alike need to remember that ADHD sometimes provides special qualities that can enrich the lives of all.

REFERENCES

Adler L, Cohen J: Diagnosis and evaluation of adults with attention-deficit/hyperactivity disorder. Psychiatr Clin North Am 27:187–201, 2004

American Academy of Pediatrics Committee on Drugs: Transfer of drugs and other chemicals into human milk. Pediatrics 108:776–789, 2001

American Psychiatric Association: Diagnosis and Statistical Manual of Mental Disorders, 4th Edition. Washington, DC, American Psychiatric Association, 1994

American Psychiatric Association: Diagnosis and Statistical Manual of Mental Disorders, 4th Edition, Text Revision. Washington, DC, American Psychiatric Association, 2000

Anderson CA, Hinshaw SP, Simmel C: Mother–child interactions in ADHD and comparison boys: relationship to overt and covert externalizing behaviors. J Abnorm Child Psychol 22:247–265, 1994

Arcia E, Connors CK: Gender differences in attention deficit hyperactivity disorder? J Dev Behav Pediatr 19:77–83, 1998

Barkley RA: Attention-Deficit/Hyperactivity Disorder: A Handbook for Diagnosis and Treatment. New York, Guilford, 1990

Barkley RA: A closer look at the DSM-IV criteria for AD/HD: some unresolved issues. ADHD Report 3:1–5, 1995

Barkley RA: Age dependent decline in ADHD: true recovery or statistical illusion? ADHD Report 5:1–5, 1997

Biederman J: Attention-deficit/hyperactivity disorder: a life-span perspective. J Clin Psychiatry 59 (suppl 7):4–16, 1998

Biederman J, Faraone SV, Spencer T, et al: Gender differences in a sample of adults with attention deficit hyperactivity disorder. Psychiatry Res 53:13–29, 1994

Biederman J, Faraone S, Mick E, et al: Clinical correlates of ADHD in females: findings from a large group of girls ascertained from pediatric and psychiatric referral services. J Am Acad Child Adolesc Psychiatry 38:966–975, 1999

Brown TE: Emerging understandings of attention-deficit disorders and comorbidities, in Attention-Deficit Disorders and Comorbidities in Children, Adolescents, and Adults. Edited by TE Brown. Washington, DC, American Psychiatric Press, 2000, pp 3–56

Campbell SB, Pierce EW, Moore G, et al: Boys' externalizing problems at elementary school age: pathways from early behavior problems, maternal control and family stress. Dev Psychopathol 8:701–719, 1996

Castellanos FX, Giedd JN, Berquin PC, et al: Quantitative brain magnetic resonance imaging in girls with attention deficit hyperactivity disorder. Arch Gen Psychiatry 58:289–295, 2001

Clifton DO, Nelson P: Soar With Your Strengths. New York, Dell Publishing, 1992

Csikszentmihaly M: Flow. New York, Harper & Row, 1990

Donenberg G, Baker BL: The impact of young children with externalizing behaviors on their families. J Abnorm Child Psychol 21:179–198, 1993

Ernst M, Liebenauer LL, King AC, et al: Reduced brain metabolism in hyperactive girls. J Am Acad Child Adolesc Psychiatry 33:858–868, 1994

Faraone SV, Biederman J, Spencer T, et al: Attention deficit hyperactivity disorder in adults: an overview. Biol Psychiatry 48:9–20, 2000

Gaub M, Carlson C: Gender differences in ADHD: a meta-analysis and critical review. J Am Acad Child Adolesc Psychiatry 36:1036–1045, 1997

Gershon J: Gender differences in AD/HD: an overview of research, in Gender Issues and AD/HD. Edited by Quinn PO, Nadeau KG. Silver Spring, MD, Advantage, 2002, pp 23–38

Giedd JN: Neuroimaging of pediatric neuropsychiatric disorders: is a picture really worth a thousand words? Arch Gen Psychiatry 58:443–444, 2001

Giedd J, Molloy E, Pope K: Gender differences in AD/HD: neurobiological factors, in Gender Issues and AD/HD. Edited By Quinn PO, Nadeau KG. Silver Spring, MD, Advantage, 2002, pp 40–54

Gilligan C: In a Different Voice. Cambridge, MA, Harvard University Press, 1982

Goodman D, Quinn P: Psychotropic medication use during pregnancy: a concern for women with AD/HD, in Gender Issues in AD/HD. Edited by Quinn PO, Nadeau KG. Silver Spring, MD, Advantage, 2002, pp 200–218

Grossman H, Grossman S: Gender Issues in Education. Needham Heights, MA, Allyn & Bacon, 1994

Hartmann T: ADHD Secrets of Success. New York, Select Books, 2002

Hechtman L: Families of children with attention deficit disorder: a review. Can J Psychiatry 41:350–360, 1996

Hochschild A: The Second Shift. New York, Avon Books, 1990

Huessy HR: The pharmacotherapy of personality disorders in women. Paper presented at the annual meeting of the American Psychiatric Association, New York, 1990

Johnston C, Mash EJ: Families of children with attention-deficit/hyperactivity disorder: review and recommendations for future research. Clin Child Fam Psychol Rev 4:183–207, 2001

Justice AJ, de Wit H: Acute effects of estradiol pretreatment on the response to *d*-amphetamine in women. Neuroendocrinology 71:51–59, 2000

Katz LJ, Goldstein G, Geckle M: Neuropsychological and personality differences between men and women with ADHD. J Atten Disord 2:239–247, 1998

Kessler RC, Adler L, Ames M, et al: The prevalence and effects of adult attention deficit/hyperactivity disorder on work performance in a nationally representative sample of workers. J Occup Environ Med 47:565–572, 2005

Langner H: Gender differences and AD/HD: role expectations, in Gender Issues in AD/HD. Edited by Quinn PO, Nadeau KG. Silver Spring, MD, Advantage Books, 2002, pp 70–80

Manos MJ, Moore M, Mays DA, et al: Treatment practices and satisfaction in population segments of families affected by ADHD. Poster presentation 61 at the 17th Annual U.S. Psychiatric and Mental Health Congress, San Diego, CA, November 2004

McGough JJ, Smalley SL, McCracken JT, et al: Psychiatric comorbidity in adult attention deficit hyperactivity disorder: findings from multiplex families. Am J Psychiatry 162:1621–1627, 2005

Miller A: Breaking Down the Wall of Silence. New York, Penguin Books, 1991

MTA Cooperative Group: Moderators and mediators of treatment response for children with AD/HD. Arch Gen Psychiatry 56:1088–1096, 1999

Nadeau KG: Neurocognitive psychotherapy for women with AD/HD, in Gender Issues in AD/HD. Edited by Quinn PO, Nadeau KG. Silver Spring, MD, Advantage, 2002, pp 220–254

Pipher M: Reviving Ophelia: Saving the Lives of Adolescent Girls. New York, Ballantine Books, 1994

Popper CW, Gammon GD, West SA, et al: Disorders usually first diagnosed in infancy, childhood, or adolescence, in The American Psychiatric Publishing Textbook of Clinical Psychiatry, 4th Edition. Edited by Hales RE, Yudofsky SC. Washington, DC, American Psychiatric Publishing, 2003, pp 833–974

Prince J, Wilens T: Medications used in the treatment of AD/HD, in Gender Issues and AD/HD. Edited by Quinn PO, Nadeau KG. Silver Spring, MD, Advantage, 2002, pp 144–182

Quinn PO: Hormonal fluctuations and the influence of estrogen in the treatment of women with AD/HD, in Gender Issues and AD/HD. Edited by Quinn PO, Nadeau KG. Silver Spring, MD, Advantage, 2002, pp 183–199

Rako S, Mazer H (eds): Semrad: The Heart of a Therapist. Northvale, NJ, Jason Aronson, 1980, pp 61–64

Rucklidge KJ, Kaplan BJ: Psychological functioning in women identified in adulthood with attention-deficit hyperactivity disorder. J Atten Disord 2:167–176, 1997

Rumberg C: Are you surviving or thriving in life? ADDvance 2:14–15, 1999

Schmidt R, Fazekas F, Reinhart B, et al: Estrogen replacement therapy in older women: a neuropsychological and brain MRI study. J Am Geriatr Soc 44:1307–1313, 1996

Solden S: Women With Attention Deficit Disorder. Grass Valley, CA, Underwood Books, 1995

Stein MA, Sandoval R, Szumowski E, et al: Psychometric characteristics of the Wender Utah Rating Scale (WURS): reliability and factor structure for men and for women. Psychopharmacol Bull 31:423–431, 1995

Weiss M, Jain U: Clinical perspectives on the assessment of ADHD in adolescence. ADHD Report 8:4–7, 2000

Weiss M, Hechtman LT, Weiss G: ADHD in Adulthood. Baltimore, MD, Johns Hopkins University Press, 1999, pp 231–259

Wender PH: Attention-Deficit Hyperactivity Disorder in Adults. New York, Oxford University Press, 1995

Wilens TE, Biederman J, Spencer TJ: Attention deficit/hyperactivity disorder across the lifespan. Annu Rev Med 53:113–131, 2002

Zametkin AJ, Nordahl TE, Gross M, et al: Cerebral glucose metabolism in adults with hyperactivity of childhood onset. N Engl J Med 323:1361–1366, 1990

APPENDIX

WITH ELLEN DETLEFSEN, D.L.S.
AND COLIN C. DOYLE, B.A.

INTERNET RESOURCES AND ADULT ADHD

Increasingly, patients and their family members use the Internet for medical information. On a typical day, more Americans look for health information online than see a doctor (Fox and Lee 2002). Patients and family members bring Internet information into their encounters with physicians (Murray et al. 2003). Given that fact, it makes sense for physicians to give patients and family members an electronic prescription (Fox and Fallows 2003). Such an "e-prescription" can recommend specific portals and Web sites to patients. The e-prescription can include materials that help patients evaluate Web sites for themselves (Diaz et al. 2002).

Clinicians can only recommend Internet material to patients if we know how to assess its quality and teach our patients how to do the same. The Internet is the world's largest collection of information, but it is like a library in which the books are scattered everywhere. Order will come, eventually. Web sites are like individual books. Portals are like doors to libraries: inside are Web sites that someone has reviewed and evaluated. Certain portals are consistently reliable as doors to good health information.

CRITERIA FOR EVALUATING HEALTH WEB SITES

1. Credibility/Sponsorship/Authorship

A Web site should state clearly who developed it, identifying specific authors and providing their credentials. It should provide contact information so that visitors can e-mail, call, or write the authors. An important indicator of quality is if the site has been chosen by a reputable

313

portal. Another clue is in the extension of the site address, as shown in the following examples:

- .org: Not-for-profit organization
- .edu: Educational institution
- .gov: Federal government site
- .net: Network
- .com: Commercial, for-profit site (note: includes many hospitals)

2. Currency/Links/Design/Interactivity

The site should show the date of the last update. Information should be timely. Links to other sites should still be active, and they should work. There should be information about the nature of links to other sites. Links to sites that ask for, or require, payment for access are of poor quality. Is the presentation of information clear? Is the site easy to navigate?

3. Audience and Purpose

Does the site clearly state its intended audience and its purpose? Does it specify whether information is intended for the consumer? Is the literacy level suitable? Can the visitor verify information at other sources? Does the site provide suggestions for further reading or additional Web links, images, or audiovisual material?

4. Disclosure/Disclaimers/Privacy

What information does the site collect, and why? Does the user have to subscribe, become a member, or give personal information? Do site developers tell exactly what they do with personal information they collect? Does the site have a clear privacy statement? It should have a clear disclaimer, such as "We have selected this information from varied health resources. We offer it as an information guide only; we cannot answer personal health-related or research questions. Please do not interpret information on the site as medical or professional advice. Review all information carefully with your physician or other health care provider."

5. Honors or Awards

Does the site have any "seals" or awards? Look for the red and blue Honor Code rectangle, which often appears on the home page of high-quality sites.

WEB SITES SPECIFIC TO ADHD

The following assessments of Web sites note quality on a numerical scale from 1 to 4. The higher the number, the better the rating:

1 = poor
2 = fair
3 = good
4 = outstanding

- **Attention Deficit Disorder Association (ADDA; http://www. add.org):** This informative site provides members access to a quarterly newsletter, teleclasses, and other materials. There are networking opportunities for adults with ADHD as well as professionals. The "Finding Help" section offers a directory of physicians and other ADHD professionals. Also, a "Find Local Support Groups" option lists these by state for adults with ADHD. The information, although helpful to the novice, is not all up to date.

    Accuracy and timeliness of information: 2
    Layout of site: 4
    Usefulness to lay public: 2
    Usefulness to clinicians: 1

- **ADDitude Magazine Online (http://www.additudemag.com):** Articles make up the bulk of this site's abundant information. Featured articles in the "ADD ABCs" section include basic information about ADHD. A full page of recommended Web sites is helpful. Articles in the "ADD Adults" section discuss relationships, career advice, and coaches (including a directory). The "ADD Medical Center" offers articles on medications, treatments, and comorbidity, and an adult symptoms checklist. The "ADD Bookstore" recommends a few books that apply to adults.

    Accuracy and timeliness of information: 3
    Layout of site: 3
    Usefulness to lay public: 3
    Usefulness to clinicians: 1

- **ADDvance (http://www.ADDvance.com):** Kathleen Nadeau, Ph.D., and Patricia Quinn, M.D., developed this sophisticated Web site. No site has more useful information for ADHD in girls and women than theirs; there is material about ADHD in boys and men as well. An on-line bookstore features Nadeau and Quinn's books about ADHD. There are also links to other suitable sites. Visitors can sign up for a free monthly e-mail newsletter, and they can post their own experiences and helpful hints. Visitors can arrange a telephone consult with Dr. Nadeau. The Web site encourages interaction with the sponsors and between visitors. Fresh and colorful, this site is easy to navigate.

Accuracy and timeliness of information: 4
Layout of site: 4
Usefulness to lay public: 4
Usefulness to clinicians: 3

- **AdhdNews (http://www.adhdnews.com/adult-adhd.htm):** This site includes general information, testimonials, and an extensive network of message boards for ADHD diagnosis, treatment, and coping. The message boards are public and not monitored by professionals.

Accuracy and timeliness of information: 1
Layout of site: 2
Usefulness to lay public: 2
Usefulness to clinicians: 1

- **Children and Adults With Attention-Deficit/Hyperactivity Disorder (CHADD; http://www.chadd.org):** CHADD is one of the leading nonprofit ADHD organizations. Its Web site is rich in information about ADHD in children, with less about adults. The "Support" section provides many links to articles, fact sheets, frequently asked questions, and other organizations. "En Español" has articles and information in Spanish, with links to a few organizations. "CHADD Shoppe" lists books on related topics, including some about adults. "Research" lists related projects, with a call for participants. "Professional Directory" lists professionals and providers of services and products by state and select foreign countries. The site is organized and informative.

Accuracy and timeliness of information: 4
Layout of site: 4
Usefulness to lay public: 4
Usefulness to clinicians: 2

- **ADD Consults Store (http://www.myaddstore.com):** Just for fun, this site offers everything from audiotapes to "fidget toys."

  Accuracy and timeliness of information: N/A
  Layout of site: 2
  Usefulness to lay public: 2
  Usefulness to clinicians: 1

- **My ADHD (http://www.myadhd.net):** The author is currently developing this site, which will offer resources primarily for adults with ADHD and those persons who are concerned about them. My plans include providing abundant, timely information about the disorder; links to other, suitable sites; and possibilities for visitors to interact with me about their questions, issues, and concerns.

- **Northern County Psychiatric Associates (http://www.ncpamd.com):** Northern County Psychiatric Associates, a group near Baltimore, MD, provides helpful information on this site, which includes numerous topics on adult ADHD. The articles are timely, easy to understand, and accurate. The site reviews books, including those on adult ADHD, and provides links to adult support groups.

  Accuracy and timeliness of information: 4
  Layout of site: 3
  Usefulness to lay public: 4
  Usefulness to clinicians: 2

- **"Attention Deficit Hyperactivity Disorder" (article; http://www.nimh.nih.gov/publicat/adhd.cfm):** This page on the National Institute of Mental Health Web site is a good article about ADHD. The site also adds helpful links.

  Accuracy and timeliness of information: 2
  Layout of site: 3
  Usefulness to lay public: 2
  Usefulness to clinicians: 2

- **oneADDplace (http://www.oneaddplace.com):** This site lists books, audiotapes, and other products. Its "Community Library" section cites articles, most of which pertain to children. Also provided are links to adult support groups, newsletters, and frequently asked questions. There is an extensive list of books about adult ADHD, among related topics. "Professional Services" offers listings in a few states, mostly New York and California.

Accuracy and timeliness of information: 2
Layout of site: 2
Usefulness to lay public: 2
Usefulness to clinicians: 1

- **WebMD (http://my.webmd.com/medical_information_centers/ add_adhd/default.htm):** Here the visitor can find physicians by name or location who specialize in ADHD treatment as well as those physicians with specific hospital or health maintenance organization affiliations.

Accuracy and timeliness of information: 3
Layout of site: 3
Usefulness to lay public: 2
Usefulness to clinicians: 3

Pharmaceutical Industry–Sponsored ADHD Web Sites

These Web sites often provide useful information. However, marketing and public relations pressures powerfully shape them.

- **Adderall XR (http://www.adderallxr.com):** Sponsored by Shire, this site is about Adderall XR. The site provides information about ADHD in children, teens, and adults. The "ADHD Resource Center" lists varied articles and pamphlets. A substantial list of books covers topics including adult ADHD.

Accuracy and timeliness of information: 3
Layout of site: 4
Usefulness to lay public: 2
Usefulness to clinicians: 1—only for information specific to Adderall XR

- **ADHD Support (http://www.adhdsupport.com):** At this site, Shire Pharmaceuticals, maker of Adderall and Adderall XR, offers information on common topics about ADHD, mostly for affected children and their parents. The information for adults is well presented.

Accuracy and timeliness of information: 3
Layout of site: 3

Usefulness to lay public: 2
Usefulness to clinicians: 0

- **AdultADD.com (http://www.AdultAdd.com):** Sponsored by Eli Lilly Company, the manufacturers of atomoxetine (Strattera), this site contains an Adult Self-Report Scale Screener and an outline of treatment. "Ask Lilly" allows consumers to send questions via e-mail or a hotline (800-Lilly-Rx). "Information for Physicians" connects the visitor to continuing medical education and patient education materials, medical society Web sites, Lilly product sites, and clinical trials.

  Accuracy and timeliness of information: 2
  Layout of site: 3
  Usefulness to lay public: 2
  Usefulness to clinicians: 1

- **Concerta (http://www.Concerta.net):** McNeil Pharmaceuticals' site offers information for parents of ADHD children but not for adults with ADHD. There is specific material on Concerta. "Learn About ADHD" gives concise information about the disorder, especially in children. The site also offers information in Spanish.

  Accuracy and timeliness of information: 4
  Layout of site: 4
  Usefulness to lay public: 1
  Usefulness to clinicians: 1

HIGH-QUALITY GENERAL HEALTH SITES AND PORTALS

- **MedlinePlus (http://medlineplus.gov):** This portal links visitors to authoritative information on desired topics and to a preformulated *MEDLINE* search. The site includes physician and hospital directories and consumer drug information. This portal is a fine place for patients or their family members to learn about adult ADHD.
- **New York Online Access to Health (NOAH; http://www.noah-health. org/en/mental):** This site includes information about adult ADHD in both Spanish and English.
- **Healthfinder (http://www.healthfinder.gov):** This site, developed by the U.S. Department of Health and Human Services, links visitors to Web sites from more than 1,500 health-related organizations. However, little information is provided about ADHD in children or adults.

- **Medem (http://medem.com/medlb/medlib_entry.cfm):** This collaborative project of leading American medical societies includes the American Psychiatric Association. It provides credible, comprehensive clinical information and secure, confidential communications.

HIGH-QUALITY MENTAL HEALTH WEB SITES AND PORTALS

These sites do not all address ADHD, but they are excellent for learning about general issues related to mental health.

- **HealthyMinds (http://www.healthyminds.org):** This Web site provides fine information from the nation's oldest national medical specialty society, the American Psychiatric Association.
- **American Psychological Association Help Center (http://helping.apa.org):** The brochures, tips, and articles at this Web site provide user-friendly information about ADHD in all populations.
- **National Institute of Mental Health (http://www.nimh.nih.gov/healthinformation/index.cfm):** This site contains a useful pamphlet but little else about adult ADHD.
- **Center for Mental Health Services (http://www.mentalhealth.samhsa.gov/cmhs):** This site, offered by the U.S. Substance Abuse and Mental Health Services Administration of the Department of Health and Human Services, offers little information about ADHD.
- **National Mental Health Association (http://www.nmha.org):** This Web site serves as an information and referral center for those seeking mental health information.
- **Mayo Foundation for Medical Education and Research (http://www.mayoclinic.com/invoke.cfm?id=MH00008):** This site has a few ADHD-related articles.
- **Intelihealth (http://www.intelihealth.com):** At this site, there is scanty information about ADHD. It is a joint project of Harvard Medical School and the Aetna health insurance company.

MENTAL HEALTH WEB SITES RECOMMENDED FOR SPECIAL POPULATIONS

- **For children:** The Web site of the Advanced Center for Intervention and Services Research for Early-Onset Mood and Anxiety Disorders (http://www.moodykids.org) was created by a National Institute of Mental Health–funded center at Western Psychiatric Institute and Clinic, University of Pittsburgh.

- **For young adults:** Go Ask Alice! (http://www.goaskalice.columbia. edu/index.html) is a question and answer Internet service produced by Columbia University's Health Promotion Program. It is a good source of information about ADHD, among other topics. The questions and answers, written in college student style, make for vivid reading.
- **For women:** The National Women's Health Information Center (http://www.4women.gov) is a gateway to selected women's health information and has reliable, timely resources. ADHD is among the health topics.
- **For those who speak Spanish:** Acceso Computerizado de la Salud en Nueva York (NOAH; http://noah-health.org) is a good source of information in Spanish, although many of the links provided are to sites in English only.
- **For those with low literacy:** The site for the Texas Medication Algorithm Project (TMAP; http://www.dshs.state.tx.us/mhprograms/ PtEd.shtm) offers one-page patient and family education materials in English and in Spanish. The materials help the patient monitor, manage, and cope with illness. However, there is little information about ADHD.

SUMMARY: AN "E-PRESCRIPTION" FOR ADHD

Patients are using the Internet for health information. Encourage them to use high-quality Web sites about mental health and adult ADHD by providing specific recommendations.

REFERENCES

Diaz JA, Griffith RA, Ng JJ, et al: Patients' use of the Internet for medical information. J Gen Intern Med 17:180–185, 2002

Fox S, Fallows D, Pew Internet and American Life Project: Internet health resources: health searches and e-mail have become more commonplace, but there is room for improvement in searches and overall Internet access. Available at: http://www.pewinternet.org/pdfs/PIP_Health_Report_ July_2003.pdf. Accessed February 7, 2006.

Fox S, Lee R: Vital decisions: how Internet users decide what information to trust when they or their loved ones are sick. Washington, DC, Pew Internet and American Life Project, May 2002. Available at: http://www.pewinternet. org/pdfs/PIP_Vital_Decisions_May2002.pdf. Accessed May 28, 2005.

Murray E, Lo B, Pollack L, et al: The impact of health information on the Internet on the physician-patient relationship: patient perceptions. Arch Intern Med 163:1727–1734, 2003

INDEX

Page numbers printed in **boldface** type refer to tables or figures.